Cerebrovascular Disease, Cognitive Impairment and Dementia

Second Edition of Cerebrovascular Disease and Dementia

Cerebrovascular Disease, Cognitive Impairment and Dementia

Second Edition

Edited by

John O'Brien BM BCh MA MRCPsych Dm
Professor of Old Age Psychiatry
Institute for Ageing and Health
University of Newcastle upon Tyne, UK

David Ames BA MD FRCPsych FRANZCP
Associate Professor of Psychiatry of Old Age
Academic Unit for Psychiatry of Old Age
University of Melbourne
Victoria, Australia

Lars Gustafson MD PhD
Professor of Geriatric Psychiatry
Department of Psychogeriatrics
University Hospital Lund, Sweden

Marshal Folstein MD
Professor of Psychiatry
New England Medical Center
Boston MA, USA

Edmond Chiu AM MBBS DPM FRANZCP
Professor of Psychiatry of Old Age
Academic Unit for Psychiatry of Old Age
University of Melbourne
Victoria, Australia

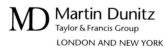

Martin Dunitz
Taylor & Francis Group
LONDON AND NEW YORK

© 2004 Martin Dunitz, an imprint of the Taylor & Francis Group plc

First published in the United Kingdom in 2004
by Martin Dunitz, an imprint of the Taylor & Francis Group plc, 11 New Fetter Lane, London EC4P 4EE

Tel: +44 (0)20 7583 9855
Fax: +44 (0)20 7842 2298
E-mail: info@dunitz.co.uk
Website: http://www.dunitz.co.uk

Although every effort has been made to ensure that all owners of copyright material have been acknowledged in this publication, we would be glad to acknowledge in subsequent reprints or editions any omissions brought to our attention.

A CIP record for this book is available from the British Library.

ISBN 1 84184 266 4

Distributed in the USA by
Fulfilment Center
Taylor & Francis
10650 Toebben Drive
Independence, KY 41051 USA
Toll Free Tel: 1-800-634-7064
E-mail: taylorandfrancis@thomsonlearning.com

Distributed in Canada by
Taylor & Francis
74 Rolark Drive
Scarborough, Ontario M1R 4G2, Canada
Toll Free Tel: +1-877 226 2237
E-mail: tal_fran@istar.ca

Distributed in the rest of the world by
Thomson Publishing Services
Cheriton House, North Way
Andover, Hampshire SP10 5BE, UK
Tel: +44 (0)1264 332424
E-mail: salesorder.tandf@thomsonpublishingservices.co.uk

Composition by Wearset Ltd, Boldon, Tyne & Wear, UK

Printed and bound in Great Britain by The Cromwell Press, Trowbridge.

Contents

Contributors

David Ames
Associate Professor of Psychiatry of
Old Age
Academic Unit for Psychiatry of
Old Age
University of Melbourne, Australia

Olafur Aevarsson
Neuropsychiatric Epidemiology
Unit
Institute of Clinical Neurosciences
Sahlgrenska Academy
Gothenburg University, Sweden

Clive Ballard
Professor of Old Age Psychiatry
Institute for Ageing and Health,
Wolfson Research Centre,
Newcastle General Hospital,
Newcastle upon Tyne, UK

Robert Barber
Consultant Psychiatrist & Honorary
Clinical Senior Lecturer
Centre for the Health of the Elderly
Newcastle General Hospital
Newcastle upon Tyne, UK

Michael Bradbury
Assistant Psychologist
Institute for Ageing and Health
Wolfson Research Centre
Newcastle General Hospital
Newcastle upon Tyne, UK

Henry Brodaty
Professor of Psychogeriatrics
Academic Department for Old Age
Psychiatry
School of Psychiatry
University of New South Wales,
Australia

Arne Erik Brun
Professor of Neuropathology
Lund University
Institute of Pathology, Sweden

Edmond Chiu
Professor of Psychiatry of Old Age
Academic Unit for Psychiatry of
Old Age
University of Melbourne, Australia

Jennifer A Court
Joint MRC/Newcastle University
Development in Clinical Brain
Ageing
Newcastle General Hospital
Newcastle upon Tyne, UK

Stephen M Davis
Director of Neurology
Royal Melbourne Hospital and
Professor of Neurology
University of Melbourne, Australia

Martin Dichgans
Department of Neurology
Grosshadern Clinic
Marchioninistr. 15
81377 Munich, Germany

Robin Eastwood
Consultant Psychiatrist
Nuffield Hospital
Plymouth
Devon, UK

Elisabet Englund
Associate Professor &
Senior Consultant
Department of Pathology
University Hospital Lund
Sweden

Leon Flicker
Professor of Geriatric Medicine
University of Western Australia
School of Medicine and
Pharmacology
Royal Perth Hospital, Australia

Marshal Folstein
Professor of Psychiatry
New England Medical Center
Boston MA, USA

Alisa Green
Research Psychologist
Formerly at Academic Department
for Old Age Psychiatry
Prince of Wales Hospital
Randwick, NSW Australia

Lars Gustafson
Professor of Geriatric Psychiatry
Department of Psychogeriatrics
University Hospital Lund, Sweden

Kazuo Hasegawa
Honorary Professor
Chief Executive Officer
St. Marianna University School of
Medicine
Kanagawa, Japan

Akira Homma
Professor
Leader, Dementia Intervention
Research Group
Tokyo Metropolitan Institute of
Gerontology, Japan

Anthony F Jorm
Director
Centre for Mental Health Research
Australian National University
Canberra, Australia

Raj N Kalaria
Professor of Cerebrovascular
Pathology
Wolfson Research Centre
Newcastle General Hospital
Newcastle upon Tyne, UK

Rajeev Kumar
Lecturer & Senior Staff Specialist
Department of Psychological
Medicine
The Canberra Clinical School
The Australian National University
Canberra, Australia

Nicola T Lautenschlager
Senior Lecturer in Psychiatry of Old
Age
School of Psychiatry and Clinical
Neurosciences
University of Western Australia
Perth, WA, Australia

Lee-Fay Low
Research Psychologist
Academic Department for Old Age
Psychiatry
Prince of Wales Hospital
Randwick, NSW, Australia

Kjell Martin Moksnes
Medical Director
Geropsychiatric Department
Psychiatric Division
Ullevaal University Hospital
Oslo, Norway

John O'Brien
Professor of Old Age Psychiatry
Institute for Ageing and Health
Newcastle General Hospital
Newcastle upon Tyne, UK

Ulla Passant
Associate Professor
Department of Psychogeriatrics
University Hospital Lund
Sweden

Elaine Perry
Professor of Neurochemical
Pathology
Joint MRC/University of Newcastle
Development in Clinical Brain
Ageing
Newcastle General Hospital
Newcastle upon Tyne, UK

Elise Rowan
Institute for Ageing and Health
Wolfson Research Centre
Newcastle General Hospital
Newcastle upon Tyne, UK

Stuart Sadler
Assistant Psychologist
Institute for Ageing and Health
Wolfson Research Centre
Newcastle General Hospital
Newcastle upon Tyne, UK

Tammy M Scott
Assistant Professor of Psychiatry
School of Nutrition Science and
Policy
Tufts University and Department of
Psychiatry
New England Medical Center
Boston, MA, USA

Ingmar Skoog
Professor
Neuropsychiatric Epidemiology Unit
Institute of Clinical Neurosciences
Sahlgrenska Academy
Gothenburg University, Sweden

Sally Stephens
Assistant Psychologist
Institute for Ageing and Health
Wolfson Research Centre
Newcastle General Hospital
Newcastle upon Tyne, UK

Rob Stewart
Senior Lecturer
Institute of Psychiatry
Kings College
London, UK

Yucun Shen
Professor of Psychiatry
Institute of Mental Health
Peking University
Beijing, PR China

Joe Stratford
Specialist Registrar
Department of Old Age
Psychiatry
Charlton Lane Centre
Gloucestershire, UK

Alan J Thomas
Senior Lecturer and Consultant in
Old Age Psychiatry
Institute for Ageing and Health
Newcastle General Hospital
Newcastle upon Tyne, UK

Katherine L Tucker
Director, Epidemiology and Dietary
Assessment Program
Jean Mayer USDA
Human Nutrition Research
Center
Tufts University
Boston, MA, USA

Anders Wallin
Professor of Geriatric
Neuropsychiatry
Institute of Clinical Neuroscience
Sahlgrenska University Hospital
Molndal, Sweden

David G Wilkinson
Consultant in Old Age Psychiatry
Honorary Senior Lecturer,
University of Southampton
Memory Assessment and Research
Centre
Moorgreen Hospital, Southampton,
UK

Yu Xin
Associate Professor of Psychiatry
Institute of Mental Health
Peking University
Beijing, PR China

Foreword

The field of vascular dementia welcomes the second edition of this book, one of the best available on this discipline. As a reflection of progress in the field in the three years that elapsed since the first edition in 2000, the title has changed to *Cerebrovascular Disease, Cognitive Impairment and Dementia;* there is a distinguished new senior editor, John O'Brien, Professor of Old Age Psychiatry at Newcastle upon Tyne, UK, and a number of new collaborators. Despite these changes, the book remains eminently clinically oriented and easy to read by the uninitiated; most importantly, it provides clinical acumen and practical advice for the practitioner while continuing to make available information at the cutting edge of research in this rapidly moving field. Most of the contributors use the term *vascular dementia* in their chapters, although the editors have been reluctant to accept this time-honored term and have settled, diplomatically, on the less controversial Cerebrovascular Disease and Dementia, adding now the name (vascular) cognitive impairment (VCI). The latter term was initially coined to signify any degree of cognitive loss caused by cerebrovascular disease (including vascular dementia); however, by analogy with mild cognitive impairment (MCI) due to Alzheimer's disease, VCI should be reserved for patients with risk factors for cerebrovascular disease and some degree of cognitive loss short of dementia. Intrinsic to the VCI concept is the hope that appropriate prevention and treatment of the vascular brain burden could prevent the development of vascular dementia. Although this is an appealing undertaking, there have been difficulties in providing a strict definition of VCI and operational diagnostic criteria. The concept of VCI suffers from the same problems once criticized in vascular dementia: the notion is too wide and too vague for a precise operative definition. Furthermore, as demonstrated in the Canadian Study on Health and Aging, some patients with diagnosis of VCI improve over time, indicating that progression from VCI to vascular dementia may not always be a unidirectional pathway.

The boundaries between vascular dementia and Alzheimer's disease have become indistinct in these past few years. The notion that cerebrovascular disease may lead to cognitive decline and dementia in the elderly has been around since 1672 when Thomas Willis first described cases of post-apoplectic dementia. Less well recognized is the fact that *silent* strokes and incomplete white matter ischemia – documented by modern brain imaging – are also strongly associated with cognitive loss, behavioral changes, and vascular dementia. Lars Gustafson, in his scholarly introductory chapter reminds us that during most of the past century it was widely held that atherosclerotic dementia was the sole cause of senile dementia, and that it was only in the 1980s that Alzheimer's disease was declared the most common form of dementia in the elderly. In their chapters on the epidemiology of VaD, Anthony Jorm, John O'Brien, and others, remark that both cerebrovascular disease and Alzheimer's disease increase exponentially with advancing age. Therefore, as explained by neuropathologist Arne Brun in his superb chapter on *The neuropathology of vascular dementia and its overlap with Alzheimer's disease,* most elderly patients with dementia coming to autopsy will have brain lesions of Alzheimer's disease coexisting with often silent cerebrovascular lesions, such as large and small strokes, hemorrhages, arteriolosclerosis, lacunes, microinfarcts, and ischemic leucoencephalopathy. Is this "mixed" dementia predominantly Alzheimer's disease? Or, is the mixture formed by equal parts of Alzheimer's disease plus cerebrovascular disease? Alternatively, is this senile dementia mostly vascular dementia?

A review of Heiko and Eva Braak's fundamental studies on the neuropathological progression of neurofibrillary tangles in Alzheimer's disease (Braak and Braak, 1997) offers tentative answers to these questions (Duyckaerts and Hauw, 1997). The Braak categories range from Stage 0, no Alzheimer's disease pathology, to Stage VI with pan cortical involvement. The hippocampus is involved at about Stage III causing amnestic MCI, while clinical dementia of the Alzheimer's type occurs at about Stages V–VI. In a reanalysis of André Delacourte's cohort (1998) performed by Donald Royall and colleagues (2002, 2003) we found that – in the absence of vascular lesions – dementia is usually recognized when Alzheimer's disease pathology reaches a few specific cortical regions involved in control of executive functions. These regions of interest are Brodmann's areas 9 and 10 in the frontal cortex, the gyrus angularis (area 39), the cingulate cortex (areas 23, 24), and the superior temporal gyrus (area 22). These areas are part of a single cortical circuit related to executive control. More frequently, however, ischemic vascular disease interrupts the cortico-subcortical connections of the circuits. Ischemic lesions, such as lacunes in the caudate, anterior thalamus, or lower genu of the internal capsule, alone or in combination with frontal white matter lesions, sever the cortical projections. Evidence from the Nun Study (Snowdon et al, 1997), corroborated by other data, concluded that lacunes increase more than 20 times the risk of clinical expression of dementia at early Braak stages insufficient to produce dementia. Moreover, there is a significant *inverse* relationship between Braak stage and the severity of cerebrovascular disease (Zekry, Hauw & Gold, 2002; Zekry et al, 2002, 2003; Goulding et al, 1999). Therefore, it would appear that cerebrovascular disease is required to "amplify" the clinical expression of Alzheimer's disease pathology beyond the stage of amnestic MCI (Braak Stage III). This explains why almost 20% of cases pathologically defined by CERAD criteria as Alzheimer's disease do not have clinical dementia. Conversely, more than half of *non-demented* octogenarians meet CERAD criteria for pathologically confirmed Alzheimer's disease (Polvikowski et al, 2001). On the other hand, studies of post-stroke dementia by Hénon and colleagues (1997, 2001) have also shown that in patients with *bona fide* post apoplectic vascular dementia, preexisting amnestic deficits occurred in about 16% of cases, suggesting that the underlying Alzheimer's disease had not progressed beyond Stage III, clearly insufficient to produce clinical dementia. In these patients, cerebrovascular disease is the defining cause of the dementia.

Population-based studies have shown that silent lacunes are extremely common in the elderly. Longstreth et al (1988) showed the presence of one or more silent lacunes in about one-fourth of the 3660 participants in the CHS, aged 65 and older that underwent cerebral MRI. Quite recently, in the Rotterdam cohort, Vermeer et al (2003) demonstrated that silent lacunes, particularly in the thalamus, more than doubled the risk of dementia [hazard ratio = 2.26, 95% CI, 1.09–4.70]. Small-vessel disease may be the commonest mechanism by which MCI evolves into Alzheimer's disease in persons over the age of 70 years (Royall, 2003).

In conclusion, in response to the questions posed earlier, the weight of the evidence seems to validate the hypothesis that cerebrovascular disease is the most important cause of dementia in the elderly, both by itself and as a catalyst for the conversion of low-grade Alzheimer's disease to dementia. As customarily done in neuroepidemiological studies (Rocca et al, 1991) the latter group of patients should be included among the vascular dementias and not in the Alzheimer's disease category. Moreover, to this group of patients we must add the thousands of cases with cognitive loss and vascular dementia resulting from cerebral hypoperfusion complicating cardiac and circulatory diseases (Román, 2003).

The current edition of this book continues to make an important contribution to the effort to educate all health providers on the need to recognize and treat patients with vascular cognitive impairment and vascular dementia, and most importantly, by emphasizing reduction of the vascular burden on the brain, it will contribute to prevent the late-life tragedy of dementia from occurring.

Gustavo C. Román MD, FACP, FRSM (Lond), FAAN
Professor of Medicine/Neurology
University of Texas Health Science Center at San Antonio,
San Antonio, Texas, USA

References

Braak H, Braak E, Frequency of stages of Alzheimer-related lesions in different age categories, *Neurobiol Aging* (1997) **18**:351–57.

Duyckaerts C, Hauw J-J, Prevalence, incidence and duration of Braak's stages in the general population: Can we know? *Neurobiol Aging* (1997) **18**:362–9.

Goulding JM, Signorini DF, Chatterjee S et al, Inverse relation between Braak stage and cerebrovascular pathology in Alzheimer predominant dementia, *J Neurol Neurosurg Psychiatry* (1999) **67**:654–7.

Hénon H, Pasquier F, Durieu I *et al,* Pre-existing dementia in stroke patients: baseline frequency, associated factors and outcome, *Stroke* (1997) **28**:2429–36.

Hénon H, Durieu I, Guerouaou D *et al,* Post-stroke dementia: incidence and relationship to pre-stroke cognitive decline, *Neurology* (2001) **57**:1216–22.

Polvikowski T, Sulkava R, Myllykangas L et al, Prevalence of Alzheimer's disease in very old people: A prospective neuropathological study, *Neurology* (2001) **56**:1690–6.

Rocca WA, Hofman A, Brayne C et al, The prevalence of vascular dementia in Europe: facts and fragments from 1980–1990 studies, *Ann Neurol* (1991) **30**:817–24.

Román GC, Stroke, cognitive decline and vascular dementia: the silent epidemic of the 21st century, (Editorial), *Neuroepidemiology* (2003) **22**:161–4.

Royall DR, A new "silent" epidemic, (Editorial), *JAGS* 2003.

Royall DR, Palmer R, Mulroy A et al, Pathological determinants of clinical dementia in Alzheimer's disease, *Exp Aging Res* (2002) **28**:143–62.

Royall DR, Román GC, Delacourte A, Pathological determinants of clinical dementia in Alzheimer's disease, (Letter to the Editor) *Exp Aging Res* (2002) **29**:107–10.

Snowdon DA, Grenier LH, Mortimer JA et al, Brain infarction and the clinical expression of Alzheimer disease. The Nun study, *J Am Med Asoc* (1997) **277**: 813–7.

Skoog I, Andreasson L-A, Landahl S, Lernfelt B, A population-based study on blood pressure and brain atrophy in 85-year-olds, *Hypertension* (1998) **32**:404–9.

Sourander P, Wålinder J, Hereditary multi-infarct dementia. Morphological and clinical studies of a new disease, *Acta Neuropathol (Berl)* (1977) **39**:247–54.

Tomlinson BE, Blessed G, Roth M, Observations on the brains of demented old people, *J Neurol Sci* (1970) **11**:205–42.

Tomonaga M, Yamanouchi H, Tohgi H, Kameyama M, Clinicopathologic study of progressive subcortical vascular encephalopathy (Binswanger type) in the elderly. *J Am Geriatr Soc* (1982) **30**:524–9.

Tournier-Lasserve E, Joutel A, Melki J et al, Cerebral autosomal dominant arteriopathy with subcortical infarcts and leukoencephalopathy maps on chromosome 19q12, *Nat Genet* (1993) **3**:256–9.

Van Bogart L, Encéphalopathie sous-corticale progressive (Binswanger) à évolution rapide chez deux soeurs, *Med Hellen* (1955) **24**:961–72.

Van Broeckhoven C, Haan J, Bakker E et al, The genetic defect in hereditary cerebral hemorrhage with amyloidosis of Dutch type is tightly linked to the β-amyloid gene on chromosome 21, *Science* (1990) **248**:1120–2.

Wallin A, Brun A, Gustafson L, Swedish consensus on dementia diseases, *Acta Neurol Scand Suppl* (1994) **90**.

Wallin A, Gottfries CG, Karlsson I, Svennerholm L, Decreased myelin lipids in Alzheimer's disease and vascular dementia, *Acta Neurol Scand* (1989) **80**:319–23.

Wattendorff AR, Bots GT, Went LN, Endtz LJ, Familial cerebral amyloid angiopathy presenting as recurrent cerebral haemorrhage, *J Neurol Sci* (1982) **55**:121–35.

Willis T, *De Anima Brutorum Quae Hominis Vitalis ac Sensitiva est* (Ric. Davis, Oxonii, 1672). (Transl Pordage S in Dr Willis' *Practice of Physick, Two Discourses Concerning the Soul of Brutes*. T Dring, C Harper & J Leigh, London, 1684.)

Wolf PA, Dawber TR, Thomas HE, Kannel WB, Epidemiological assessment of chronic atrial fibrillation and risk of stroke: The Framingham Study, *Neurology* (1978) **28**:973.

World Health Organization, *ICD-10*, 10th revision of the International Classification of Diseases (WHO: Geneva, 1992).

Yamamoto H, Bogousslavsky J, Mechanisms of second and further strokes, *J Neurol Neurosurg Psychiatry* (1998) **64**:771–6.

chapter 2

Classification and diagnostic criteria

Robert Stewart

'Diagnosis' – historical influences

It is fair to say that 'measurement' has been a Holy Grail for mental health research throughout its history. Early in the 20th century, the path to enlightenment seemed to lie in the science of phenomenology. Pioneering clinical researchers such as Kraepelin and Bleuler, faced with a 'sea' of mental illness, sought to differentiate subtypes with distinguishable symptomatology and outcome. Parallel, seminal work by Jaspers and others focused on symptoms rather than syndromes, seeking to distinguish and describe these in a way that could be understood and communicated between clinicians – a new 'language' in effect.

Communication

These issues (distinguishing symptomatology, linking syndromes with course and communication between health professionals) are central to the idea of diagnosis. The purpose of a diagnosis is to define a collection of symptoms, signs or results of investigations which can be easily understood (by other health professionals at least) and have some meaning, sometimes with respect to etiology/pathology but definitely with respect to response to treatment and prognosis. The process of making a diagnosis is central to clinical practice which in turn, has traditionally had a strong influence on research: because the rationale for most health research is its relevance to clinical practice and because many researchers originally trained as clinicians.

Re-evaluation

Diagnoses are rarely set in stone. If a research field is active, it should be expected that traditional definitions for disorders are called into question as new findings arise. For mainstream mental health research, the 1960s were an important period since there was a concerted attack on frail psychiatric diagnoses whose validity was becoming taken for granted. The basis for some of the criticisms may not have stood the test of time but they undoubtedly constituted a healthy wake-up call which led to a large amount of work re-evaluating and standardizing the process of diagnosis.

Categories and dimensions

Diagnoses generally involve an attempt to impose categories on dimensions of physiological disturbance. Hypertension is therefore defined as blood pressure above predefined levels, diabetes as glucose tolerance which has become impaired beyond a given point, and cancer as cellular dysplasia of a particular severity. The problem that has always faced mental health research has been in identifying and measuring its 'dimensions'. If one response to the challenges of the 1960s was to stabilize clinical diagnostic procedures, another was an ever more intensive search for dimensions, particularly through biological research.

Diagnosis in vascular dementia

Historical processes have shaped the way in which 'vascular' dementia has been conceptualized. Although Alois Alzheimer's work coincided with the development of phenomenology in other mental health fields, the neuropathological studies that brought 'his' disease to the fore were carried out in the late 1960s and early 1970s, at a time when the basis for clinical psychiatric diagnoses was under threat. Dementia has an advantage over schizophrenia and affective disorder in its reasonably well established pathological basis. This has led to the elevated status of pathological diagnoses and the possible/probable/definite levels in most diagnostic systems.

Clinical studies lagged behind neuropathology but a gradual growth in interest led, by the mid-1980s, to research diagnostic criteria for Alzheimer's disease (AD) which could be applied in life. A need for other clinical diagnoses continued the use of the Hachinski Ischemic Scale (HIS) for some time in the field of vascular dementia, and led eventually to the publication of ADDTC and the NINDS-AIREN criteria in the early 1990s. These coincided with a rapid expansion in international epidemiological research, and the

NINDS-AIREN criteria in particular passed into widespread use. Although the validity of vascular dementia as a diagnosis had been questioned from the outset, it was not until the late 1990s that accepted systems began to receive more concerted criticism. Broadly, this has reflected a shift of interest from descriptive studies of prevalence and incidence towards risk factors and causation, and from clinical to early or preclinical disease. More specifically, the distinction between AD and vascular dementia has become less tenable in the light of findings from epidemiology, neuroimaging and neuropathology, suggesting that cerebrovascular and Alzheimer processes are not as distinguishable as was once thought. These issues will be considered further after the principal diagnostic systems are reviewed in more detail.

Clinical diagnostic criteria for vascular dementia syndromes and related diagnoses

Hachinski Ischemic Scale (1975, 1980)

Interestingly, for a widely used research instrument, this scale was originally assembled for an investigation of cerebral blood flow in dementia and only briefly described in the paper reporting these findings (Hachinski et al, 1975). It was devised simply by listing and scaling 13 features of 'arteriosclerotic psychosis' from a widely read textbook of psychiatry (Mayer-Gross et al, 1969). Some features refer to the course of the dementia (e.g. abrupt onset, stepwise deterioration, fluctuation), some to symptoms (e.g. nocturnal confusion, depression, somatic complaints) and some to the likely presence of or risk for cerebrovascular disease (e.g. history of strokes or hypertension, focal neurological signs). No attempt was made to validate the instrument or to investigate its scaling properties or the validity of the different weights given to some items. A later paper suggested that these criteria could be reduced to eight – the 'revised HIS' (Rosen et al, 1980). However, further clinicopathological research found only six items of the original HIS to be significantly increased in multi-infarct dementia (MID) compared to AD and discriminant function analysis only supported two of these – fluctuating course and focal neurological symptoms; (Mölsa et al, 1985) – although a recent study found that the original HIS gave a higher inter-rater reliability than all subsequent attempts to define vascular dementia (Chui et al, 2000).

DSM criteria (1980–94)

The parallel development of ICD and DSM diagnostic criteria were largely driven by a need for consensus on disorders such as schizophrenia rather than dementia syndromes. The third edition of the *Diagnostic and Statistical Manual of Mental Disorders* (DSM-III; American Psychiatric Association, 1980) was an influential development in this field. Criteria for MID were:

1. dementia
2. stepwise course with 'patchy' deficits at early stages
3. focal neurological signs and symptoms
4. evidence of significant cerebrovascular disease judged to be etiologically related.

These were not altered in the revised third edition (DSM-III-R; American Psychiatric Association, 1987). In the fourth edition (DSM-IV; American Psychiatric Association, 1994) the syndrome name is changed to vascular dementia. Three criteria are generic to dementia (multiple cognitive deficits, functional impairment/evidence of decline, exclusion of delirium), criterion 2 above is dropped and *either* (rather than both) criteria 3 and 4 are permissible. DSM-III-R criteria formed the basis for EURODEM analyses (Andersen et al, 1999).

NINCDS-ADRDA criteria for Alzheimer's disease (1984)

Not very long after the publication of the DSM-III criteria, a work group was established by the National Institute of Neurological and Communicative Disorders and Stroke (NINCDS) and the Alzheimer's Disease and Related Disorders Association (ADRDA) to draw up criteria for AD which could be applied in clinical research (McKhann et al, 1984). An important aspect of the criteria was a drive to improve reliability in a research setting by focusing on a relatively 'pure' syndrome. Therefore a requirement for the 'probable' level of diagnosis is the absence of systemic disorders or other brain diseases that in themselves could account for the dementia syndrome. This last criterion involves a considerable degree of subjective judgment. AD cases with comorbid vascular risk factors or cerebrovascular disease may be excluded or not, depending on how these criteria are applied.

ADDTC criteria (1992)

By the beginning of the 1990s, demand had increased for a systematized diagnosis for 'vascular' dementia. Two sets of criteria were proposed. The first of these to be published was from the State of California Alzheimer's Disease Diagnostic and Treatment Centers (ADDTC; Chui et al, 1992). These criteria focused on 'ischemic vascular dementia'. Like the NINCDS-ADRDA criteria for AD, 'definite', 'probable' and 'possible' levels were proposed. The 'definite' level requires histopathological confirmation. The 'probable' level requires dementia, CT/MRI evidence of at least one infarct outside the cerebellum and then *either* clinical evidence of two or more ischaemic stokes *or* a single stroke with a clear temporal relationship to the onset of dementia. Further support is allowed if there is evidence of multiple infarcts in brain regions known to affect cognition, multiple transient ischaemic attacks, a history of vascular risk factors and an elevated HIS score. A 'possible' level includes dementia with a single stroke of uncertain temporal relationship or with features of 'Binswanger's syndrome' (unexplained urinary incontinence or gait disturbance with vascular risk factors, and extensive white matter changes on neuroimaging). ADDTC criteria have been used in the large Honolulu–Asia Aging Study (Ross et al, 1999).

NINDS-AIREN criteria (1993)

A second response to the diagnostic challenge arose from an international workshop held in 1991 between the neuroepidemiology branch of the National Institute of Neurological Disorders and Stroke and the Association Internationale pour la Recherche et l'Enseignement en Neurosciences (NINDS-AIREN; Roman et al, 1993). The NINDS-AIREN criteria for a 'probable' level of diagnosis require dementia defined similarly to ADDTC. Evidence of cerebrovascular disease both clinical and from neuroimaging is also required but less specifically defined, and includes multiple basal ganglia and white matter lacunes or extensive periventricular white matter lesions. A further requirement is a relationship between cerebrovascular disease and dementia, specified as an onset of dementia within three months following a stroke, or an abrupt deterioration in cognitive function or fluctuating, stepwise progression. These criteria have perhaps had the most widespread application including large international studies (Yoshitake et al, 1995; Ott et al, 1995; Posner et al, 2002).

ICD-10

The International Classification of Diseases (ICD) criteria have developed in parallel with the DSM diagnostic systems in the USA, the two systems becoming gradually more harmonized over successive revisions but with important disagreements in some fields. Criteria for vascular dementia in the tenth ICD revision (WHO, 1992) are:

1. dementia
2. uneven distribution of cognitive deficits
3. evidence of focal brain damage (unilateral spastic limb weakness or unilateral increased tendon reflexes or extensor plantar response or pseudobulbar palsy)
4. evidence of cerebrovascular disease judged to be etiologically related to the dementia.

These criteria were used in the Canadian Study of Health and Aging (Lindsay et al, 1997).

Vascular dementia subcategories

The potential for subcategorization in vascular dementia is large and some attempt to describe a multitude of causal pathways is made in most reviews. In the description of NINDS-AIREN criteria, six groups of 'lesions' are described:

1. multi-infarct dementia
2. strategic infarct dementia
3. small vessel disease with dementia
4. hypoperfusion
5. haemorrhagic dementia
6. 'other mechanisms' (including combinations of the previous ones).

A more formal eight-category system was proposed by Konno et al (1997) but has not passed into general use. Of the diagnostic systems described above, only ICD-10 formally recognizes subtypes, all of which require the generic criteria summarized earlier. These categories are:

- F01.0 'Vascular dementia of acute onset (rapid onset within 3 months of one or more strokes)'
- F01.1 Multi-infarct dementia (gradual onset following minor ischemic episodes'
- F01.2 Subcortical vascular dementia (with a history of hypertension and evidence of deep white matter vascular disease with cortical preservation)

- F01.3 'Mixed cortical and subcortical vascular dementia'
- F01.8 'Other vascular dementia'
- F01.9 'Vascular dementia, unspecified'.

Although all these systems describe potential pathways linking cerebrovascular disease and dementia, there is little evidence that these can be reliably defined and distinguished as categories in life.

Problems with the vascular dementia diagnosis

Most diagnoses have an arbitrary basis and serve particular agendas which will inevitably change over time and demand re-evaluation. Vascular dementia has received criticism throughout its existence as a diagnosis, although this has intensified more recently. Several factors underlie this.

A shift in focus towards mild/preclinical disease

People dying in the 1960s (and therefore contributing to early clinicopathological studies) would have had much more florid cerebrovascular disease than would occur in today's older generations, at least in developed nation settings. With increased longevity, mixed states of relatively mild pathology have become more common. These mixed states have also become more readily identified in life with advances in neuroimaging and other technology. Furthermore, there is increasing evidence that cerebrovascular and Alzheimer processes overlap to a large extent (Neuropathology Group of the Medical Research Council Cognitive Function and Ageing Study, 2001), may interact in their effects (Stewart, 1998) and cannot be considered as truly distinct. These are poorly characterized by mutually exclusive diagnoses, or indeed by any categorical system.

Assumed causation

Whatever qualifications are made, vascular dementia as a diagnosis will always convey the impression of a syndrome with discrete etiology and outcome. Diagnoses based on assumed causation are frail constructs since understanding of causal processes inevitably changes and nature rarely operates in ways that are convenient for taxonomists. Cerebrovascular disease can now be measured at levels which may contribute to dementia but are unlikely to be a sufficient *cause* in isolation. Cerebrovascular disease may frequently precipitate dementia in the presence of comorbid Alzheimer pathology (Snowdon et al, 1997; Esiri et al, 1999), questioning the extent to which the two processes can be separated. It is also doubtful whether any clinician or pathologist can ever identify the cause of dementia with certainty, particularly where processes may be occurring within the bounds of what is 'normal for age'.

Problems applying criteria

Chui et al (2000) found very poor agreement between diagnostic instruments with proportions of case vignettes identified as vascular dementia varying from 5% (NINDS-AIREN probable) to 26% (DSM-IV). Poor inter-rater reliability scores have also been found for most diagnostic instruments (Lopez et al, 1994; Chui et al, 2000). Furthermore, clinical diagnoses using the systems described above show poor agreement with pathological diagnoses in several studies (Gold et al, 1997; Holmes et al, 1999; Gold et al 2002), in particular poor detection of vascular pathology.

The meaning of the diagnosis

The diagnosis of vascular dementia essentially involves ascertaining whether dementia is present, ascertaining whether cerebrovascular disease is present and, in some systems, deciding on whether or not there might be a causal link between the two in any given individual. All of these, but particularly the last, involve subjective judgments which give rise to poor inter-rater and between-instrument agreement. Certain aspects of the dementia syndrome, such as the course characteristics and an unequal distribution of cognitive deficits, have traditionally been used to define likely causation in individuals. However these do not stand up well to clinical or clinicopathological investigation (Fischer et al, 1990; Boston et al, 2001). Even histopathological examinations cannot establish causation at an individual level and 'validation' of clinical criteria concerns their ability to predict levels of a particular pathology (e.g. cerebrovascular disease) rather than the actual *cause* of the dementia, particularly now that traditional thresholds for Alzheimer and cerebrovascular pathology have been called into question (Neuropathology Group of the Medical Research Council Cognitive Function and Ageing Study, 2001). If causation cannot be established at an individual level, vascular dementia as a diagnosis merely defines a group of people who have both dementia and cerebrovascular disease. This may not communicate anything more than the presence of two commonly comorbid conditions.

The meaning of 'dementia'

A particular criticism of vascular dementia as a diagnosis concerns the way in which 'dementia' has been defined (Hachinski, 1992; Bowler and Hachinski, 2000). All criteria refer to a definition of dementia which might be called generic but was in fact defined with Alzheimer's disease in mind, placing emphasis on memory impairment. This is important both for research (e.g. investigating domain-specific cognitive function in dementia where this has been pre-defined as part of the diagnosis) and for clinical practice (because people with deterioration in other cognitive functions may fail to receive appropriate services from AD-focused 'memory clinics').

The importance of diagnoses

Diagnostic systems are principally devised with researchers and clinicians in mind. These two groups may have the same needs but this is not always necessarily the case. For dementia, research agendas have principally shaped current diagnoses, particularly the need to maximize comparability between studies. This was achieved for Alzheimer's disease by restricting the profile of the disorder to one which could be agreed on. The same was attempted for vascular dementia although this involved broadening rather than restricting the syndrome and has not stood up well to critical evaluation. The problems for research are self-evident. From a clinical perspective, it has been traditional to subcategorize dementia for many years but this has had few real implications until recently. What was being communicated clinically by a diagnosis of vascular dementia or MID was that the patient concerned might have vascular risk factors such as hypertension or diabetes which required consideration, that they might experience further strokes and possibly that they had a higher mortality than if they had AD. A diagnosis of dementia has been sufficient for most aspects of care and service delivery, with subcategories generally of little further relevance.

This situation has changed with the advent of agents that may modify the course of dementia. Diagnoses determine inclusion criteria for clinical trials and, ultimately, treatment eligibility. If a large proportion of people with dementia and cerebrovascular disease have comorbid AD, should cerebrovascular disease be considered an exclusion criterion for clinical trials? Should cerebrovascular disease preclude a given intervention if trials have only been conducted in its absence? For a given agent, are separate trials required for

Alzheimer's disease and vascular dementia if underlying pathological processes cannot be separated or easily distinguished?

Potential solutions

If diagnoses serve conflicting agendas in research and clinical practice, it is reasonable to consider each separately before deciding whether 'one size fits all'. In some respects, clinical practice comes with less 'baggage' and can be considered first.

Potential solutions for clinical practice

Firstly, it is important to bear in mind the limited value of subcategorizing dementia in most areas of clinical decision-making. It is also important to consider whether assigning vascular dementia as a diagnosis imparts any more information than saying 'This patient has some cerebrovascular disease which may or may not have contributed to their dementia'. Etiology has limited relevance in clinical practice if the outcome has already developed, unless response to treatment, course or prognosis can be predicted. Cerebrovascular disease is recognized as an important risk factor for dementia but there has so far been little evidence of a substantial effect on the course of dementia once this has developed (Lee et al, 2000; Mungas et al, 2001). What impact it may have (e.g. on mortality or risk of depression) may not be substantially different from that in someone without dementia. Assumed etiology is more appropriately considered in the formulation rather than the diagnosis (there is no perceived need to define 'life event depression' or 'obstetric complication schizophrenia'). Dementia is then the primary diagnosis and cerebrovascular disease considered as one of several potential predisposing or precipitating factors. Where an intervention has been shown to be specific to a particular pathological process (and this has yet to be conclusively demonstrated for any pharmacological intervention to date), it may then be appropriate to come to an opinion on what might be causing a particular aspect of cognitive and/or functional decline at a given point and intervene accordingly.

Potential solutions for research

The problem for research is that the more a particular system of measurement or classification is used, the more background literature accumulates and the less easy it is to evaluate critically. There is also a need in many areas of investigation to communicate findings to clinicians or other interested parties. What better way of doing this than to use a system which may be flawed but at least is understood by most people? The problem is that it may not be possible to continue to ignore the flaws when they begin to compromise the validity of results. Furthermore, it is not clear how well vascular dementia is actually understood. If new measurements are to be devised, there are various possible avenues.

Syndrome restriction

A criticism of vascular dementia as it is currently conceptualized is that it tries to include too many separate syndromes under one label and is therefore heterogeneous and meaningless. One possibility would be to carry out further investigation with a view to identifying more discrete entities. Vascular dementia certainly includes syndromes for which a diagnosis is reasonable, such as strategic single infarct syndromes or specific genetic disorders such as CADASIL (cerebral autosomal dominant arteriopathy with subcortical infarcts and leukoencephalopathy). However, to date, these account for very few cases of dementia. A focus on subcortical vascular dementia has also been proposed (Erkinjuntti et al, 2000).

Syndrome expansion

Another approach might be to forget any attempts to deduce causation and to apply a category to anyone with dementia and a given level of cerebrovascular disease, regardless of other suspected pathology. This has some pragmatic advantages and was the approach taken in a recent trial of an acetylcholinesterase inhibitor, targeting people both with 'probable vascular dementia' and 'AD combined with cerebrovascular disease' (Erkinjuntti et al, 2002). Of course there is then the criticism that heterogeneous 'subgroup effects' may not have been detected (Schneider, 2002) but this is essentially a no-win situation with current diagnostic systems.

Forget subclassification

Another approach is to abandon attempts to classify dementia, at least with respect to AD/vascular dementia, in the first place. One alternative would be to adopt a dimensional rather than categorical system of 'measuring' underlying disease, for example the degree of cortical infarction, degree of white matter damage or the degree of primary degeneration. This would in theory provide a more valid means to assess the contributions of overlapping

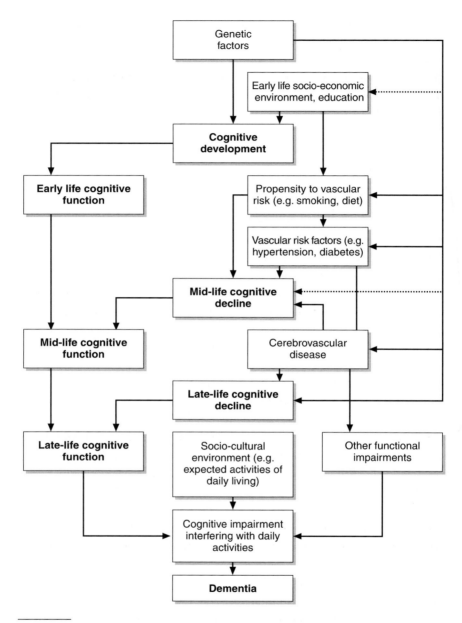

Figure 2.1 *Potential causal pathways underlying cerebrovascular disease and dementia.*

pathological processes. It is uncertain whether current techniques can quantify causal processes *in vivo* with sufficient accuracy for this approach, although this may not be too distant a prospect. An approach which is increasingly adopted in epidemiological research is to treat dementia as the primary outcome for most analyses and then to include, possibly, secondary analyses for specific subcategories.

Forget dementia

The approaches discussed above assume that dementia is itself an appropriate outcome for research. Causal pathways underlying associations between cerebrovascular disease and dementia may operate over an entire life course (Figure 2.1) and many of these are best investigated by focusing on cognitive impairment, or longitudinally on cognitive decline, at a much earlier stage and in younger age groups. Although there are important reasons to support this line of research, it has to be recognized that, to some extent, it breaks the line of communication with clinical practice. Effects on levels of (or change in) performance on one or more of a legion of cognitive tests have little meaning for most clinicians. This is not necessarily a problem but it requires an acceptance that clinical practice and research may have to go their own ways for a while.

As discussed above, definitions of dementia have been conceptualized with AD in mind and may poorly reflect cognitive decline associated with cerebrovascular disease because of their focus on memory impairment. This is also the case with respect to mild cognitive impairment since many definitions require evidence of memory impairment (Ritchie and Touchon, 2000); vascular cognitive impairment has been proposed as an alternative (Hachinski and Bowler, 1993; Rockwood et al, 2000; O'Brien et al, 2003). This allows a more broad spectrum of cognitive deficits and gets away from definitions of dementia which may be influenced by a number of factors apart from the absolute level of cognitive impairment (see Figure 2.1) and may involve, at early stages, highly subjective judgments (e.g. as to whether the perceived effects of cognitive impairment constitute grounds for diagnosis). The problem with this approach is that it may, like vascular dementia, be difficult to operate in a research setting because of assumed etiology, involving a (strongly subjective) decision whether someone's level of cognitive function is or is not related to their level of cerebrovascular disease.

Summary

Diagnoses in the field of vascular dementia have evolved over time but may have reached a stage where they have little further usefulness. In clinical settings, it is doubtful whether the vascular dementia diagnosis ever was useful, and it may now even be harmful with the advent of pharmacotherapy in dementia and indications for treatment. In research settings, the categorization of pathology in dementia is now seriously out of step with the complex, overlapping systems which are actually being observed. A dimensional approach makes intuitive sense and is possibly just beginning to come within the reach of technology. However categorical diagnoses remain fundamental in clinical practice. If new 'measurement' systems are to be developed in the future, an important question will be whether research and clinical practice can find common ground.

References

American Psychiatric Association, *Diagnostic and Statistical Manual of Mental Disorders*, 3rd edn., (APA: Washington DC, 1980).

American Psychiatric Association, *Diagnostic and Statistical Manual of Mental Disorders*, 3rd edn rev, (APA: Washington DC, 1987).

American Psychiatric Association, *Diagnostic and Statistical Manual of Mental Disorders*, 4th edn, (APA: Washington DC, 1994).

Andersen K, Launer LJ, Dewey ME et al, Gender differences in the incidence of AD and vascular dementia, *Neurology* (1999) **53**:1992–7.

Boston PF, Dennis MS, Jagger C et al, Unequal distribution of cognitive deficits in vascular dementia – is this a valid criterion in the ICD-10? *Int J Geriatr Psychiatry* (2001) **16**:422–6.

Bowler JV, Hachinski V, Criteria for vascular dementia: replacing dogma with data, *Arch Neurol* (2000) **57**:170–1.

Chui HC, Victoroff JI, Margolin D et al, Criteria for the diagnosis of ischemic vascular dementia proposed by the state of California Alzheimer's Disease Diagnostic and Treatment Centers, *Neurology* (2000) **42**:473–80.

Chui HC, Mack W, Jackson JE et al, Clinical criteria for the diagnosis of vascular dementia, *Arch Neurol* (2000) **57**:191–6.

Erkinjuntti, T., Inzitari, D., Pantoni, L. et al, Research criteria for subcortical vascular dementia in clinical trials. *Journal of Neural Transmission Supplementum* (2000) **59**: 23–30.

Erkinjuntti T, Kurz A, Gauthier S et al, Efficacy of galantamine in probable vascular dementia and Alzheimer's disease combined with cerebrovascular disease: a randomised trial, *Lancet* (2002) **359**:1283–90.

Esiri MM, Nagy Z, Smith MZ et al, Cerebrovascular disease and threshold for dementia in the early stages of Alzheimer's disease, *Lancet* (1999) **354**:919–20.

Fischer P, Gatterer G, Marterer A et al, Course characteristics in the differentiation of dementia of the Alzheimer type and multi-infarct dementia, *Acta Psychiatr Scand* (1990) **81**:551–3.

Gold G, Giannakopoulos P, Montes-Paixao CJ et al, Sensitivity and specificity of newly proposed clinical criteria for possible vascular dementia, *Neurology* (1997) **49**:690–4.

Gold G, Bouras C, Canuto A et al, Clinicopathological validation study of four sets of clinical criteria for vascular dementia, *Am J Psychiatry* (2002) **159**:82–7.

Hachinski V, Preventable senility: a call for action against the vascular dementias, *Lancet* (1992) **340**:645–8.

Hachinski VC, Bowler JV, Vascular dementia, *Neurology* (1993) **43**:2159–60.

Hachinski VC, Iliff LD, Zilhka E et al, Cerebral blood flow in dementia, *Arch Neurol* (1975) **32**:632–7.

Holmes C, Cairns N, Lantos P, Mann A, Validity of current clinical criteria for Alzheimer's disease, vascular dementia and dementia with Lewy bodies, *Br J Psychiatry* (1999) **174**:45–50.

Konno S, Meyer JS, Terayama Y et al, Classification, diagnosis and treatment of vascular dementia, *Drugs Ageing* (1997) **11**:361–73.

Lee JH, Olichney JM, Hansen LA et al, Small concomitant vascular lesions do not influence rates of cognitive decline in patients with Alzheimer disease, *Arch Neurol* (2000) **57**:1474–9.

Lindsay J, Hebert R, Rockwood K, The Canadian Study of Health and Aging: risk factors for vascular dementia, *Stroke* (1997) **28**:526–30.

Lopez OL, Larumbe MR, Becker JT et al, Reliability of NINDS-AIREN clinical criteria for the diagnosis of vascular dementia, *Neurology* (1994) **44**:1240–5.

Mayer-Gross W, Slater E, Roth M, *Clinical Psychiatry*, 3rd edn (Baillière, Tindall & Carsell: London, 1969).

McKhann G, Drachman D, Folstein M et al, Clinical diagnosis of Alzheimer's disease. Report of the NINCDS-ADRDA Work Group under the auspices of the Department of Health and Human Services Task Force on Alzheimer's Disease, *Neurology* (1984) **34**:939–44.

Mölsa PK, Paljärvi L, Rinne JO et al, Validity of clinical diagnosis in dementia: a prospective clinicopathological study, *J Neurol Neurosurg Psychiatry* (1985) **48**:1085–90.

Mungas D, Reed BR, Ellis WG, Jagust WJ, The effects of age on rate of progression of Alzheimer's disease and dementia with associated cerebrovascular disease, *Arch Neurol* (2001) **58**:1243–7.

Neuropathology Group of the Medical Research Council Cognitive Function and Ageing Study, Pathological correlates of late-onset dementia in a multicentre, community-based population in England and Wales, *Lancet* (2001) **357**:169–75.

O'Brien JT, Erkinjuntti T, Reisberg B et al, Vascular Cognitive Impairment, *Lancet Neurology* 2003 (in press).

Ott A, Breteler MMB, van Harskamp F et al, Prevalence of Alzheimer's disease and vascular dementia: association with education. The Rotterdam Study, *BMJ* (1995) **310**:970–3.

Posner HB, Tang M-X, Luchsinger J et al, The relationship of hypertension in the elderly to AD, vascular dementia, and cognitive function, *Neurology* (2002) **58**:1175–81.

Ritchie K, Touchon J, Mild cognitive impairment: conceptual basis and current nosological status, *Lancet* (2000) **355**:225–8.

Rockwood K, Wentzel C, Hachinski V et al, Prevalence and outcomes of vascular cognitive impairment, *Neurology* (2000) **54**:447–51.

Roman GC, Tatemichi TK, Erkinjuntti T et al, Vascular dementia: diagnostic criteria for research studies: Report of the NINDS-AIREN International Workshop, *Neurology* (1993) **43**:1609–11.

Rosen WG, Terry RD, Fuld PA et al, Pathological verification of ischemic score in differentiation of dementias, *Ann Neurol* (1980) **7**:486–8.

Ross GW, Petrovitch H, White LR et al, Characterization of risk factors for vascular dementia. The Honolulu–Asia Aging Study, *Neurology* (1999) **53**:337–43.

Schneider LS, Galantamine for vascular dementia: some answers, some questions, *Lancet* (2002) **359**:1265–6.

Snowdon DA, Greiner LH, Mortimer JA et al, Brain infarction and the clinical expression of Alzheimer's disease, *JAMA* (1997) **277**:813–17.

Stewart R, Cardiovascular factors in Alzheimer's disease, *J Neurol Neurosurg Psychiatry* (1998) **65**:143–7.

World Health Organization (2002), *International Classification of Diseases and Health Related Problems*, 10th revision (World Health Organization: Geneva).

Yoshitake T, Kiyohara Y, Kato I et al, Incidence and risk factors of vascular dementia and Alzheimer's disease in a defined elderly Japanese population: the Hisayama Study, *Neurology* (1995) **45**:1161–8.

Part II

Epidemiology and Risk Factors

chapter 3

Epidemiology of vascular dementia in Europe

Ingmar Skoog and Olafur Aevarsson

Introduction

Vascular dementia (VaD) may be caused by several different cerebrovascular disorders, the most common being stroke and ischemic white matter lesions. Almost all population-based studies, however, use the term to describe the prevalence and incidence of VaD related to small and large strokes. The only population study that examined VaD related to ischemic white matter lesions suggested that this may be the most common cause of all dementias (Skoog et al, 1994). Seventy percent of demented 85-year-olds in that study had ischemic white matter lesions compared to 35% in the non-demented group.

Prevalence of vascular dementia

VaD related to stroke is generally believed to be the second most common cause of dementia after Alzheimer's disease (AD). As may be seen in Table 3.1, the proportion of demented individuals diagnosed with VaD varies, while there is no substantial difference in the age-stratified prevalence of dementia. The proportion diagnosed with VaD is believed to be lower in Western Europe and among North Americans of European ancestry than in Asia and Eastern Europe (Jorm et al, 1987; Rocca et al, 1991). One Swedish study (Skoog et al, 1993), and two Italian studies (Rocca et al, 1990, Ravaglia et al, 2002) reported a higher proportion of VaD than otherwise reported in western countries. The Swedish study, which concerned 85-year-olds in Gothenburg, also had a higher proportion of VaD than reported in another Swedish study from Stockholm published at about the same time (Fratiglioni

Table 3.1 Prevalence of dementia and vascular dementia (VaD) in Europe

	Country	Age (yrs) Gender	All dementias					Proportion (%) with VaD among the demented
			70–74 %	75–79 %	80–84 %	85–89 %	90+ %	
Fratiglioni et al (1991)	Sweden	men		5	10	14	22	26
		women		6	10	22	34	24
Ott et al (1995)	Holland	men	2	6	14	28	41	18
		women	2	6	19	33	41	15
Rocca et al (1990)	Italy	men	4	9	26	43		40
		women	3	8	11	33		35
O'Connor et al (1989)	Britain	all		4	11	19	33	21
Aevarsson & Skoog (1997)	Sweden	men				27[e]/25[f]		44[e]/44[f]
Skoog et al (1993)	Sweden	women				31[e]/46[f]		44[e]/45[f]
Livingston et al (1990)	Britain	men	2[b]		9>			13 (both sexes)
		women	4[b]		18>			
Sulkava et al (1985)	Finland	men	5[a]	8[d]		12[g]		42
		women	3[a]	12[d]		20[g]		37
Manubens et al (1995)	Spain	men		9	14	24		16
		women		14	19	26		11
Brayne & Calloway (1989)	Britain	women	0	3				31
Ravaglia et al (2002)	Italy	all	6[c]					45

[a] = 65–74, [b] = 65–80, [c] = 65–97, [d] = 75–84, [e] = age 85, [f] = age 88, [g] = this age group and above.

et al, 1991). However, the crude prevalence of AD in the same age group was similar in these two studies (13.0% in Gothenburg vs 11.8% in Stockholm), while the prevalence of VaD differed considerably (14.0% in Gothenburg vs 4.9% in Stockholm). It is not clear whether the difference corresponds to differences in risk factors for VaD between these two Swedish cities, to differences in assigning a diagnosis of VaD in cases of stroke, or to any other methodological factor as described below.

The prevalence of dementia increases with age. Most studies find, however, that the prevalence of VaD rises less sharply with age than that of AD (O'Connor et al, 1989; Brayne and Calloway, 1989; Rocca et al, 1991; Åkesson, 1969) and at very high ages the prevalence of VaD may even level off. Therefore most studies report that the relative proportion of VaD among the dementias decreases with increasing age, while that of AD increases (O'Connor et al, 1989; Sulkava et al, 1985; Brayne and Calloway, 1989; Rocca et al, 1991; Magnússon, 1989). These findings are counterintuitive considering that the prevalence of stroke increases with age (Di Carlo et al, 2000).

The prevalence of AD is generally reported to be higher in women than in men (Rocca et al, 1990; O'Connor et al, 1989; Sulkava et al, 1985; Ravaglia et al, 2002; Åkesson, 1969; Kay et al, 1964; Mölsä et al, 1982), especially after age 80. VaD, on the other hand, is reported to be more common in men (Rocca et al, 1990; O'Connor et al, 1989; Sulkava et al, 1985; Jorm et al, 1987; Rocca et al, 1991; Magnússon, 1989; Kay et al, 1964), especially before the age of 75 years.

There are no indications that the prevalence of VaD is decreasing, despite the steady decline in stroke incidence, and better treatment of hypertension. One reason may be that more patients survive after severe stroke. The paradox may be that better treatment of stroke leads to a higher prevalence of VaD.

Incidence of vascular dementia

Prevalence rates are influenced by disease incidence but also by the duration of the disease. Incidence rates therefore provide a better measure of disease risk. However, very few studies have calculated incidence rates for VaD. The incidence of dementia and VaD is shown in Table 3.2. A meta-analysis regarding age-specific incidence of all dementias including VaD was published by Jorm and Jolley (1998). They used a loess-curve fitting to analyze

Table 3.2 Incidence of dementia

	Country	Age (yrs) Gender	70–74	75–79	80–84	85–89	90+	Proportion (%) with VaD among the demented
				Rate per 1000 person-years				
Jorm & Jolley (1998)	Europe mild	all	18	33	60	104	180	
	East Asia mild	all	7	15	33	72		
	Europe moderate	all	6	12	22	38	66	
	USA moderate	all	5	11	18	28		
Fratiglioni et al (1997)	Sweden	men		12	33	25	15	38
		women		20	43	72	87	12
Ott et al (1998)	Holland	men	5	15	25	29	26	23
		women	4	18	25	50	77	11
Aevarsson & Skoog (1996)	Sweden	men				90		46
		women				103		46
Paykel et al (1994)	Britain	men		15	71	29	0	25 (both sexes)
Brayne et al (1995)	Britain	women		27	36	112	89	
Boothby et al (1994)	Britain	all	6	37	39[c]			24
Copeland et al (1992)	Britain	all	4[a]	12[b]		29[c]		21

[a] = 65–74, [b] = 75–84, [c] = this age group and above,

data from 23 published studies reporting age-specific incidence data; the incidence of dementia increased exponentially with age. However, most of the increase seems to be accounted for by an increase in the incidence of AD. Few incidence studies have analyzed VaD separately. The incidence of VaD varies widely between studies but it seems clear that it increases less rapidly with age as compared to AD. Men tend to have a higher incidence of VaD at younger ages and women in very old age.

Two large European incidence studies confirm these findings. The Rotterdam Study (Ott et al, 1998) examined 7046 subjects aged 55 years and older with a mean follow-up time of 2.1 years. The incidence of AD increased steeply with age, while that of VaD increased somewhat up to the oldest age categories where it leveled off. Men had a tendency to develop VaD more often than women. The Kungsholmen Project (Fratiglioni et al, 1997) examined 1473 individuals aged 75 and above. The incidence of VaD was 2.3 per 1000 person-years for women and 3.1 for men in the age group 75 to 79, 7.5 for women and 13.7 for men in the age group 80 to 84, 6.8 for women and 12.3 for men in the age-group 85 to 89, whereas in those above age 90 the figures were 3.9 for women and 0 for men. These figures were much lower than those obtained for AD and the incidence rate increased much more steeply with age for AD than for VaD. As in the other studies, women had a higher incidence of AD in all age groups, while men tended to have a higher incidence of VaD. Two large analyses with pooled data from several European studies (Andersen et al, 1999; Fratiglioni et al, 2000) also reported that the incidence rate of AD increased much more steeply with age than that of VaD but the incidence of VaD was similar in men and women.

The findings that both the prevalence and incidence of VaD appear to level off with age despite the fact that the incidence of stroke increases with age (Hollander et al, 2003) are counterintuitive. One reason may be that the proportion of cerebral infarcts that are clinically silent increases dramatically with age (Vermeer et al, 2002). In traditional epidemiological studies, these cases might be diagnosed as AD.

Methodological factors affecting the proportion diagnosed with vascular dementia

As described in Table 3.3, several methodological factors may influence the proportion diagnosed with VaD.

Auxiliary examinations

Most epidemiological studies have relied mainly on history to obtain information regarding symptoms of cerebrovascular disease. Three European studies (Rocca et al, 1990; Skoog et al, 1993; Livingston et al, 1990) used detailed clinical diagnostic procedures, including computed tomography (CT)-scanning in some cases, on subjects diagnosed as demented in population surveys. In two of these studies (Rocca et al, 1990; Skoog et al, 1993) the relative proportion of VaD was higher than previously reported. In a three-year follow-up study of the 85-year-olds examined by Skoog et al (1993), the proportion of VaD increased from 47% at age 85 to 54% at age 88 despite a higher mortality rate in VaD than in other dementias (Aevarsson and Skoog, 1997). One reason for the increased proportion of vascular dementia was that new episodes of focal neurological symptoms and signs and new infarcts on CT scans were detected during the follow-up in demented individuals with a cause of dementia other than vascular at the age of 85. Diagnosis changed to VaD in 9 out of 31 cases with a diagnosis of AD at age 85. Thus, the more information that is gathered (e.g. from close informants, medical records or brain imaging) and the longer the subjects

Table 3.3 Causes for differences between studies in the proportion diagnosed with vascular dementia (VaD)

- The amount of information collected
- Differential mortality
    - screening
    - prevalence day
- Inclusion of institutionalized individuals
- Diagnostic criteria and their application
- Clinical similarities between AD and VaD
- Cognitive decline after severe stroke
    - dementia or not?
    - AD, VaD or mixed?

are followed, the more cerebrovascular factors are likely to be found. It could be argued whether the classification in these cases should be mixed dementia or AD. However, the new episodes could be an expression of previously silent cerebrovascular disease, which might have already contributed to the dementia at baseline. Cerebrovascular diseases may also increase the possibility that individuals with Alzheimer lesions in their brains will express a dementia syndrome (Snowdon et al, 1997).

Differential mortality

The mortality rate is higher in VaD than in AD (Aevarsson et al, 1998), which may influence the relative proportion diagnosed with VaD in population studies. Many population studies use a screening procedure to identify individuals with dementia. In those screened positive a more comprehensive examination is performed to diagnose the type of dementia. The time between screening and actual examination may strongly affect the proportions of different types of dementia due to the higher mortality rate in VaD. Even in studies not using a screening procedure, the relative proportion of VaD will be affected by differential mortality. Most studies select a certain prevalence day and include all people that are alive on that date. The actual examinations are, however, generally performed some time afterwards. During this time, those with high mortality (e.g. VaD) may be lost disproportionally more often due to death (Skoog et al, 1993). This may be especially important in the very old where mortality rate is high, and may be one explanation for the finding that the frequency of VaD rises less sharply with age than that of AD.

Inclusion of institutionalized individuals

Many population studies do not examine individuals in institutions. This may be especially important at high ages where the institutionalization rate is high. Individuals with VaD are reported to have a higher institutionalization rate than those with AD (Skoog et al, 1993; Fratiglioni et al, 1994). It may be that individuals with VaD more often suffer from other handicaps, such as paresis or aphasia. Studies not including institutionalized individuals may thus yield lower relative proportions of VaD.

The importance of these factors is shown in Table 3.4 where a comparison between the Gothenburg study (Skoog et al, 1993) and the East Boston study (Evans et al, 1989) is performed. The Gothenburg study had a comparatively high proportion with VaD, while the East Boston study had the opposite. In

Table 3.4 A comparison of dementia prevalence in East Boston and Gothenburg

	East Boston	*Gothenburg*
Alzheimer's disease	84	43
Vascular dementia	4	48
Including institutions	No	Yes
Screening	Yes	No
Interval screening → examination	16 months	0
CT-scan	No	Yes
After modifications		
Alzheimer's disease	84	61
Vascular dementia	4	25

Evans et al (1989); Skoog et al (1993).

contrast to the Gothenburg study, the East Boston study used a screening procedure, did not include brain imaging in the diagnostic process and did not include institutionalized individuals. To compensate for the 16-month interval between screening and examination in the East Boston study, all individuals who died during the 16 months after examination are excluded from the Gothenburg study in Table 3.4. Second, diagnoses in Gothenburg are recalculated without using information from CT scans, and finally all individuals in institutions are excluded. By this approach the proportion of VaD in Gothenburg decreased from 47% to 25%.

Diagnostic criteria

In epidemiological studies the criteria for VaD are mainly based on the presence of significant stroke or cerebrovascular disease. The National Institute of Neurological Disorders and Stroke and the Association Internationale pour la Recherche et l'Enseignement en Neurosciences (NINDS-AIREN criteria) (Roman et al, 1993) suggest that a diagnosis of 'possible' vascular dementia may be made in the presence of dementia with focal neurological signs if brain imaging studies are missing or in the absence of a clear temporal relationship between dementia and stroke. Thus, by using these criteria, the dementias will often be divided into one group with and one without stroke. The temporal relationship between stroke and the onset of dementia is often used to strengthen the possibility that the two disorders are etiologically related. The NINDS-AIREN criteria (Roman et al, 1993) suggest a limit of three months for the onset of dementia after stroke. This is difficult to apply in population studies, in which dementia often has had its onset many years before examination and where the exact time of onset of dementia and stroke may be difficult to determine. Most criteria leave much room for the researcher to decide when a stroke is related to a dementia. In studies using brain imaging, the NINDS-AIREN criteria suggest that a diagnosis of probable vascular dementia requires that focal signs consistent with stroke *and* relevant cerebrovascular disease by brain imaging should be present. In the study by Skoog et al (1993), the use of the NINDS-AIREN criteria for probable VaD, requiring a history of stroke *and* brain imaging findings of infarcts, yielded a proportion of 13% for vascular dementia, while the use of the possible VaD criteria gave a proportion of 47%.

Wetterling et al (1996) applied different criteria to 167 elderly patients admitted with probable dementia. Forty-five were classified as VaD according to DSM-IV, 21 according to ICD-10, 12 according to the NINDS-AIREN criteria and 23 according to the criteria of the State of California Alzheimer's Disease Diagnostic and Treatment Centers (ADDTC). Only five cases met criteria for VaD in all diagnostic guidelines. This study illustrates that the proportion of different forms of dementia reported in the literature relies heavily on the criteria used.

Similarities in the clinical expression of AD and VaD

It is possible that VaD may be underdiagnosed and AD may be overdiagnosed in population studies because of the similarities in the clinical expression of these disorders. Firstly, VaD may have an insidious onset and gradual course (Erkinjuntti and Sulkava, 1991; Fischer et al, 1990; O'Brien, 1988) and may be mistaken for AD. Secondly, many infarctions are clinically silent, without evidence of stroke or focal neurological symptoms and signs (Vermeer et al, 2002, Del Ser et al, 1990). Thirdly, even if CT has been used, many infarcts are not detectable by CT (Mohr et al, 1978; Radue et al, 1978), and cerebral areas can be damaged and non-functional although CT-scan imaging remains normal (Harsch et al, 1988).

Stroke

It is not always clear whether individuals with dementia symptoms after one or two major strokes are included in the demented group. It is possible that some population studies have not diagnosed individuals with severe cognitive impairment after a major stroke as having dementia. Furthermore, a diagnosis of dementia may be especially difficult to make in stroke patients suffering from severe aphasia. Thus, if individuals with severe stroke are already excluded at the stage of classification where the presence or absence of dementia is determined, this may explain why the proportion of VaD is often far lower than would be expected considering the frequency of stroke in the population.

Mixed dementias

The brains of a large percentage of cognitively normal individuals contain numerous histopathologic signs of AD (Esiri et al, 2001) and only a small percentage are relatively free of these changes (Esiri et al, 2001; Davis et al, 1999). Similar findings relate to cerebrovascular disease (Esiri et al, 2001). On the other hand, in cases with a typical picture of AD or VaD only minor pathological brain changes are detected (Esiri et al, 2001). This may be one reason why several recent neuropathological studies report that a high proportion of individuals fulfilling the neuropathological diagnosis of AD also exhibit significant cerebrovascular lesions (Esiri et al, 2001; Holmes et al, 1999; Lim et al, 1999; Nagy et al, 1997; Heyman et al, 1998). The contribution of cerebrovascular lesions to the clinical symptoms of dementia are not easy to elucidate. These changes may be the main cause of dementia, they may be the factor that overcomes the brain's compensatory capacity in a subject whose brain is already compromised by Alzheimer encephalopathy and minor manifestations of both disorders, each of which would not be enough to produce dementia alone, may produce it together (Erkinjuntti and Hachinski, 1993). Cerebrovascular diseases may thus increase the possibility that individuals with AD lesions in their brains will express the clinical symptoms of dementia (Skoog et al, 1995), and individuals with a stroke may have increased risk for dementia if they already have subclinical AD lesions in their brains.

In living individuals, several biological markers for AD, such as increased τ-protein levels (Hollander et al, 2003) and decreased levels of β-amyloid (Skoog et al, 2003) in cerebrospinal fluid (CSF), are also found in VaD, and markers for cerebrovascular pathology, such as an increased CSF/blood albumin ratio (Skoog et al, 1998) and white matter lesions on brain imaging

(Skoog et al, 1994) are often seen in AD. These clinical and neuropathological findings suggest that there is a large co-occurrence of AD and VaD in old-age dementias. The proportion of dementias with mixed etiologies is probably underrated. The best approach at present may be to search for treatable vascular causes of cognitive decline in spite of arbitrary borders between VaD and AD. Prevention of cerebrovascular disease may thus be one way to prevent the clinical expression of AD (Skoog, 1999).

Vascular factors in AD

Several population studies from Europe have reported that vascular risk factors may be important also in AD (Skoog et al, 1999; Kivipelto et al, 2001, Ott et al, 1999; Hofman et al, 1997; Skoog et al, 1996). The finding from the Syst-Eur trial (Forette et al, 1998) that treatment of isolated systolic hypertension reduces the incidence of dementia (which in most cases was diagnosed as AD) by 50% emphasizes vascular risk factors as possible targets for prevention. Recently, it was reported that the reduced incidence of dementia in the treated group was maintained two years after the double-blind trial was terminated. It was suggested that antihypertensive treatment of 1000 patients for five years may prevent 20 cases of dementia (Forette et al, 2002). Finally, as already mentioned, other types of VaD than the form associated with stroke, such as white matter dementia, have generally not been examined in population studies. All this indicates that not only the frequency of VaD (i.e. cerebrovascular disease causing dementia) but also the frequency of vascular risk factors in AD have been underestimated during recent decades.

References

Aevarsson O, Skoog I, A population-based study on the incidence of dementia disorders between 85 and 88 years of age, *J Am Geriatr Soc* (1996) **44**:1455–60.

Aevarsson O, Skoog I, Dementia disorders in a birth cohort followed from age 85 to 88. The influence of mortality, non-response and diagnostic change on prevalence, *Int Psychogeriatrics* (1997) **9**:11–23.

Aevarsson O, Svanborg A, Skoog I, Seven-year survival after age 85 years. Relation to Alzheimer disease and vascular dementia, *Arch Neurol* (1998) **55**:1226–32.

Åkesson H, A population study of senile and arteriosclerotic psychoses, *Hum Hered* (1969) **19**:546–66.

Andersen K, Launer LJ, Dewey ME et al, Gender differences in the incidence of AD and vascular dementia: the EURODEM Studies. EURODEM Incidence Research Group, *Neurology* (1999) **53**:1992–7.

Boothby H, Blizard R, Livingston G, Mann AH, The Gospel Oak Study stage III: the incidence of dementia, *Psychol Med* (1994) **24**:89–95.

Brayne C, Calloway P, An epidemiological study of dementia in a rural population of elderly women, *Br J Psychiatry* (1989) **155**:214–19.

Brayne C, Gill C, Huppert FA et al, Incidence of clinically diagnosed subtypes of dementia in an elderly population. Cambridge Project of Later Life, *Br J Psychiatry* (1995) **167**:255–62.

Copeland JRM, Davidson IA, Dewey ME et al, Alzheimer's disease, other dementias, depression and pseudodementia: prevalence, incidence and three-year outcome in Liverpool, *Br J Psychiatry* (1992) **161**:230–9.

Davis DG, Schmitt FA, Wekstein DR, Markesbery WR, Alzheimer neuropathologic alterations in aged cognitively normal subjects, *J Neuropathol Exp Neurol* (1999) **58**:376–88.

Del Ser T, Bermejo F, Portera A et al, Vascular dementia. A clinicopathological study, *J Neurol Sci* (1990) **96**:1–17.

Di Carlo A, Launer LJ, Breteler MM et al, Frequency of stroke in Europe: a collaborative study of population-based cohorts. ILSA Working Group and the Neurologic Diseases in the Elderly Research Group. Italian Longitudinal Study on Aging, *Neurology* (2000) **54** (Suppl 5):S28–S33.

Erkinjuntti T, Sulkava R. Diagnosis of multi-infarct dementia, *Alzheimer Dis Assoc Disord* (1991) **5**:112–21.

Erkinjuntti T, Hachinski V, Dementia post stroke. In: *Physical Medicine and Rehabilitation: State of the Art Reviews*, Vol 7. (Hanley & Belfus Inc: Philadelphia, 1993) 195–212.

Esiri MM, Matthews F, Brayne C, Ince PG for the Neuropathology Group of the Medical Research Council Cognitive Function and Ageing Study (MRC CFAS), Pathological correlates of late-onset dementia in a multicentre, community-based population in England and Wales, *Lancet* (2001) **357**:169–75.

Evans DK, Funkenstein H, Albert MS et al, Prevalence of Alzheimer's disease in a community population of older persons. Higher than previously reported, *JAMA* (1989) **262**:2551–6.

Fischer P, Gatterer G, Marterer A et al, Course characteristics in the differentiation of dementia of the Alzheimer type and multi-infarct dementia, *Acta Psychiatr Scand* (1990) **81**:551–3.

Forette F, Seux M-L, Staessen JA et al, Prevention of dementia in randomised double-blind placebo-controlled Systolic Hypertension in Europe (Syst-Eur) trial, *Lancet* (1998) **352**:1347–51.

Forette F, Seux ML, Staessen JA et al, The prevention of dementia with antihypertensive treatment: new evidence from the Systolic Hypertension in Europe (Syst-Eur) study, *Arch Intern Med* (2002) **162**:2046–52.

Fratiglioni L, Forsell Y, Torres HA, Winblad B, Severity of dementia and institutionalization in the elderly: prevalence data from an urban area in Sweden, *Neuroepidemiology* (1994) **13**:79–88.

Fratiglioni L, Grut M, Forsell Y et al, Prevalence of Alzheimer's disease and other dementias in an elderly urban population: relationship with age, sex and education, *Neurology* (1991) **41**:1886–92.

Fratiglioni L, Viitanen M, von Strauss E et al, Very old women at highest risk of dementia and Alzheimer's disease: incidence data from the Kungsholmen Project, Stockholm, *Neurology* (1997) **48**:132–8.

Fratiglioni L, Launer LJ, Andersen K et al, Incidence of dementia and major subtypes in Europe: a collaborative study of population-based cohorts. Neurologic Diseases in the Elderly Research Group, *Neurology* (2000) **54**:(11 Suppl 5):S10–S15.

Harsch HH, Tikofsky RS, Collier BD, Single photon emission computed tomography imaging in vascular stroke, *Arch Neurol* (1988) **45**:375–6.

Heyman A, Fillenbaum GG, Welsh-Bohmer KA et al, Cerebral infarcts in patients with autopsy-proven Alzheimer's disease: CERAD, Part XVIII. Consortium to Establish a Registry for Alzheimer's Disease, *Neurology* (1998) **51**:159–62.

Hofman A, Ott A, Breteler MMB et al, Atherosclerosis, apolipoprotein E, and the prevalence of dementia and Alzheimer's disease in the Rotterdam Study, *Lancet* (1997) **349**:151–4.

Hollander M, Koudstaal PJ, Bots ML et al, Incidence, risk, and case fatality of first ever stroke in the elderly population. The Rotterdam Study, *J Neurol Neurosurg Psychiatry* (2003) **74**:317–21.

Holmes C, Cairns N, Lantos P, Mann A, Validity of current clinical criteria for Alzheimer's disease, vascular dementia and dementia with Lewy bodies, *Br J Psychiatry* (1999) **174**:45–50.

Jorm AF, Jolley D. The incidence of dementia: a meta-analysis, *Neurology* (1998) **51**:728–33.

Jorm AF, Korten AE, Henderson AS, The prevalence of dementia: a quantitative integration of the literature, *Acta Psychiatr Scand* (1987) **76**:465–79.

Kay DWK, Beamish P, Roth M, Old age mental disorders in Newcastle upon Tyne. Part I: A study of prevalence, *Br J Psychiatry* (1964) **110**:146–58.

Kivipelto M, Helkala E-L, Laakso M et al, Midlife vascular risk factors and Alzheimer's disease in later life: longitudinal, population-based study, *BMJ* (2001) **322**:1447–51.

Lim A, Tsuang D, Kukull W et al, Clinico-neuropathological correlation of Alzheimer's disease in a community-based case series, *J Am Geriatr Soc* (1999) **47**:564–9.

Livingston G, Sax K, Willison J et al, The Gospel Oak study stage II: the diagnosis of dementia in the community, *Psychol Med* (1990) **20**:881–91.

Magnússon H, Mental health of octogenarians in Iceland. An epidemiological study, *Acta Psychiatr Scand* (Suppl) (1989) **79**:1–112.

Manubens JM, Martinez-Lage JM, Lacruz F et al, Prevalence of Alzheimer's disease and other dementing disorders in Pamplona, Spain, *Neuroepidemiology* (1995) **14**:155–64.

Mohr JP, Caplan LR, Melski JW et al, The Harvard cooperative stroke registry: a prospective registry, *Neurology* (1978) **28**:754–62.

Mölsä PK, Marttila R, Rinne UK, Epidemiology of dementia in a Finnish population, *Acta Neurol Scand* (1982) **65**:541–52.

Nagy Z, Esiri MM, Jobst KA et al, The effects of additional pathology on the cognitive deficit in Alzheimer disease, *J Neuropathol Exp Neurol* (1997) **56**:165–70.

O'Brien MD, Vascular dementia is under diagnosed, *Arch Neurol* (1988) **45**:797–8.

O'Connor DW, Pollitt PA, Hyde JB et al, The prevalence of dementia as measured by the Cambridge Mental Disorders of the Elderly examination, *Acta Psychiatr Scand* (1989) **79**:190–8.

Ott A, Breteler MMB, van Harskamp F et al, Incidence and risk of dementia. The Rotterdam Study, *Am J Epidemiol* (1998) **147**:574–80.

Ott A, Breteler MMB, van Harskamp F et al, Prevalence of Alzheimer's disease and vascular dementia: association with education. The Rotterdam Study, *BMJ* (1995) **310**:970–3.

Ott A, Stolk RP, van Harskamp F et al, Diabetes mellitus and the risk of dementia: The Rotterdam Study, *Neurology* (1999) **53**:1937–42.

Paykel ES, Brayne C, Huppert FA et al, Incidence of dementia in a population older than 75 years in the United Kingdom, *Arch Gen Psychiatry* (1994) **51**:325–32.

Radue E-W, Du Boulay GH, Harrison MJ, Thomas DJ, Comparison of angiographic and CT findings between patients with multi-infarct dementia and those with dementia due to primary neuronal degeneration, *Neuroradiology* (1978) **16**:113–15.

Ravaglia G, Forti P, Maioli F et al, Education, occupation, and prevalence of dementia:

findings from the Conselice study. *Dement Geriatr Cogn Disord* (2002) **14:** 90–100.

Rocca WA, Bonaiuto S, Lippi A et al, Prevalence of clinically diagnosed Alzheimer's disease and other dementing disorders: a door-to-door survey in Appignano, Macerata Province, Italy, *Neurology* (1990) **40:**626–31.

Rocca WA, Hofman A, Brayne C et al, The prevalence of vascular dementia in Europe: facts and fragments from 1980–1990 studies, *Ann Neurol* (1991) **30:**817–24.

Roman GC, Tatemichi TK, Erkinjuntti T et al, Vascular dementia: diagnostic criteria for research studies. Report of the NINDS-AIREN international workshop, *Neurology* (1993) **43:**250–60.

Skoog I, Possibilities for secondary prevention of Alzheimer's disease. In: Mayeux R, Christen Y, eds, *The Epidemiology of Alzheimer's Disease: From Gene to Prevention* (Springer Verlag: Berlin, 1999).

Skoog I, Kalaria RN, Breteler MM, Vascular factors and Alzheimer disease, *Alzheimer Dis Assoc Disord* (1999) **13:**S106–S14.

Skoog I, Palmertz B, Andreasson L-A, The prevalence of white matter lesions on computed tomography of the brain in demented and non-demented 85-year-olds, *J Geriatr Psychiatry Neurol* (1994) **7:**169–75.

Skoog I, Nilsson L, Palmertz B et al, A population-based study of dementia in 85-year-olds, *New Engl J Med* (1993) **328:**153–8.

Skoog I, Vanmechelen E, Andreasson L-A et al, A population-based study of tau protein and ubiquitin in cerebrospinal fluid in 85-year-olds: relation to severity of dementia and cerebral atrophy, but not to the apolipoprotein E4 allele. *Neurodegeneration* (1995) **4:**433–42.

Skoog I, Lernfelt B, Landahl S et al, A 15-year longitudinal study on blood pressure and dementia, *Lancet* (1996) **347:**1141–5.

Skoog I, Wallin A, Fredman P et al, A population study on blood–brain barrier function in 85-year-olds. Relation to Alzheimer's disease and vascular dementia, *Neurology* (1998) **50:**966–71.

Skoog I, Davidsson P, Aevarsson O et al, Cerebrospinal fluid beta-amyloid 42 is reduced before the onset of sporadic dementia: a population-based study in 85-year-olds, *Dement Geriatr Cogn Disord* (2003) **15:**169–76.

Snowdon DA, Greiner LH, Mortimer JA et al, Brain infarction and the clinical expression of Alzheimer disease. The Nun Study, *JAMA* (1997) **277:**813–17.

Sulkava R, Wikström J, Aromaa A et al, Prevalence of severe dementia in Finland, *Neurology* (1985) **35:**1025–9.

Vermeer SE, Koudstaal PJ, Oudkerk M et al, Prevalence and risk factors of silent brain infarcts in the population-based Rotterdam Scan Study, *Stroke* (2002) **33:**21–5.

Wetterling T, Kanitz R-D, Borgis K-J, Comparison of different diagnostic criteria for vascular dementia (ADDTC, DSM-IV, ICD-10, NINDS-AIREN), *Stroke* (1996) **27:**30–6.

chapter 4

Epidemiology of vascular dementia in North America

Robin Eastwood and John O'Brien

History

The early studies of epidemiology of dementia in North America, now primarily of historical interest, have been reviewed elsewhere (Eastwood et al, 1991). The early mental hospital studies dealt mainly with such diagnostic categories as senile psychoses and cerebral arteriosclerosis. Studies in Massachusetts and New York state in the first part of the 20th century suggested that cerebral arteriosclerosis was increasing (Elkind and Taylor, 1936; Malzberg, 1935; Landis and Page, 1938). These authors recognized that there were nosocomial effects and that the differential diagnosis of these disorders was often difficult and that the conditions frequently coexisted.

Subsequently, community cross-sectional studies (Pfeffer et al, 1987; Evans et al 1989) showed that Alzheimer's disease (AD) and cognitive impairment were more prevalent than previously reported. Longitudinal studies obviously give more interesting information than cross-sectional studies, and can provide data on incidence and risk factors. One example was a New York study of volunteers (Katzman et al, 1989) which looked at the incidence of dementia over a five-year period. Fifty-six cases out of 434 subjects, all 75–85 years on entry, developed dementia with 32 (57%) meeting diagnostic criteria for AD and 15 (27%) for multi-infarct dementia (MID) or mixed dementia; eight (14%) had other disorders or were undiagnosed. The observed incidence of dementia was 3.53 per 100 person-years at risk and for AD alone was about two per 100 person-years at risk. Risk factors for MID and mixed dementia were diabetes, left ventricular hypertrophy and a history of stroke.

However, several methodological issues limit the interpretation of these early studies. The recognition that mixed dementia occurs more commonly than expected by chance alone (Rockwood, 1997), together with the growing consensus that there is a spectrum of disease from pure AD to pure vascular dementia (VaD) (O'Brien et al, 2003), has greatly influenced the way epidemiological studies should be conducted and how their results are interpreted. These facts substantially complicate the calculation of estimated rates and investigation of risk factors. For example, previous formulations of VaD as purely 'multi-infarct' dementia have almost certainly led to a significant underestimation of VaD in most epidemiological studies to date (see 'Classification').

Classification

It is important to consider the historical perspective on diagnosis (see also Chapter 1). During the 20th century there was an initial interest in 'hardening of the arteries' producing chronic hypoperfusion but interest waned when AD became *au courant* in the mid- and late-century. What was left was a belief in North America that VaD was the second most common dementia, at around 10–20% of all dementias. Hachinski, who has had such a significant role in this field, developed the terms 'multi-infarct dementia' (MID) (Hachinski et al, 1974) and 'leukoaraiosis' (Hachinski et al, 1987), and described the Hachinski scale (Hachinski et al, 1975) to separate AD and MID. In 1992 he made a 'call for action against the vascular dementias' (Hachinski, 1992). It was realized that the term 'multi-infarct dementia' was too limited and that conceptually the term 'vascular dementia' (VaD) was an improvement. This allowed for such mechanisms as single, strategic strokes, small vessel disease and white matter changes, hypoperfusion and other non-stroke cardiovascular causes. Nevertheless, the tussle between the cerebral infarct argument and the hypoperfusion viewpoint has so far not been settled.

Several sets of criteria for VaD have been proposed and are described in more detail in Chapter 2. These are:

- the Hachinski ischemic score (Hachinski et al, 1975)
- the ICD-9 definition of arteriosclerotic dementia and the ICD-10 definition of VaD (World Health Organization, 1992)
- the DSM-III, DSM-III-R and DSM-IV definitions of multi-infarct dementia (American Psychiatric Association, 1994)
- the CAMDEX definition of multi-infarct/VaD (Roth et al, 1988)

- the California Alzheimer Treatment Centers definition (Chui et al, 1990)
- NINDS-AIREN Consensus Group criteria (Roman et al, 1993)
- the criteria for Subcortical Ischemic Vascular Dementia (SIVD) (Erkin-juntti et al, 2000).

These sets of criteria are 'conceptually similar but differ in detail' and, apart from those for SIVD, are each rooted in the multiple infarct model for VaD and the AD model for cognitive impairment. The sensitivity and specificity of these criteria vary and they are not interchangeable (Gold et al, 2002). The NINDS-AIREN criteria (Roman et al, 1993), often considered the most rigorous, have high specificity (>80%) though sensitivity can be low (40–50%) (Gold et al, 2002). As such, interpretation of the data from epidemiological studies is very dependent on the criteria used. There are three very important points to make. Firstly, that the low sensitivity means that epidemiological measures of prevalence and incidence of VaD using such criteria will be underestimates compared with AD, for which the criteria have higher sensitivity. Secondly, that the current criteria do not recognize mixed dementias, yet mixed pathology is almost certainly the most common cause of cognitive impairment in epidemiologically representative samples (MRC/CFAS, 2001). Finally, the emphasis on dementia, with the need for significant memory impairment, which is often absent in those with VaD, as a requirement for 'caseness' in epidemiological studies, will also lead to underestimates of prevalence and incidence rates for significant cognitive impairment due to cerebrovascular disease. A possible solution to these particular issues has been by the suggested use of the term, 'vascular cognitive impairment' (VCI), which recognizes the full spectrum of vascular contribution to cognitive impairment (Bowler and Hachinski, 1995; O'Brien et al, 2003). One current difficulty with the term VCI is that some authors use it to include all cognitive impairment (i.e. including VaD) whilst others reserve it to describe cognitive impairments falling short of the traditional definition of dementia. Any distinction between these two uses is somewhat arbitrary as a continuum exists. However, it is important to note that VCI, as used in the epidemiological studies referred to below, excludes VaD.

Cross-sectional (prevalence) studies

More recent epidemiological studies confirm the higher prevalence rates for VaD compared to AD in North American samples and show both disorders to be highly age-related. The Canadian Study of Health and Aging is a prevalence and incidence study of 10 253 randomly selected community and institution dwelling subjects over the age of 65 from five centers. Prevalence rates for AD were 5.1% (ranging from 1% for those 65–74 to 26% for over 85) while rates for VaD were 1.5% (ranging from 0.6% in those 65–74 to 4.8% in those over 85) (CSHA, 1994). Similar findings are reported from the Cache County Study on Memory in Aging, which has studied 5092 residents 65 and older from Cache County, Utah. Of the 6.5% with dementia, 65% had AD and 19% VaD (Lyketsos et al, 2000). This study also provided some of the first data on the frequency and prevalence of non-cognitive features of dementia, often known as Behavioral and Psychological Symptoms of Dementia (BPSD), in an epidemiologically representative cohort. Of those with dementia, 61% had one or more behavioral symptoms with apathy, depression and agitation/aggression being the most common. Overall, there were surprisingly few differences in types or frequency of BPSD between VaD and AD, though AD subjects were more likely to have delusions (22.4% vs 8.1%) and less likely to have depression (20.1% vs 32.3%) than those with VaD (Lyketsos et al, 2000).

One of the most interesting epidemiological puzzles has been the finding of higher rates for AD than VaD in Western (including USA) studies and vice versa for Japanese and Asian studies. The Honolulu–Asia Aging study has specifically examined prevalence rates in Japanese-American men. Rates of dementia were 9.3% (the sample was aged over 70) with 5.4% AD and 4.2% VaD (White et al, 1996). Of those with VaD, 50% cases were attributed to small vessel disease, 23% to large vessel infarcts and 16% to both (Ross et al, 1999). Interestingly, rates for VaD were lower than in Japan but higher than expected in Europe-ancestry US populations. This study also examined risk factors, finding that age, coronary heart disease and elevated glucose were associated with VaD while a preference for the Western diet and the use of vitamin E were protective. This suggests that environmental as well as genetic factors might explain some of the differences in prevalence rates for VaD between countries.

VCI, being a somewhat more recent concept, has not been well investigated in many epidemiological studies. However, the Canadian Study on Health and Aging used the term 'cognitive impairment no dementia' (CIND) and divided this into different types, including vascular CIND (Rockwood et al, 2000). Vascular CIND had a higher prevalence than VaD (2.6% vs 1.5%) and was also age related (prevalence 1.4% in 65–74 years but 3.8% in 85+); there were no clear sex differences. Similar high prevalence rates (3.6% of all those over 65) for cognitive impairment due to stroke, and so presumably vascular, have also been reported from other populations (Unverzagt et al, 2001). While further studies are awaited with interest from the limited evidence to date it appears that VCI will be at least twice as common as VaD, just as 'amnestic' mild cognitive impairment (a risk factor for AD) is at least twice as common as AD.

Relatively recently neuroimaging investigations performed on large samples have made data available on the prevalence of cerebral pathology in the general population, including the frequency of infarcts and white matter lesions. One such study investigated magnetic resonance imaging (MRI) changes in 3324 older subjects who were part of the Cardiovascular Health Study. Infarcts, defined as lesions greater than 3 mm in size, were present in 31% of subjects, including 28% with no prior history of stroke (Longstreth et al, 1998). They were associated with cognitive impairment and neurological abnormalities. Most were small and the most common location was the basal ganglia. Silent infarcts were an independent predictor of subsequent symptomatic stroke over a 4-year follow-up (Bernick et al, 2001), as were white matter lesions, with the highest stroke risk seen in those with a combination of the two (Longstreth et al, 2001). Risk factors for silent stroke and white matter change were similar, including advancing age, low income and hypertension. A subgroup with no infarcts at baseline were rescanned five years later (Longstreth et al, 2002). Incidence of new infarction was 18%, but only 11% of these had experienced a stroke or transient ischemic attack. New infarctions were associated with white matter lesions at baseline and cognitive decline over the follow-up. Such large prospective imaging studies provide important data on the high prevalence and incidence of 'silent' infarction in epidemiological samples and help define risk factors, including the presence of white matter changes. The association with cognitive decline means that small infarcts, such as white matter change, should not really be considered 'silent' but an important substrate of cognitive impairment.

Longitudinal (incidence) studies

Dementia after stroke

Several studies have shown that stroke is an extremely important risk factor for subsequent dementia. Tatemichi et al (1990) from Columbia, New York, determined the prevalence of dementia in 927 patients over the age of 60 who had suffered an acute ischemic stroke. Of 726 testable patients, 116

(16%) were demented as ascertained by the clinical judgment of a neurologist. Regarding risk factors, the prevalence of dementia was related to age, reduced alertness, aphasia and hemi-neglect but not to gender, race, handedness, education level or employment status prior to the stroke. Previous stroke and previous myocardial infarction were also related to stroke but not hypertension, diabetes mellitus, atrial fibrillation and a previous use of antithrombotic drugs. Prevalence was most linked to infarcts following large vessel disease. The authors use the generic term 'dementia' and, in actuality, over one-third of their cases were vascular, over one-third were AD and a quarter were mixed. From CT findings, it was shown that the number of old and new lesions, cortical atrophy and hydrocephalus were significantly associated with prevalence but not infarct volume. Regarding site, dementia was more frequent when the lesion was in the occipital, temporo-occipital and temporoparietal areas. Incidence was determined on 610 patients not demented at stroke onset and was found to be 5.4% for a 60-year-old and 10.4% for a 90-year-old. Age, but not gender, previous stroke and cortical atrophy were risk factors at stroke onset.

Two years later, the same group (Tatemichi et al, 1992) asked the following research question: does cerebrovascular disease increase the risk of dementia and, if so, to what extent? They repeated their previous study but added refinements. The subjects were examined in much more detail and were rated on the clinical dementia rating (CDR) scale. There had to be a temporal link between the dementia syndrome and stroke. Of the 297 subjects enrolled, 251 (84.5%) were testable and examined at three months. Using DSM-III-R criteria, 66 patients (26.3%) proved to be demented. Stroke caused about half of the cases and, as a complication of AD, about another third. Compared to stroke-free controls the risk of dementia in the stroke group was nine times greater. Risk factors were age, less education and to some extent being non-white. This rate means that in 1988 there were almost half a million Americans with stroke and dementia.

Two years later, in 1994, the same group (Tatemichi et al, 1994) then asked the question: is there a delayed dementia following well-defined stroke, the incidence of which is greater than in a control group? The patients were from the previous study with a longer follow-up. Those without dementia in the 1992 paper were followed up for four years or until death if earlier (18.4%). Over four years, 36 went on to develop dementia (incidence rate of 8.4 cases per 100 person-years) compared to eight or an incidence of 1.3 in the controls (all AD). The authors noted that, even after adjusting for key variables and allowing for potential biases, the incidence of dementia in the stroke group was exceptionally high. Most were mild with a CDR of 1. Eight had new strokes, eight had significant medical comorbidity and a few had smooth deteriorations as found in AD. Expressed differently, about one-third became demented following stroke, giving a relative risk of 5.5. Older age at stroke, fewer years of education and a low score on the mini-mental state examination were significantly related. The authors concluded that

'...ischemic stroke in elderly persons increases the long-term risk of developing dementia by approximately five fold compared to those without stroke. Age, education, and baseline intellectual function contribute independently to that risk *and* our results are at least consistent with the thesis that a stroke may accelerate the cognitive consequences of aging, including the effects of Alzheimer's Disease.'

Slooter et al (1997) examined the role of apolipoprotein E genotypes in dementia and stroke and found that APOE ε4 was more common than in normal controls. The attributable risk of APOE ε4 among dementia patients with stroke was 41% overall, 33% among those with VaD and 44% among those with AD and cerebrovascular disease. This may imply a common genetic susceptibility. In the well-known Nun Study (Snowdon et al, 1997) post-mortem data showed that those who met the neuropathological criteria for AD *and* had brain infarcts had poorer cognition and higher prevalence of dementia in life, particularly if the infarcts were in the basal ganglia, thalamus or deep white matter. Conversely, in those not meeting the criteria for AD, the presence of lacunar infarcts was not particularly relevant.

It has to be remembered that North America has three parts: the USA, Canada and Mexico, which are all different. Similarly the main ethnic groups in the USA – Caucasian, African-American, Hispanic-American and Asian-American – are also different. First, comparison of stroke incidence worldwide shows modest variation (Alter et al, 1986). Second, cerebrovascular disease in the USA started to increase in the 1980s, especially in older people, men and African-Americans (Gillum, 1986). The increase may have been due to better detection by neuroimaging. In earlier decades, the stroke incidence had decreased, thought to be due to better treatment of hypertension (Higgins and Thom, 1993). There are ethnic differences: African-, Japanese- and Chinese-Americans have more intracranial and Caucasians more extracranial cerebrovascular disease. There also appears to be a persistent 'stroke belt' in the southern USA. Risk factors are older age, male sex, black race, lower socioeconomic status, heart disease, hypertension, diabetes, smoking, alcohol and diet (Feldmann et al, 1990). Better living standards, reduced smoking and drinking and better diet have helped lower rates, but have been offset by better detection, increase in longevity and better survival from coronary heart disease. In contrast (Gillum, 1995), older Hispanics have lower rates thought to be due to lower blood pressure, and this is true also of Native Americans. By comparison, Canada has one of the lowest death rates from cerebrovascular disease (Petrasovits and Nair, 1994). However, in both the USA and Canada the rates are comparable for cerebrovascular disease, which in each country is the third leading cause of death (Feinleib et al, 1993). Finally, a survey showed that the overall incidence rate for first ever and recurrent stroke, excluding transient ischemic attacks, was 411 per 100 000 among black patients and 179 per 100 000 among white for all age groups except for those over 75 years (Broderick et al, 1998). This gave 731 100 first ever or recurrent strokes in the USA in 1996. It is, therefore, important to consider ethnic mix when considering epidemiological studies from North America, as exemplified by the high rates for VaD reported in the Honolulu–Asia study (White et al, 1996).

Incidence of VaD in population studies

Few true incidence studies of VaD have been conducted. Longitudinal studies in Rochester, New York, have allowed approximate rates to be calculated and also illustrate the methodological difficulties inherent in the actual choice of criteria used (Knopman et al, 2002). They report 482 incident cases of dementia with 18% classified as VaD (10% having onset or worsening within three months of stroke and 11% fulfilling imaging criteria for VaD, though only 4% had both). In keeping with prevalence data, incidence rates increased markedly with age though did not differ between sexes. This study also provides a striking demonstration of the effect diagnostic criteria have on determining incidence rates. The Canadian Study of Health and Aging found incidence rates of VaD to be 2.5 per 1000 per year (Hebert et al, 2000). Risk factors were found to be age, rural residence, living in an institution, diabetes, depression, heart disease and apolipoprotein E4. Protective factors were eating shellfish and regular exercise.

chapter 5

Epidemiology of vascular dementia in Japan

Akira Homma and Kazuo Hasegawa

Introduction

According to a recent report from the National Institute of Population and Social Security Research (2002), the proportion of people aged over 65 years was 17.4% of the total Japanese population in 2000. It is estimated that this proportion will rise to 22% in 2010, and 28% in 2030 (Figure 5.1). This percentage, in particular, that of the old-old population, is expected to increase at the highest speed in the world until the year 2020. The number of the aged with dementia will increase concomitantly (Figure 5.2) (Otsuka, 2001). Approximately 70% to 80% of the aged with dementia are living in the community (Karasawa, 1988). Local governments in Japan have been greatly concerned with the various problems of the aged because of the rapid increase in their number, and they have investigated living conditions and the need for welfare services, especially for disabled elderly persons with dementia. In the last two decades, 45 surveys on dementia in the community have been conducted in Japan. Methodological features of epidemiological surveys on dementia and some recent results showing changing prevalence rates of vascular dementia will be described here.

Methodological features of surveys in Japan

Sites of previous investigations are distributed nationwide and in some areas surveys have been repeated. In all surveys, clinical diagnoses were made through interviews by psychiatrists on door-to-door visits. Japan offers special advantages for epidemiological studies as all residents eligible to take part in surveys are registered in the office of their local government. This

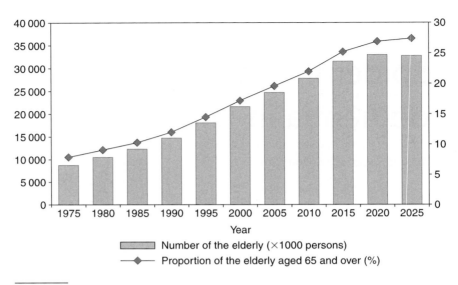

Figure 5.1 *Past and projected increases in the population of Japan.*

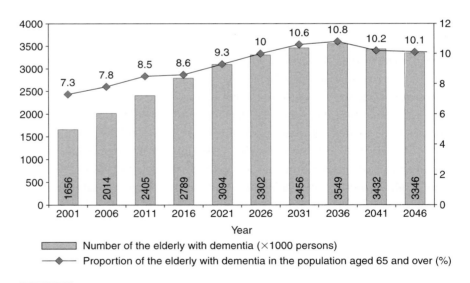

Figure 5.2 *Estimated increases in the elderly with dementia in Japan.*

system makes it easy to select subjects by random sampling with governmental co-operation. The system, however, has a drawback. Financial sponsorship from local governments to conduct surveys is limited by the stipulation that surveys must be completed within one fiscal year. For this reason, large, population-based incidence studies have been difficult to conduct in Japan.

There is a tendency towards decrease in the response rate in surveys, especially in urban areas. In 1980, for instance, the response rate to a secondary door-to-door survey by psychiatrists in the Tokyo metropolis was as high as 96.8%, while in 1988, it was 91.6% (Homma, 1992) and only 69.6% in 1995 (Department of Welfare, Tokyo Metropolis, 1996) – a decrease of 27.2%. In Kanagawa prefecture, which is adjacent to the Tokyo metropolis, epidemiological surveys have been conducted three times. The response rates of the secondary surveys were 83.7% in 1982, 74.0% in 1985 and 78.0% in 1993, respectively (Homma, 1992; Imai et al, 1994).

There is great concern about the problems of the aged in general. However, it seems that the concerns are not always accompanied by an increased understanding of elderly people, even by their caregivers. In 2000 long-term care insurance started to share the financial burden of care for disabled elderly persons, including the aged with dementia. In a questionnaire survey on awareness of dementia among 1115 randomly selected inhabitants over the age of 20 years living in the metropolitan areas and major cities of Japan (Homma, 2001), approximately one half of the respondents answered that dementia was not an illness. Although long-term care insurance actually made issues relating to dementia more visible, awareness of dementia was still low in the general population. It is obvious that more extensive enlightening activities are needed to improve the low response rate to epidemiological surveys on dementia, as well as to progress to early detection of the elderly with dementia in the community.

Another characteristic of Japanese surveys is that two-step survey procedures have been used in all surveys except for the two surveys conducted in Tochigi prefecture and in Fukui prefecture (Katsuyama city). Japanese elderly persons are not accustomed to being recruited or asked to volunteer for research purposes – it has been considered difficult to administer even a simple psychometric test to elderly people in a screening survey. Consequently, in most surveys, subjects with suspected dementia have been screened mainly based on information concerning activities of daily living (ADL) and on the behavioral symptoms of dementia, obtained from their relatives. Although such a screening procedure is not efficient, it seems unlikely that cases with suspected dementia will be overlooked and it helps to improve the response rate.

In 1992 an epidemiological survey on the demented elderly living in the community was conducted (Imai et al, 1994). Criteria including ADL, past medical histories, present physical status, the degree of care required, mental and physical decline as judged by relatives, and behavioral symptoms were used in the screening survey (Table 5.1). No psychometric examinations were included in the screening process. Five thousand randomly selected subjects from approximately 350 000 elderly persons in Kanagawa prefecture were subjected to the screening survey using these criteria; 408 elderly people with suspected dementia were identified by screening. Of these, 116 persons were diagnosed as demented in a secondary survey by psychiatrists using a semistructured interview form. No cases of suspected dementia were found in 102 randomly selected subjects in the rest of the total sample, i.e. there were approximately 4600 subjects without suspected dementia. The results confirmed that the screening criteria were likely to be valid and practical, taking into account the reluctant attitude of the Japanese elderly to participate in such surveys.

In the results from an epidemiological survey conducted in a rural area of Japan in 1997 (Nakamura et al, 2000), the Mini-Mental State Examination (MMSE) (Folstein et al, 1975) was administered to the total elderly population ($N = 7847$) of that area to screen for suspected dementia. Of 7847 subjects, 1453 (18.5%) refused administration of the MMSE. Also, in an epidemiological survey where 2516 elderly persons were approached in a rural area of the northern part of Japan, Ishizaki et al (1998) reported that the MMSE was successfully administered to 2266 subjects (90.0%). In addition, 94.6% of 887 subjects were examined by a simple psychometric test in the initial screening survey of an incidence study (Yoshitake et al, 1995). It seems that the administration of a psychometric test is feasible as a screening instrument. Thus, considering that the number of elderly persons will increase, the development of administrative procedures for psychometric tests which are easily acceptable to elderly people in Japan will be more important than before in conducting epidemiological surveys in the Japanese community.

Table 5.1 Screening criteria for the elderly with suspected dementia in the Kanagawa survey 1992

I. Both A and B
A. General activity or mobility less than getting out independently
B. One of the following
    1. Marked physical decline
    2. Marked mental decline
    3. Concomitant cerebral vascular disorders
    4. Previous episode of cerebral vascular disorder
    5. Care required: always or occasionally
    6. Assistance required in eating
    7. Assistance required in dressing
    8. Assistance required in bathing
    9. Assistance required in urinating
    10. Assistance required in defecating
II. In cases with neither A nor B, one of the following
    1. Getting lost
    2. Delusions
    3. Rejecting bathing or dressing with no reason
    4. Marked forgetfulness (meals, etc.)
    5. Doing/saying that where he/she lives is not really his/her home
    6. Misidentification of his/her spouse or children living together
    7. Nocturnal confusion
    8. Confusing night-time with daytime
    9. Hallucinations

Diagnostic criteria for vascular dementia (VaD)

Diagnostic criteria for VaD have been a long-standing source of disagreement and are also the major barrier to obtaining consensus results on the epidemiology of VaD. Rocca and Kokmen (1999) indicate four problems that may be responsible for differences in incidence or prevalence across studies:

- classification of patients with so called 'mixed' dementia in whom the etiology appears to include both cerebrovascular and primary degenerative features
- disagreement about criteria and evaluation tools
- the use of imaging findings in the definition of VaD
- how to define the range of severity of VaD to be detected in the survey.

Ikeda et al (2001) and Meguro et al (2002) reported contrasting results for the prevalence rate of Alzheimer's disease (AD) and VaD in Nakayama town, Ehime prefecture, and Tajiri town, Miyagi prefecture, respectively. In both surveys, imaging findings by computed tomography or magnetic resonance imaging were used and AD was diagnosed by NINCDS-ADRDA criteria (McKhann et al, 1984), while VaD was diagnosed by modified DSM-IV criteria (American Psychiatric Association, 1994) in Nakayama town and by NINDS-AIREN criteria (Roman et al, 1993) in Tajiri town. Apart from these two studies, there is only one report in which CT and autopsy data were used to estimate the prevalence rate of dementia (Ueda et al, 1992). DSM-IV criteria for VaD originally allowed focal neurological signs or laboratory evidence indicating cerebrovascular disease. Only the latter were adopted in the study in Nakayama town. As shown in Table 5.2, the prevalence rate of VaD diagnosed by NINCDS-AIREN, which is more specific than DSM-IV, is lower than that by DSM-IV. Although the actual prevalence rate of VaD was different in both regions, it seems likely that the use of diverse diagnostic criteria has influenced these rates. The aim of the study in Tajiri town was to see whether VaD had been overdiagnosed in previous surveys. It seems to be confirmed to some extent by the results of Meguro et al (2002) that the prevalence rates of VaD previously reported in Japan were not overestimates. This conclusion seems to be compatible with the report by Rocca and Kokmen (1999) that the prevalence rate of VaD diagnosed with imaging findings is higher than that found without imaging. Most previous surveys

Table 5.2 Prevalence rates (%) of dementia subtypes in Nakayama and Tajiri towns

Diagnosis	Nakayama town (N = 1162)	Tajiri town (N = 1654)
Probable Alzheimer's disease	1.7	1.5
Possible Alzheimer's disease with cerebrovascular disorders	0.1	4.0
Vascular dementia	2.2	1.6
Other/unspecified dementia	0.8	1.4

Cranial computed tomography was used in the diagnosis of subtypes of dementia in Nakayama town and MRI in Tajiri town. Probable Alzheimer's disease was diagnosed by NINCDS-ADRDA criteria in both regions. For vascular dementia, modified DSM-IV criteria were used in Nakayama town and NINDS-AIREN in Tajiri town.

in Japan employed similar diagnostic criteria to DSM-IV which does not require imaging findings in the diagnosis of AD or VaD. This raises the possibility that VaD was underdiagnosed in the community surveys. However, a possibility still remains that VaD patients with white matter lesions and no neurological signs, who are commonly encountered in routine clinical practice, were diagnosed as having AD, resulting in overdiagnosis of AD.

Prevalence rate of vascular dementia in Japan

As shown in Table 5.3, 45 epidemiological surveys on age-associated dementia have been conducted in the Japanese community. The elderly aged over 65 years were the subject of all the surveys. The overall prevalence rates of dementia range from 3.0% to 10.6% with marked variation. The institutionalized and elderly people in hospitals were included in the three surveys in Tochigi, and Toyama prefectures and in the second survey of Fukuoka city. The prevalence rates were 5.5%, 5.7% and 4.7%, respectively, but these were not always related to where the elderly lived. Higher prevalence rates were not found in the surveys that included the institutionalized and elderly in hospital as subjects. This observed variation is partly due to differences in study design, inclusion criteria, sample characteristics, and the definitions and diagnostic criteria used, although no one factor can account for all of the variance (Jorm et al, 1987).

However, a trend is seen when the 45 surveys are divided into two groups: 26 surveys conducted before 1989 and 19 surveys conducted after 1990. In the former group, a relative predominance of AD is reported in 6 surveys (23.0%), while in the latter the results of 15 surveys (78.9%) show that AD is more predominant than VaD. Figure 5.3 shows overall prevalence rates and AD/VaD ratios from 1956 to 1998 in the 45 surveys. Although statistical calculations are not made, it seems that AD/VaD ratios increase with time, especially after 1990. Also, Figure 5.4 illustrates the change in the proportions of AD and VaD in each overall prevalence rate. It seems that the predominance of VaD is reversed after 1990. In these surveys, the prevalence rates of VaD varied from 1.1% in Yamanashi prefecture to 5.0% in Yamato town, Niigata prefecture; the average rate was 2.0%. In contrast, rates of AD varied from 0.6% in the second survey of Tokyo metropolis to 6.0% in Itoigawa city, Niigata prefecture; 2.0% on average. Of course, it is problematic to compare overall prevalence rates because of differences in the age distribution of the subjects of each survey. However, as pointed out by Homma (1994) and Graves et al (1994), VaD has

Table 5.3 Prevalence rates of age-associated dementia in the community in Japan

Area investigated	Year	Number of subjects	Prevalence rate (%)	Etiological diagnosis		VaD/AD
				AD	VaD	
Hokkaido	1986	9274	3.4	1.2	1.5	1.3
Akita Yuwa Town	1984	1144	7.3	1.2	2.5	2.1
Gumma pref.	1992	2242	3.0	1.4	1.2	0.8
Chiba pref.	1987	5000	3.2	1.8	1.2	0.7
Tochigi pref.	1990	2016*	5.5*	0.9*	3.0*	3.2*
Tokyo metropolis	1973	4716	4.5	1.2	2.7	2.3
Tokyo metropolis	1980	4502	4.6	0.6	1.7	2.9
Tokyo metropolis	1988	4586	4.0	0.9	1.3	1.3
Tokyo metropolis	1995	4343	4.1	1.8	1.2	0.7
Yokohama City	1982	2287	4.8	1.0	1.7	1.6
Yokohama City	1990	4550	3.7	1.7	1.5	0.9
Kanagawa pref.	1982	1507	4.8	1.2	2.0	1.7
Kanagawa pref.	1987	2232	4.9	2.0	2.0	1.0
Kanagawa pref.	1992	4259	3.8	1.8	1.5	0.8
Kawasaki City+	1985	1607	4.7	1.5	2.2	1.5
Yamanashi pref.	1985	2509	3.1	1.4	1.1	0.8
Nagano pref.	1987	1923	5.7	1.9	2.7	1.4
Niigata pref. (3 areas)	1983	2511	3.5	1.1	1.9	1.8
Niigata Yamato Town	1989	2446	7.9	1.2	5.0	4.3
Toyama pref.	1982	913	5.6	2.7	1.6	0.6
Toyama pref.	1985	1327	4.5	2.6	1.7	0.8
Fukui Katsuyama City	1990	5160	5.0	2.0	1.8	0.9
Toyama pref.	1990	1550*	5.7*	2.5*	2.2*	0.9*
Aichi pref.	1983	3106	5.8	2.4	2.8	1.1
Aichi pref.	1990	2992	4.7	2.0	2.4	1.2
Aichi pref.	1996	3302	4.8	2.8	1.8	0.6
Gifu pref. (3 areas)	1983	1649	3.5	0.9	1.6	1.7
Osaka-fu	1983	1844	4.3	1.6	2.3	1.4
Nara Yagi Town	1956	696	4.5	2.2	2.3	1.1
Hiroshima pref.	1991	5000	4.5	2.1	1.4	0.7
Tottori Ooyama Town	1982	1236	4.4	1.8	2.2	1.2
Fukuoka City	1984	3883	3.4	1.3	1.5	1.2
Fukuoka City	1991	5269*	4.7*	1.4*	2.3*	1.6*
Fukuoka Hoshino Village	1983	782	3.5	1.0	1.7	1.7
Fukuoka Hisayama Town	1985	887	6.7	1.4	2.4	1.8
Okinawa Sashiki Village	1975	708	3.8	1.0	2.5	2.4
Okinawa pref.	1991	3524	7.0	3.3	2.2	0.7

* institutionalized & admitted subjects included, AD: Alzheimer-type dementia, VaD: vascular dementia

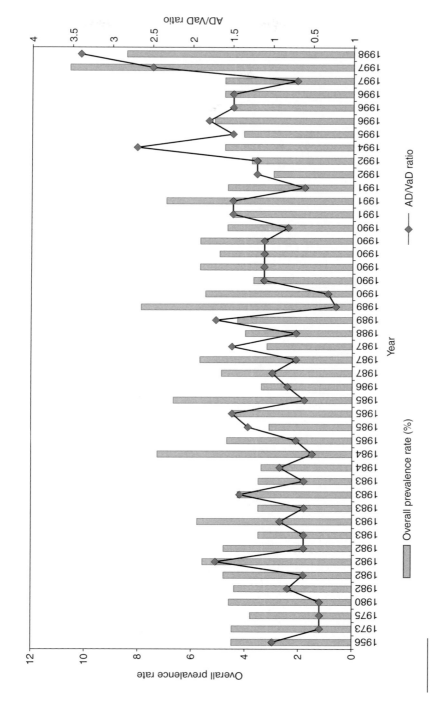

Figure 5.3 Overall prevalence rates and AD/VaD ratio 1956–98.

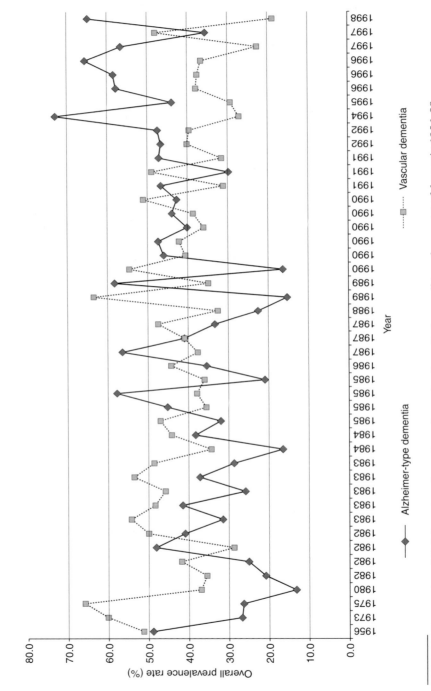

Figure 5.4 Percentages of Alzheimer-type dementia and vascular dementia in overall prevalence rates of dementia 1956–98.

been a major cause of dementing illnesses in the elderly in Japan, while the composition of dementia subtypes seems to have changed recently.

Compared with AD, it is quite difficult to compare epidemiological results for VaD cross-nationally because of a lack of established common diagnostic criteria. Recently Graves et al (1996) conducted an epidemiological survey of the Japanese-American population in Washington State, USA. The prevalence rates of VaD and AD were 1.4% and 3.5%, respectively. In comparison with the average prevalence rates in Japan, the prevalence rate of VaD was slightly higher than that of Japan, and the difference in prevalence for VaD between Japan and the USA was smaller than that for AD. Comparing the results for age-specific prevalence of VaD and AD in King County, Washington, and the Tokyo metropolis in 1995, where the survey was conducted with the identical diagnostic criteria to those of the survey in King County (Larson et al, 1998), it was shown that although age-specific prevalence rates of VaD and AD in Japan were slightly lower than those in the USA, the overall tendency seems to be quite similar. Also, similar results were reported in a cross-cultural comparative epidemiological study of Nigerian Africans and African-Americans of similar ethnic origin (Hendrie et al, 1995, 2001). Taking into consideration that the difference in prevalence rates between Japan and the USA, or Nigeria and the USA are bigger for AD than for VaD, it may be possible that the prevalence rates of VaD are less susceptible to environmental factors than those of AD.

Incidence studies of age-associated dementia in Japan

Few studies on incidence rates of age-associated dementia, especially disease-specific incidence rates, have been reported in Japan. Miyanaga et al (1994) reported an overall dementia incidence rate of 1.8% (that of AD was 0.5% and that of VaD 1.0%) in a population of 2255 individuals aged 65 years and over of Yamato town, Niigata prefecture, located in the center of Japan. The incidence rates of VaD were 0.95% for men and 1.07% for women, and those of AD were 0% for men and 0.8% for women. No incident male case of AD was found in the study period. In this report, the incidence rate of VaD was still higher than that of AD. In the results of a Hisayama town, Fukuoka prefecture (located in the southern part of Japan) (Yoshitake et al, 1995), the incidence rates of VaD were 1.22% for men and 0.90% for women, and for AD, 0.51% for men and 1.1% for women. In the USA (Katzman et al, 1989) incidence rates of VaD and AD were 0.9% and 2.0%, respectively, and in France (Forette et al, 1991) they were 0.7% and 1.6%, respectively. It is interesting that differences among incidence rates of VaD are smaller than those for AD across studies. It is not possible to examine any change of incidence rates in Japan because of a lack of reports.

Summary

Despite numerous methodological difficulties, some patterns seem to emerge from epidemiological studies of VaD. However, the results to date are uncertain and tentative. The results on VaD from studies in Japan remain far more limited than those we can now draw on in AD. In this chapter, prevalence rates of age-associated dementia, some methodological features of the surveys in Japan, and diagnostic issues relating to VaD were described. A possible increasing prevalence rate of AD and decreasing prevalence rate of VaD were indicated in surveys conducted after 1990 as a recent trend of epidemiological findings in Japan. Taking into account a role of environmental or cultural factors in the difference of prevalence rates of AD in two culturally different regions with similar ethnic origin (Hendrie et al 1995, 2001), it cannot be ruled out that changes in the environment – excluding decreased mortality due to cerebrovascular disorders, nutrition and life style – may affect the recent pattern of the prevalence of dementia in Japan.

References

American Psychiatric Association, *Diagnostic and Statistical Manual of Mental Disorders,* 4th edn (American Psychiatric Association Press: Washington DC, 1994.)

Department of Welfare, Tokyo Metropolis, *A Report on Health and Living Conditions of the Elderly in the Tokyo Metropolis* (Department of Welfare, Tokyo Metropolis: Tokyo, 1996.)

Folstein MF, Folstein SE, McHugh PR, 'Mini-Mental State': a practical method for grading the cognitive state for the clinician, *J Psychiatr Res* (1975) **12**:189–98.

Forette F, Amery A, Staessen J et al, Is prevention of vascular dementia possible? The Syst-Eur Vascular Dementia Project, *Aging Milano* (1991) **3**:373–82.

Graves AB, Larson EB, White LR et al, Opportunities and challenges in international collaborative epidemiologic research of dementia and its subtypes: studies between Japan and the US, *Int Psychogeriatr* (1994) **6**:209–23.

Graves AB, Larson EB, Edland SD et al, Prevalence of dementia and its subtypes in the Japanese American population of King County, Washington State: the Kame Project, *Am J Epidemiol* (1996) **144**:760–71.

Hendrie HC, Osuntokun BO, Hall KS et al, Prevalence of Alzheimer's disease and dementia in two communities: Nigerian Africans and African Americans, *Am J Psychiatry* (1995) **152**:1485–92.

Hendrie HC, Ogunniyi A, Hall KS et al, Incidence of dementia and Alzheimer disease in 2 communities: Yoruba residing in Ibadan, Nigeria, and African Americans residing in Indianapolis, Indiana, *JAMA* (2001) **285**:739–47.

Homma A, Epidemiology and risk factors of age-associated dementia, *Clin Psychiatry* (1992) **21**:1877–87.

Homma A, Mental illness in elderly persons in Japan, In: Copeland JRM, Abou-Saleh MT, Blazer DG, eds, *Principles and Practice of Geriatric Psychiatry* (John Wiley & Sons: Chichester, 1994.) 857–63.

Homma A, Recognition and awareness of age-associated dementia in the community, *Jpn J Gerontol* (2001) **23**:340–51.

Ikeda M, Hokoishi K, Maki N et al, Increased prevalence of vascular dementia in Japan. A community-based epidemiological study, *Neurology* (2001) **57**:839–44.

Imai Y, Homma A, Hasegawa K et al, An epidemiological study on dementia in Kanagawa prefecture, *Jpn J Geriatr Psychiatry* (1994) **5**:855–62.

Ishizaki J, Meguro K, Ambo H et al, A normative, community-based study of Mini-Mental State in elderly adults: the effect of age and educational level, *J Gerontol* (1998) **53B**:B359–B363.

Jorm AF, Korten AE, Henderson AS, The prevalence of dementia: a quantitative integration of the literature, *Acta Psychiatr Scand* (1987) **76**:465–79.

Karasawa A, Prevalence of dementia among the elderly in Japan, *Biomed Ther* (1988) **13**:598–601.

Katzman R, Aronson M, Fuld P et al, Development of dementing illnesses in an 80-year-old volunteer cohort. *Ann Neurol* (1989) **25**:317–24.

Larson EB, McCurry SM, Graves AB et al, Standardization of the clinical diagnosis of the dementia syndrome and its subtypes in a cross-national study: the Ni-Hon-Sea Experience, *J Gerontol* (1998) **53A**:M313–M319.

McKhann G, Drachman D, Folstein M et al, Clinical diagnosis of Alzheimer's disease: report of the NINCDS-ADRDA Work Group under the auspices of Department of Health and Human Services Task Force on Alzheimer's Disease, *Neurology* (1984) **34**:939–44.

Meguro K, Ishii H, Yamaguchi S et al, Prevalence of dementia and dementing diseases in Japan. The Tajiri Project, *Arch Neurol* (2002) **59**:1109–14.

Miyanaga K, Yonemura K, Kuroiwa T et al, An epidemiological study on dementia in Yamato town, *Jpn J Geriatr Psychiatr* (1994) **5**:323–32.

Nakamura S, Iwamoto M, Tsuno N et al, Prevalence of dementia in Itoigawa city, Niigata prefecture. Presented at the *15th Annual Meeting of the Japanese Gerontopsychiatric Society* (2000) June 5–6, 2000, Yokohama, Japan.

National Institute of Population and Social Security Research, *Projection of the Population in Japan* (National Institute of Population and Social Security Research: Tokyo, 2002.)

Otsuka T, Future projection of the elderly with dementia in Japan, *J Jpn Psychiatr Hosp Ass* (2001) **20**:65–9.

Rocca W, Kokmen E, Frequency and distribution of vascular dementia, *Alzheimer Dis Assoc Disord* (1999) **13** (Suppl 3):S9–S14.

Roman GC, Tatemichi TK, Erkinjuntti T et al, Vascular dementia: diagnostic criteria for research studies. Report of the NINDS-AIREN International Workshop, *Neurology* (1993) **43**:250–60.

Ueda K, Kawano H, Hasuo Y, Fujishima M, Prevalence and etiology of dementia in a Japanese community, *Stroke* (1992) **23**:798–803.

Yoshitake T, Kiyohara Y, Kato I et al, Incidence and risk factors of vascular dementia and Alzheimer's disease in a defined elderly Japanese population. *Neurology* (1995) **45**:1161–8.

chapter 6

Epidemiology of vascular dementia in China

Xin Yu and Yucun Shen

The problem of population aging in China

The rate of aging has accelerated in recent years while the proportion and absolute number of elderly people in the total population has increased. (Table 6.1). The life expectancy of the Chinese reached 70 years by 1993. In 2000, the elderly comprised 10.81% of the population, i.e. 129 million elderly persons. In Beijing and Shanghai, almost one in five residents is elderly (Lu, 1994).

Through the successful implementation of the 'one child per family' policy, the proportion of aging persons in China is constantly increasing. China became an elderly nation by the end of the last century but professional and social infrastructures have yet to be organized to meet the challenge of this aging problem (Table 6.2).

The 1% sampling survey showed that the average family size in 1995 was 3.7, a 0.3 reduction compared to the 1990 national population survey (Chinese National Statistical Bureau, 1996). Thus in China, the traditionally

Table 6.1 Data from four population surveys in China

Population Survey	Aged population (million)	Total population (million)	Aged/total population (%)
1953	41.54	567.44	7.32
1964	42.20	694.58	6.08
1982	76.65	1003.79	7.64
1990	98.21	1143.33	8.59

Table 6.2 Prediction of the aging population in China

	1985	*1990*	*1995*	*2000*	*2025*	*2050*
Total population (million)	1049.00	1143.33	1197.00	1270.00	1498.00	1547.00
Aged population (million)	86.00	98.21	116.00	129.00	264.00	331.00
Aged/total population (%)	8.20	8.59	9.69	10.18	17.63	21.40

valued extended family in which three or even four generations live together is weakened. There are many attributions for this change. Firstly, with the fast growth of population density, living conditions are deteriorating, especially in urban areas. The standard apartments, which were built by the government, obviously cannot accommodate a large family. Secondly, the accelerating industrialization process and relatively loose political control in the last 20 years made mobility both necessary and easy. Young people, especially from rural areas, tend to move away from their parents' home town to try to find jobs in cities. Thirdly, the family planning policy inevitably influences family size. Furthermore, in the final quarter of the last century, many unpredicted changes occurred in China. For the first time in thousands of years, the authority of the elderly is being questioned, especially when they are living on a limited pension while their children are enjoying the fruits of the market economy. 'Reverence to the elderly' is repeatedly emphasized in the media, not because the Chinese are still proud of it but because it is felt that this virtue is threatened by social reform. Chinese traditional values are struggling to survive within these tremendous social changes. Numerous elderly people are still playing important roles in family life. They are the main force binding the whole family closely together and contributing significantly to both the society and their family by looking after their grandchildren. Furthermore, some senior citizens (most of them are well educated) are still very active in social and political life, including the academic world. An important issue is raised: what can Chinese society do for the welfare of the elderly, and what can the elderly continue to contribute to Chinese society?

With the astonishing change in society and public health, Chinese psychiatrists also face a great challenge never before met. In 1997, there were 485 psychiatric hospitals in China, with 107 362 beds and 13 912 doctors working in psychiatric hospitals. Unfortunately, facilities for elderly patients are very limited. Accurate statistical figures are not available, but it is estimated that fewer than 10% of beds in each psychiatric hospital serve the elderly. Qualified geriatric psychiatrists are proportionally even fewer.

In response to the urgency of health service facilities for the elderly, in the last five years nursing homes and hospices for the elderly have been established in both rural and urban areas. Some are funded by local government and some are run privately for profit. Most of them mainly admit the elderly without caregivers or the elderly with terminal illnesses. They all face similar problems – shortage of expertise and of policy guidance. Sometimes they even face a shortage of patients as, under the influence of the old Chinese tradition, the elderly are not willing to go into nursing homes because they believe that these are for the childless, and their children are not willing to send their parents to nursing homes because they are afraid of losing face.

One point that should be highlighted is the gap between the Chinese urban and rural areas becoming wider. With the rapid growth of the economy, the well-to-do elderly city dwellers are becoming more self-reliant and tend to formulate their own aging plan such as employing or adopting a 'country girl' as a carer instead of disturbing their busy children. The reverse is that 900 million people who live in the country are not covered by any medical or social insurance. It is almost impossible for China to structure a paradigm for elderly care which is applicable to the whole nation.

Epidemiological studies of vascular dementia in China

Useful information about the epidemiology of vascular dementia (VaD) was not available until the last 20 years. The first set of Chinese psychiatric diagnostic criteria were published in 1957, and did not include 'VaD'. In 1980, the first edition of a psychiatric textbook edited by Beijing Medical College mentioned Alzheimer's disease under 'Senile dementia', and VaD under mental disorder due to cerebral VaD.

A search of the literature published before 1980 for epidemiological studies on VaD did not generate any valuable data, with only a few case reports related to 'dementia symptoms after severe strokes'.

The first study that met with all requirements of epidemiological research was conducted in 1982, led by the Institute of Mental Health, Beijing Medical University. This study adopted a standard sampling method, a survey instrument whose validity and reliability were tested, and ICD-9 used as the diagnostic criteria. Twelve areas with 51 982 people were involved in this study. This survey found that the life-time prevalence rate of 'senile dementia' was 0.29% (in 38 136 people aged 15 and above) and 'mental disorders induced by cerebral vascular disease' was 0.50%. However, no data on VaD are available since cases were included in the category of 'mental disorders induced by cerebral vascular disease' (Twelve Areas Coordinating Group, 1986).

Incidence rate of VaD

In epidemiological research, an incidence study often offers more useful information about the disease, especially the risk factors. However, incidence research needs more funding and a higher standard of expertise. For these reasons, incidence research on VaD is relatively rare in China. So far, only two such incidence studies have been conducted.

In 1989, Shen et al completed a three-year follow-up study on dementia in an urban community of Beijing (Shen et al, 1994), in which 812 people aged over 60 who did not have dementia by mini-mental state examination (MMSE) evaluation were followed up for three years. MMSE was used to detect possible cases. DSM-III was adopted for diagnostic criteria and Dementia Differential Diagnostic Schedule (DDDS) for differential diagnosis. During the three-year period, seven elderly patients developed moderate-to-severe dementia, and six were diagnosed as having mild dementia. The average annual incidence rate of total dementia was 5.6%. In the seven moderate-to-severe dementia patients, three were classified as having VaD. The VaD incidence rate was 1.23%. The classification in six mild dementia patients was not available. Further analysis demonstrated that low education level, previous unemployment and reduced physical mobility were possible risk factors for the development of dementia. However, the relatively small sample made this analysis less useful. A few years later, an incidence study was conducted in the same community with similar screening and evaluation instruments except that diagnostic criteria were changed to ICD-10. After two years' follow-up, investigators found that the incidence rate of VaD was 0.32% while the incidence of AD was 0.54% in 1403 elderly people aged over 60, which was virtually no change compared to the first study (Yan et al, 2002).

The Mental Health Center of Shanghai and the University of California at San Diego collaborated on a study of dementia in an urban community of Shanghai, where 1970 elderly aged 65 and over who did not have dementia at the baseline were followed up for five years. The incidence rate of dementia was 1.15%. In new dementia cases, there were more patients with AD than with VaD (one-quarter of total dementia patients). The incidence rate in females was slightly higher than that in males (1.27% vs 0.98%). It was also higher in the older age groups (65–69 years old: 0.68%; 80–84: 3.37%) and in the illiterate elderly when compared to educated subjects. This survey was conducted by the application of ADRC laboratory tests and computed tomographic examinations to differentiate VaD and AD, hence the results were relatively reliable (Zhang et al, 1998).

Prevalence rate of VaD in China

In 1986 the first epidemiological study of age-related dementia on a population aged 60 and over was conducted in China in an urban area of Beijing (Li et al, 1989). In this study, 1090 elderly people were screened by MMSE, the suspected cases were interviewed by psychiatrists, DSM-III was adopted for diagnostic criteria and DDDS for differential diagnosis. Fourteen cases of dementia of moderate and severe degree were identified, with the prevalence rates 1.28% ($\geq$60) and 1.82% ($\geq$65). Among 14 cases of dementia, eight were VaD, three were PDD and one was due to carbon monoxide intoxication.

All the studies listed in Table 6.3 demonstrated that dementia was more prevalent in older age and in illiterate groups. All studies suggested that AD was more common in women, and most of these studies demonstrated that men were more vulnerable to VaD. Lai et al (2000) reported a survey in a group of people older than 75 and showed that the prevalence rate of dementia, especially AD, was much higher in this age group. Zhang et al (1990) indicated that loss of spouse and lower economical status were more common in dementia patients.

Except for two prevalence rate studies on VaD conducted in Beijing in the early 1990s, all studies indicate that the prevalence rate of VaD is lower than that of AD.

A national survey on the epidemiology of dementias included 42 890 people aged 55 and over in both rural and urban areas in six areas of China. Although the final paper has not yet been published, sections have been published and some of results are listed in Table 6.3. This survey suggests that AD is a major type of dementia in old age and more prevalent in men.

Table 6.3 Prevalence rates of VaD in China

Author	Year	Location	Population	Diagnostic criteria	Differential diagnostic instruments or diagnostic criteria for AD	Results: VaD/ (Alzheimer's disease)
Li et al	1989	Beijing, urban area	1090 (≥60)	DSM-III	DDDS	0.83% (0.37%)
Zhang et al	1990	Shanghai, urban area	5055 (≥55)	DSM-III-R	NINCDS-ADRDA Hachinski Ischemic Scale	>55: 0.74% (1.50%) >65: 1.26% (2.90)
Chen et al	1992	Beijing, urban community	5172 average age: 68.9±6.6	DSM-III	DDDS	0.50% (0.2%)
Gao et al	1993	Shanghai, rural and urban areas	3779 rural/urban: 2560/1219	DSM-III-R	Hachinski Ischemic Scale	0.85% (3.15%)
Zhang et al	1998	Beijing, urban area	1243	DSM-III-R	Hachinski Ischemic Scale	0.96% (1.37%)
Fan et al	2000	Nanjing, urban and rural areas	3268 (≥60)	DSM-III-R	NINCDS-ADRDA Hachinski Ischemic Scale	0.49% (0.95%)
Lai et al	2000	Guangzhou urban area	3825 (>75)	DSM-III-R,	NINCDS-ADRDA for AD	1.16% (7.49%)
Qu et al	2001	Xian, rural and urban areas	4850 ≥55)	DSM-IV, NINCDS/ AIREN	NINCDS-ADRDA Hachinski Ischemic Scale	1.11% (2.06%)
Zhou et al	2001	Shanghai, rural and urban areas	17 018 (≥55)	DSM-IV, NINCDS/ AIREN	NINCDS-ADRDA Hachinski Ischemic Scale	0.42% (1.46%)
Zhang et al	2001	Beijing, rural and urban areas	5743 (≥55)	DSM-IV, NINCDS/ AIREN	NINCDS-ADRDA Hachinski Ischemic Scale	1.5% (2.0%)
Tang et al	2002	Beijing, rural and urban areas	2788 (≥60)	DSM-III-R, NINCDS/ AIREN	NINCDS-ADRDA	1.06% (4.43%)

VaD seems more common in rural areas. The survey did not find any correlation between education level and the prevalence of dementias.

Other relevant factors and problems in epidemiological studies on VaD in China

As the majority of the demented elderly are currently looked after by their families in China, some researchers conducted studies that focused on the burden and health/psychological status of caregivers. A pilot study (Li et al, 1990) showed that 50% of caregivers were spouses of demented patients. Relatives' Stress Scale and SCL-90 assessments indicated that caregivers reported higher stress levels and more negative feelings such as depression, anxiety, hostility and paranoia compared to a control group. Although female caregivers reported more stress in caring for demented patients, they reported fewer negative symptoms than male caregivers. The authors proposed that females in China were expected to undertake more household work and were more liable to accept the role of caregiver.

Another study completed more recently in Shanghai (Wu et al, 1995) reported that 56% caregivers were children of demented patients and 30% were spouses. The severity of dementia, impairment of ability of daily life and gender were correlated to the psychological status of caregivers. Caregivers reported more negative responses when they looked after male, severely demented and more disabled elderly people.

One study (Zhu et al, 1997) analyzed the mortality rate of VaD in follow-up. The annual mortality rate of VaD was 25.7%, i.e. higher than AD. In the group over 75 years old, with the estimated relative risk of dementia contributing to death consensus, VaD was ranked the highest.

Summary

The epidemiological studies on VaD conducted in China so far have several problems:

- Comparisons are difficult because of the use of different diagnostic criteria and screening instruments.
- The sample size was often too small.
- Most of the studies were conducted in urban areas and limited to big cities such as Beijing or Shanghai.

One very important issue to consider in the evaluation of epidemiological data on VaD is the homogeneity of subjects. Since China is a huge country, it encompasses diverse geographical characteristics. The demographic features of the Chinese people, including physical appearance, dialects, customs and diets vary considerably according to geographic areas, the Chinese are more heterogeneous than was previously supposed. This difference is reflected in the epidemiology of environment-related diseases.

It should be pointed out that all risk factors of VaD have increased in the last five years. A recent study on the epidemiology of hypertension investigated 280 000 subjects aged 35 and over in both rural and urban areas. They reported the prevalence of hypertension as 31.7% in cities and 32.9% in rural areas respectively (Hu et al, 2000). It is estimated that the prevalence of hypertension is rising rapidly. Wang et al (2001) analyzed the acute stroke events in Beijing in the last 15 years and indicated that the incidence of acute stroke increased year by year, and more significantly in elderly people. Another study estimated that more than 30% of the total population of China is overweight. Obesity used to be a condition that nobody was concerned about. However it is becoming a visible reality. A national surveillance system on dementias needs to be set up to monitor the changes and to analyze relevant risk factors regularly if we wish to know more about the epidemiology of VaD in China.

Reference

Chen C, Shen Y, Li S et al, The investigation on prevalence rates of elderly dementia in an urban area of Beijing, *Chin Mental Health J* (1992) **6**:49–52.

Chinese National Statistical Bureau, *Statistical report on 1995 1% Sampling Survey of China*. (Chinese National Statistical Bureau, 1996.)

Fan J, Yan J, Chen Z et al, An epidemiological report of senile dementia in Nanjing area, *J Clin Psychiatry* (2000) **10**:137–8.

Gao Z, Liu F, Fang Y et al, A study of morbidity rate of senile dementia among the aged in urban and rural areas, *J Neurol Psychiatry Chin* (1993) **26**:209–11.

Hu Y, Li L, Cao W et al, Community-based comprehensive prevention and control of hypertension in China (CCPACH Study) – prevalence and epidemiological characteristics in urban and rural areas, *Chin J Epidemiol* (2000) **21**:177–80.

Lai S, Wen Z, Liang W et al, Prevalence of dementia in an urban population aged 75 and over in Guangzhou, *Chin J Geriatr* (2000) **19**:450–5.

Li G, Shen Y, Chen C et al, An epidemiological survey of age-related dementia in an urban area of Beijing. *Acta Psychiatr Scand* (1989) **79**:557–63.

Li Y, Chen C, Luo H et al, The psychological well-being of caregivers of the elderly with dementia, *Chin Mental Health J* (1990) **4**:1–5.

Lu Z, Current status of the elderly and its development tendency in China, *Chin J Geriatr* (1994) **14**:194–8.

Qu Q, Qiao J, Yang J et al, Study of the prevalence of senile dementia among elderly people in Xian, China, *Chin J Geriatr* (2001) 20:283–6.

Shen Y, Li G, Li S et al, The 3-year follow-up study on elderly dementia in an urban area of Beijing, *Chin Mental Health J* (1994) 8:165–6.

Tang Z, Meng S, Dong H et al, Prevalence of dementia in rural and urban parts of Beijing, *Chin J Geriatr* (2002) 22:244–6.

Twelve Areas Epidemiological Investigation on Mental Disorders Coordinating Group, The summary of prevalence rates of various mental disorders from 12 areas epidemiological investigation, *Chin J Neurol Psychiatry*, (1986): 19:80–2.

Wang W, Zhao D, Wu G et al, The trend of incidence rates of acute stroke events in urban areas: Beijing from 1984 to 1999, *Chin J Epidemiol* (2001) 22:269–72.

Wu W, Zhang M, He Y et al, A study on the well-being and related factors of caregivers of dementia patients, *Chin Mental Health J* (1995) 9:49–52.

Yan F, Li S, Liu J et al, Incidence of senile dementia and depression in the elderly population in Xicheng District, Beijing; an epidemiological study, *Chin Med J* (2002) 82:1025–8.

Zhang J, Zhang H, Tao G et al, An epidemiological study on senile dementia among 1390 elderly people in Haidian District, Beijing *Chin J Epidemiol* (1998): 19:18–20.

Zhang M, Katzman R, Chen P et al, The incidence of dementia and Alzheimer's disease, *Chin J Psychiatry* (1998) 31:195–8.

Zhang M, Katzman R, Liu W et al, Prevalence study on dementia and Alzheimer's disease. *Chin Med J* (1990): 70:424–8.

Zhang Z, Wei J, Hong X et al, Prevalence of dementia and major subtypes in urban and rural communities of Beijing, *Chin J Neurol* (2001) 34:199–203.

Zhou B, Hong Z, Huang M et al, Prevalence of dementia in Shanghai urban and rural areas, *Chin J Epidemiol* (2001) 22:368–71.

Zhu Z, Zhang M, Katzman R et al, Mortality of dementia and other medical conditions in a five-year follow-up survey in the community, *Chin J Psychiatry* (1997) 30:231–4.

chapter 7

Epidemiology of vascular dementia: meta-analysis

Anthony F Jorm and Rajeev Kumar

Introduction

Meta-analysis is simply the use of statistical methods to aid a review of the literature. It has been applied in a number of reviews of the epidemiology of dementia to estimate prevalence rates, incidence rates and the strength of risk factors. Most of this work has been focused on the dementia syndrome or on Alzheimer's disease, with much less done on vascular dementia (VaD). The reasons for the dearth of work on VaD relate primarily to inadequacies in the data available. The results of a meta-analysis are only as good as the data it is based on. In considering the results of meta-analyses on VaD, there are important limitations on the available data which must be borne in mind:

1. The diagnosis of VaD has changed considerably over time. Earlier studies used the term 'arteriosclerotic dementia', which was eventually replaced by 'multi-infarct dementia' and then 'vascular dementia'. Diagnostic criteria were not available for the early studies and have gradually evolved over time. For this reason, earlier studies are difficult to compare with more recent ones.

2. The diagnosis of VaD was originally based on clinical examination, but more recently brain imaging techniques have played an important role. Such techniques are often not feasible in field surveys, so that the diagnosis of VaD in epidemiological studies is generally more basic than in clinical studies. The development of new technology has led VaD to be split into various subtypes, but these are seldom distinguished in epidemiological studies.

3. As cerebrovascular disease and Alzheimer's disease become more common with age, they are frequently found to co-occur, particularly in

the very elderly. Whereas clinical studies can select out relatively pure types by excluding these mixed dementias, epidemiological studies of representative samples must include them. Most epidemiological studies attempt to force all subjects into a pure category, but some allow a residual mixed category. If there is mixed category, it is not clear whether they should be grouped with VaD for the purposes of a meta-analysis or kept separate. Pooling them has the disadvantage that any associations found may really be attributable to co-morbid Alzheimer's disease, whereas excluding them may lead to an underestimation of the occurrence of vascular dementia.

When considering the results of the meta-analyses described below, these important limitations of the data must be kept in mind.

Prevalence of vascular dementia

The first meta-analysis of dementia prevalence was reported by Jorm, Korten and Henderson in 1987 (Jorm et al, 1987). They analyzed 47 prevalence studies, including 22 which gave age-specific rates, and found that while the prevalence rates differed significantly from study to study, they varied with age in a surprisingly consistent manner. Specifically, the prevalence of dementia was found to increase exponentially up to age 95, with a doubling in prevalence for every 5.1 years of age (95% confidence interval: 4.8–5.4 years). There was too little data after age 95 to draw any conclusions. However, it is not possible for prevalence to continue rising exponentially to extreme ages because rates would soon exceed the possible maximum of 100%. At higher ages, a logistic model may be more appropriate than an exponential one because it has a theoretical upper limit of 100% (Dewey, 1991).

Of the 22 studies which were used to fit the exponential model for dementia prevalence, only seven provided data on Alzheimer's and vascular dementias. When an attempt was made to fit an exponential model to data from these seven studies, the VaD data from one study did not fit. However, when this study was excluded, the model gave a satisfactory fit. Prevalence rates for VaD were found to double every 5.3 years of age (95% confidence interval: 4.6–6.3), while those of Alzheimer's dementia doubled every 4.5 years (95% confidence interval: 4.0–5.0). In other words, the exponential rise with age was steeper for Alzheimer's than for VaD.

In the Jorm et al (1987) meta-analysis, the relative importance of Alzheimer's and VaD was found to differ by sex and by country. When sex differences were examined, prevalence rates for Alzheimer's dementia showed a significantly higher female rate, while for VaD there was no significant sex difference. Examining country differences, VaD was found to be more prevalent than Alzheimer's in Japanese and Russian studies, there was no difference in Finnish and US studies, while British and Scandinavian studies found Alzheimer's to be more prevalent.

The country differences found in the meta-analysis could have been due to differences in diagnostic practice across countries, particularly in view of the rudimentary diagnostic procedures that are often used in field surveys. However, the case for cross-national differences can be strengthened by examining data from other sorts of studies. Clinic studies provide a more rigorous diagnosis, but at the expense of representativeness. Neuropathological studies provide the gold standard diagnosis, but the cases coming to autopsy are even less representative. Nevertheless, if clinical and neuropathological studies from various studies provide similar findings to prevalence surveys, we can have more confidence in the findings. To check for such consistency, Jorm later carried out a semi-quantitative analysis of the relative occurrence of Alzheimer's and VaD in various regions of the world (Jorm, 1991). There was consistent evidence that Alzheimer's dementia is more common than VaD in Britain and North America and, to a lesser extent, in Scandinavia. In the rest of Europe and in Australia, the evidence also favored a higher occurrence of Alzheimer's dementia, with the exception of Russian prevalence studies, which reported more VaD. However, Russian neuropathological studies have found that VaD is considerably overdiagnosed there at the expense of Alzheimer's dementia. Consequently, it was concluded that Alzheimer's dementia predominates in countries with largely Caucasian populations. In East Asia the picture was quite different, with both prevalence and neuropathological studies fairly consistently reporting a higher prevalence of vascular than Alzheimer's dementia.

The next attempt to cover VaD was the EURODEM project which pooled prevalence data from western European studies published between 1980 and 1990 (Rocca et al, 1991a). However, this attempt was hampered by the limited amount of data available and the lack of common diagnostic criteria. The only conclusions that could be drawn were that prevalence rises steeply with age, it is generally higher in men and Alzheimer's dementia is generally more common than VaD.

The most recent meta-analysis, by Fratiglioni et al (1999), reported pooled data on the prevalence rate of dementia and its subtypes from Europe, Asia and North America. It appeared that there was a difference in the prevalence of Alzheimer's dementia and VaD among these countries. Of interest were the higher percentages of VaD in Asian studies, accounting for 38% of the total demented cases based on the data in older studies. However, when only the more recent data from Asia were taken into account, VaD occurred at a frequency of 31% and Alzheimer's disease at 61%. These findings are similar to those reported in Europe, North America and Africa. However, VaD prevalence was much higher in Asian-Americans than in other ethnic groups in the USA.

Although a number of other meta-analyses have been carried out on dementia prevalence, these have either dealt with dementia as a syndrome (Hofman et al, 1991; Ritchie et al, 1992; Ritchie and Kildea, 1995) or with Alzheimer's dementia (Rocca et al, 1991b; Corrada et al, 1995; USGAO, 1998).

Incidence of vascular dementia

While prevalence rates are useful for planning services, incidence rates are better for studying risk factors. This is because differences between groups in prevalence may be due to differences in either the duration of the disease or in incidence. Because they require longitudinal data, incidence studies are much less frequently carried out than prevalence studies. It has only been very recently that enough incidence studies have become available to permit a meta-analysis. Three meta-analyses of dementia incidence have been published (Jorm and Jolley, 1998; Gao et al, 1998; Fratiglioni et al, 2000) but only two of these specifically examined VaD (Jorm and Jolley, 1998; Fratiglioni et al, 2000).

Jorm and Jolley analyzed the data from 23 studies that reported age-specific incidence data. Eleven of these studies gave data on VaD and 14 on Alzheimer's dementia. The data were analyzed using Loess curve fitting. This method uses local neighborhoods to find curves that best fit the data. Loess curves make no assumptions about the form of the incidence curve, unlike parametric methods, which assume either an exponential or logistic curve. However, if log incidence is plotted against age, and the Loess curve forms a straight line, this implies that the rise in incidence with age is exponential.

When the data on all dementias were analyzed, the Loess curve relating log incidence to age was found to be linear, implying an exponential rise. However, there were few data on persons over the age of 90, so what happens in extreme old age remains an open question. Figure 7.1 shows the data on VaD. Although the Loess curves are basically straight lines, the data points show considerable variability, reflecting the problems of assessing VaD in field surveys. As would be expected, studies assessing mild+ VaD tend to show higher incidence rates than those assessing moderate+ VaD. Figure 7.1 also shows an interesting sex difference, with steeper incidence curves for females. Males have a higher incidence at younger ages but

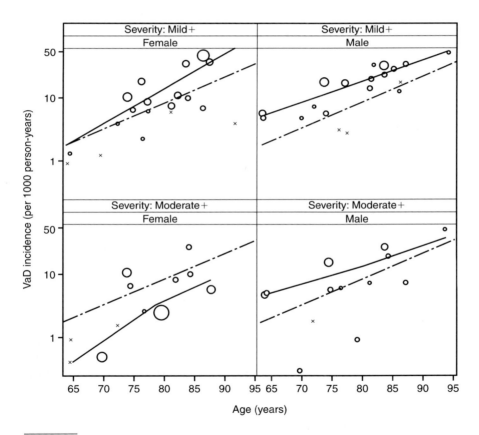

Figure 7.1 *Loess curves of log incidence by sex. The solid line is the Loess curve. The dashed line is for visual reference in making comparison across panels. The circles are data points from the various studies, with the area of the circle proportional to the weight of the point. Very small circles are shown by an X to make them more visible.*

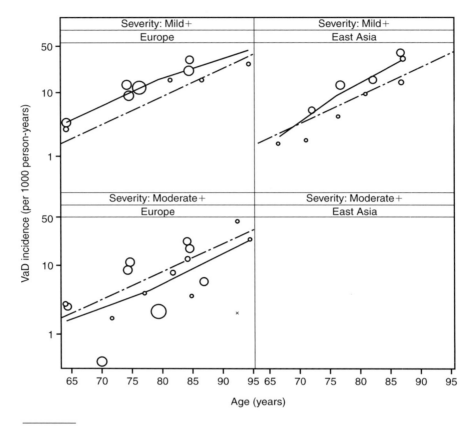

Figure 7.2 *Loess curves of log incidence by region. The solid line is the Loess curve. The dashed line is for visual reference in making comparison across panels. The circles are data points from the various studies, with the area of the circle proportional to the weight of the point. Very small circles are shown by an X to make them more visible.*

females tend to catch up at older ages. The higher incidence in males at younger ages may reflect the effects of smoking, with only non-smokers surviving to very old age.

Figure 7.2 shows the findings for Europe compared to East Asia (no data were available for other regions). The European studies are divided according to whether they assessed mild+ or moderate+ VaD. By contrast, the East Asia studies only assessed mild+ dementia. The incidence of mild+ VaD did not differ significantly between Europe and East Asia.

Jorm and Jolley carried out similar analyses for Alzheimer's dementia. Again, the rise with age appeared to be exponential up to age 90, although it tended to be steeper for Alzheimer's than for VaD. There was no sex difference at younger ages, but females tended to have a higher incidence at the older ages. The incidence of Alzheimer's dementia tended to be lower in East Asian countries at younger ages but this regional difference disappeared at the older ages.

In a more recent report on pooled data from Europe, the incidence of VaD was assessed separately from Alzheimer's dementia (Fratiglioni et al, 2000). The pooled data included 835 cases of mild to severe dementia and 42 996 person-years of follow-up. There were 147 cases of VaD. The incidence rates increased with age without any substantial gender difference. Figures 7.3 and 7.4 show the pooled incidence rates of VaD and Alzheimer's disease by age group and sex.

Summary

Although meta-analysis has provided some useful summaries of epidemiological findings on global dementia and Alzheimer's dementia, limitations of the available data make it difficult to draw firm conclusions about VaD. However, the following tentative conclusions can be offered:

1. The prevalence and incidence of VaD rise approximately exponentially with age, at least until age 90.
2. The occurrence of VaD rises less steeply with age than Alzheimer's.

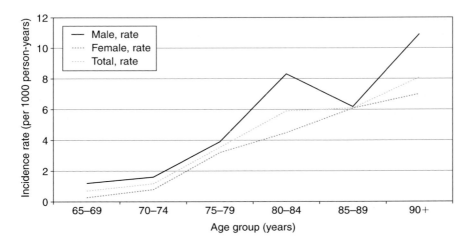

Figure 7.3 *Vascular dementia: pooled incidence rates by age group and sex.*

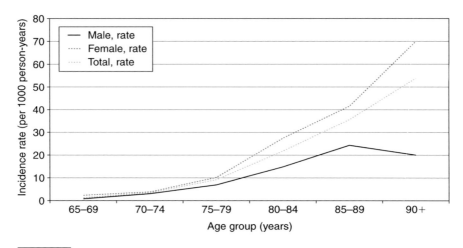

Figure 7.4 *Alzheimer's disease: pooled incidence rates by age group and sex.*

3. Cerebrovascular disease is a relatively more important cause of dementia for males than for females.
4. In the past, cerebrovascular disease was a relatively more important cause of dementia in East Asian than in Western countries. However, this appears to have changed over time, with East Asian countries becoming more like Western countries in the distribution of dementia types.

Any advance in the epidemiology of VaD beyond these basic conclusions will rest on the development of valid diagnostic methods which are feasible in field surveys and which can be applied consistently in different studies.

References

Corrada M, Brookmeyer R, Kawas C, Sources of variability in prevalence rates of Alzheimer's disease, *Int J Epidemiol* (1995) **24**:1000–5.

Dewey M, How should prevalence be modelled? *Acta Psychiatr Scand* (1991) **84**:246–9.

Fratiglioni L, Ronchi DD, Aguero-Torres H, Worldwide prevalence and incidence of dementia, *Drugs Aging* (1999) **5**:365–75.

Fratiglioni L, Launer LJ, Andersen K et al, Incidence of dementia and major subtypes in Europe: a collaborative study of population-based cohorts, *Neurology* (2000) **54**:S10–S15.

Gao S, Hendrie HC, Hall KS, Hui S, The relationship between age, sex, and the incidence of dementia and Alzheimer disease, *Arch Gen Psychiatry* (1998) **55**:809–15.

Hofman A, Rocca WA, Brayne C et al, The prevalence of dementia in Europe: a collaborative study of 1980–1990 findings, *Int J Epidemiol* (1991) **20**:736–48.

Jorm AF, Cross-national comparisons of the occurrence of Alzheimer's and vascular dementias, *Eur Arch Psychiatr Clin Neurosci* (1991) **240**:218–22.

Jorm AF, Jolley D, The incidence of dementia: a meta-analysis, *Neurology* (1998) **51**:728–33.

Jorm AF, Korten AE, Henderson AS, The prevalence of dementia: a quantitative integration of the literature, *Acta Psychiatr Scand* (1987) **76**:465–79.

Ritchie K, Kildea D, Robine J-M, The relationship between age and the prevalence of senile dementia: a meta-analysis of recent data, *Int J Epidemiol* (1992) **21**:763–9.

Ritchie K, Kildea D, Is senile dementia 'age-related' or 'ageing-related'? – evidence from meta-analysis of dementia prevalence in the oldest old, *Lancet* (1995) **346**:931–4.

Rocca WA, Hofman A, Brayne C et al, The prevalence of vascular dementia in Europe: facts and fragments from 1980–1990 studies, *Ann Neurol* (1991a) **30**:817–24.

Rocca WA, Hofman A, Brayne C et al, Frequency and distribution of Alzheimer's disease in Europe: a collaborative study of 1980–1990 findings, *Ann Neurol* (1991b) **30**:381–90.

United States General Accounting Office (USGAO), *Alzheimer's Disease: Estimates of Prevalence in the United States* (United States General Accounting Office: Washington DC, 1998).

chapter 8

The epidemiology of vascular dementia: an overview and commentary

Anthony F Jorm and John O'Brien

The first four chapters in this section have summarized the evidence on the epidemiology of vascular dementia (VaD) in different regions of the world, while the previous chapter in the section summarizes the results of meta-analyses involving all countries from which data are available. The purpose of the present chapter is to provide an integration and commentary on these varied contributions. This chapter identifies common themes raised in the previous chapters as well as areas of difference.

Diagnostic criteria and methods

At the present time, epidemiologists are unable to give anything like definitive prevalence and incidence rates for VaD by age, sex and region. There are many reasons for this, which Skoog and Aevarsson summarise well in their Table 3.2. Probably the issue of diagnostic criteria is the most important factor, which is highlighted by all authors. Criteria for VaD have changed considerably over time, have been much less well validated than those for Alzheimer's disease (AD) and vary greatly between studies. As highlighted by Skoog and Aevarsson and Eastwood and O'Brien, criteria used in most epidemiological studies are very much based on the 'infarct' model of VaD and do not adequately recognize the current broader view of VaD, particularly the recognized importance of subcortical vascular disease (lacunes and white matter lesions) in causing dementia. Recently proposed criteria, such as those of the NINDS-AIREN, are highly specific but have low sensitivity (20–50%) so their use would lead to underestimates of VaD. Another important issue is that VaD criteria do not adequately cope with mixed dementia, now recognized as a common if not the most common cause of dementia in population studies. The fact that the various criteria for VaD are not interchangeable makes it very difficult to compare studies between different countries or over time in the same country. A final problem when comparing VaD with AD is that definitions of dementia are based on the Alzheimer model, requiring the presence of memory deficit, which is not always prominent in vascular cases, and so may bias case ascertainment towards AD (Chapter 4).

There are other sources of methodological variation which are particularly important in epidemiological field studies. The existing criteria are designed primarily for use in clinical research where a wide range of investigations is possible. However, some types of investigation (for example brain imaging) are difficult to implement within the constraints of field studies. The more clinical investigations carried out when making a diagnosis, the higher the relative prevalence of VaD (Chapter 3). There are also problems in making judgments about the etiological significance of cerebrovascular lesions: the historical information available about onset may be limited; VaD may have an insidious onset in some cases, mimicking AD; and infarctions may be clinically silent (Chapter 3). The advent of large 'epidemiological imaging' studies has shown that almost one-third of elderly subjects have hitherto unsuspected cerebrovascular disease (Chapter 4).

There are also regional differences in diagnostic approach, which may be seen even where the same diagnostic criteria are being used. Homma and Hasegawa point out that elderly Japanese do not like psychometric screening tests and that subjects are not used to participating in research studies. As such, researchers must rely on relatives' reports of activities of daily living and behavioral changes. On the other hand, in other countries there may be difficulty in finding a suitable informant because of a weaker cultural commitment to caring for elderly relatives.

Cultural differences in patterns of aged care can have an effect in another way, through national differences in rates of nursing home placement. Nursing home residents are often omitted from epidemiological field studies. Even within a single region, some studies include nursing home residents and others do not (Chapter 3 and Chapter 5). The rate of nursing home placement may also vary over time, making historical comparisons difficult. However, whether these differences in sampling substantially affect prevalence and incidence rates is difficult to determine because other methodological differences have a masking effect (Chapter 5).

Differential mortality may also be a problem, in that VaD survival is shorter than AD and in large epidemiological studies patients with VaD who have been identified from a screen may die before detailed assessment can be undertaken, leading to an underestimate of VaD prevalence (Chapter 3).

Prevalence

Despite the 'noise' created by all these methodological differences, it is possible to come to some conclusions. Regional differences are discussed below, but overall VaD clearly emerges from nearly all recent studies as the second most common cause of dementia in later life after AD. Not surprisingly, the prevalence of VaD increases steeply with age, although the increase appears to be less steep for VaD than for AD (Chapter 3 and Chapter 7). This means that even though rates of VaD increase with age, the relative proportion of those with dementia who have VaD compared to AD decreases with age. There are still too few studies including subjects over 90 years old to know whether prevalence of VaD continues to increase with age or shows a plateau (Chapter 3).

There are also likely to be sex differences. Early studies showed a higher crude prevalence of VaD in men than women, and the converse for AD (Chapter 7). However, recent studies give a more refined picture of sex differences: the prevalence of AD is higher in women, especially after age 80, while VaD is more common in men, especially before 75 (Chapter 3).

For epidemiologists, incidence studies are preferable to prevalence studies. The reason is that prevalence may differ between groups because of incidence differences or because of survival differences. The mortality in VaD has been reported as very high in both Europe and China (Chapter 3 and Chapter 6), implying that VaD may appear to be a bigger contributor to dementia incidence than to dementia prevalence.

Incidence

Incidence studies are unfortunately rare. Barriers to carrying out an incidence study include not only the greater resources required but the short-term research funding policies in some countries (Chapter 5 and Chapter 6).

As with prevalence, the rates vary greatly from study to study, undoubtedly due to methodological differences (Chapter 7). Nevertheless, we can say that incidence rises steeply with age in an exponential fashion, at least up to age 90 (Chapter 7). Incidence also appears to rise less steeply for VaD than for AD, consistent with the data on prevalence (Chapter 3 and Chapter 7), showing that survival differences do not account for this effect. Sex differences are also similar for prevalence and incidence. Men tend to have a higher incidence of VaD at younger ages, and women a higher incidence of AD at higher ages (Chapter 3 and Chapter 7).

Are there true regional differences?

There is considerable interest in whether incidence or prevalence rates differ between regions. Such a difference implies a different profile of risk factors between the regions. There may be some risk factors that vary more between regions than within regions and that can only be feasibly identified by cross-regional comparisons.

A meta-analysis of early prevalence studies found that AD was the most common dementing disease in some countries, while in others such as Japan and Russia, VaD was more common (Chapter 7). Later evidence suggested that the predominance of VaD in Russian studies was due to different diagnostic practices. However, the Japanese pattern of dementia continues to arouse epidemiological interest. As discussed below, this pattern may be changing, with Japan becoming more like Caucasian populations in having a predominance of AD. The data on cross-national differences in incidence are more sparse. A meta-analysis of the available studies found no difference in VaD incidence between Europe and East Asia (Chapter 7). By contrast, the incidence of AD was lower in East Asia, at least in the young old. The difference disappeared with age as the East Asian countries caught up. This raises the interesting issue that it is AD, not VaD, that varies between countries (Chapter 5).

There may also be regional and ethnic differences within countries. In China, for example, the prevalence of VaD may be higher in urban areas and in Beijing compared to Shanghai (Chapter 6). Consistent with this observation, the prevalence of hypertension is higher in Beijing, perhaps because of the higher salt intake (Chapter 6). Both Yu and Shen, and Eastwood and

O'Brien highlight the huge cultural and geographical diversity within China and North America respectively, which also has to be considered when comparing studies between countries. For example, in the USA, there are certain regions with a higher stroke risk, although whether the VaD rates also differ is unknown (Chapter 4). Furthermore, there are ethnic differences, African-, Japanese- and Chinese-Americans having more intracranial and Caucasians more extracranial vascular disease (Chapter 4).

The study of regional and ethnic differences is made difficult because of the many methodological differences between studies. There is a clear need for studies which attempt to use identical methodology with different groups (Chapter 5 and Chapter 7). Homma and Hasegawa point to the KAME Project in Washington State, USA, which examines dementia in Japanese-Americans, as the sort of project that needs to be extended across countries.

Are there historical changes?

It is very difficult to judge whether the prevalence or incidence of VaD has changed, for several reasons. Very little information was available 20 years ago (Chapter 6) and, even where historical data are available, the changes in classification and diagnostic methods make direct comparison difficult (Chapter 4). Even societal changes like declining participation rates in epidemiological studies can have an effect (Chapter 5).

Nevertheless, despite a decline in stroke incidence and better treatment of hypertension, the limited evidence available from Europe does not support any decline in prevalence (Chapter 3). There could be other factors at work that offset these gains, such as better treatment of stroke leading to longer survival and better detection (Chapter 3). On the other hand, prevalence studies in Japan show a historical trend in the relative prevalence of VaD and AD. In studies carried out before 1989, VaD tended to predominate, whereas in more recent studies, AD has become dominant (Chapter 5). In a series of prevalence studies carried out in Tokyo, overall rates of dementia did not change, while VaD decreased and AD increased (Chapter 5). However, there were inevitable changes in assessment methods over time which complicate comparisons, and the number of nursing home beds also increased. Homma and Hasegawa speculate that there has been an historical change in exposure to environmental risk factors for AD. As with the study of regional differences, serial studies using identical methodology are needed before we will know whether dementia prevalence or incidence is changing.

Aging of the population

One conclusion that probably no one would disagree with is that the aging of the population will lead to a rapid increase in the number of VaD cases. This rapid increase is already apparent in more developed countries such as Japan (Chapter 5), but will be increasingly apparent in the less developed countries such as China in the present century (Chapter 6).

Part III

Pathophysiology of Cerebrovascular Disease – with Reference to Dementias

The neuropathology of vascular dementia and its overlap with Alzheimer's disease

Arne Brun

Introduction

Cerebrovascular lesions often cause dementia in co-operation with other brain changes. In such mixed cases the symptoms are varied and the weight of each structural component may be difficult to evaluate, which leads to classification difficulties. Vascular lesions also cause dementia on their own as shown by the many proven pathology cases with various types of pure vascular disease with dementia. The clinical profile of these cases varies, e.g. with or without neurological deficits and with or without obvious stepwise progression. Hence it is difficult to justify the clinical term 'dementia of the cerebrovascular type.' This term also fails to cover noncerebral causes such as cardiac and hypotensive/hypoperfusive forms. Multi-infarct dementia (MID), a term introduced by Hachinski et al (1974), was originally meant to cover the whole field of vascular dementia (VaD) but is now mostly used to designate dementia due to multiple large infarcts. A similar definition also limits the usefulness of the term 'post-stroke dementia.' 'Vascular cognitive impairment', suggested by Bowler and Hachinski (1998), does not explicitly imply dementia but rather may denote a stage that may or may not evolve into dementia. Here as with other designations new definitions of dementia may cause difficulties and invite various levels of impairment. Stroke dementia, conventionally defined as due to MID, does not include anoxic, hypoperfusive or extracerebral hemorrhagic etiologies. The term 'vascular dementia' chosen here might best cover the subject since it is broad, uncommitted and may be taken to encompass all forms including cardiac and hypoperfusive/anoxic–ischemic forms (O'Brien, 1994).

Aging is a confounding factor

One of the most common confounding factors in VaD is the aging process, which can be described as a combination of milder degenerative and cerebrovascular changes among which the latter may be difficult to single out from a superimposed vascular dementing disease. In the literature, VaD is usually described as VaD or VaD plus other disorders, but VaD plus aging is rarely considered. The importance of aging in this context is emphasized by the finding that VaD is the most common form of organic dementia after the age of 85 (Amar and Wilcock, 1996). Normal aging with its gray and especially white matter loss, degenerative changes and small, silent vascular lesions can be viewed as predisposing to dementia due to a reduction of brain reserve capacity. This brings an aged individual closer to the level of insufficiency where only minor additional lesions may be required to precipitate dementia.

The degenerative aging changes, though milder, repeat much of the pathology of Alzheimer's disease (AD). Senile plaques and neurofibrillary tangles are the most obvious of these. The latter are particularly pronounced in the entorhinal area of the hippocampus, an area vital to memory processing. There is also an amyloid angiopathy, sometimes as severe as that seen in AD, in which it can vary considerably in severity. More important, however, there is as in AD, a progressive loss of synapses in the cortex often amounting to as much as 40–50% in the oldest cases (Liu et al, 1996). The vascular lesions, accepted as an inevitable consequence of aging, are mainly expressed as a varying number of complete small infarcts in the gray and white matter and incomplete white matter infarcts, shown as white matter lucencies on imaging.

When sufficiently pronounced, the various lesions co-operate with the aging process to produce a dementia which may be named 'summational dementia' (Brun et al, 1992), since many of the changes are not demonstrable clinically, no single lesion can be held responsible and thus no conventional label can be applied. Before this stage is reached, however, the reduced reserve capacity may co-operate with any disease to produce dementia, which then appears to progress more quickly in the aged than in the younger patient with greater reserve capacity. Thus the more advanced the age, the less severe the lesion required to cause dementia. This then also means that even a minor stroke may seem to cause dementia, resulting in a clinical mislabeling of the condition, since the stroke is just the final straw and would not have resulted in dementia in a younger patient with greater reserve capacity. Further neuronal stress, for example in connection with narcosis, or functionally important deficiency states such as for vitamin B_{12} and folic acid, hyperhomocysteinemia (Nilsson et al, 2001) and failing function of other organs, such as an aging heart, would more easily produce cognitive impairment in the elderly, temporarily or definitely. Summational dementia of the aged may be regarded as a special subgroup of dementias in which vascular lesions play an important role.

Pathoanatomical classification of VaD

A simple basis for pathoanatomical classification of VaD is the size of the vessels responsible (Brun, 1994). This approach is rational since the large vessels comprising the aorta and carotids, the circle of Willis and its main branches and the larger meningeal arteries, are mainly afflicted with the consequences of common arteriosclerosis with atheromatous lesions. Small vessels of arteriolar size on the other hand suffer mainly from hypertensive angiopathy and fibrohyaline arteriolosclerosis. This results not only in a different pathogenesis but also a different lesion pattern and infarct size in the two categories. From this it also follows that large and small vessel disease may appear separately, resulting in pure large or small vessel dementia as demonstrated on extensive neuropathological examination. When all types of VaD were considered, almost half of them were of the pure type, and a combination of large and small vessel disease with large and small infarcts accounted for only 22% of VaD (Brun, 1994). Also, combinations with the hypoperfusive type may occur.

Physiological circulation and metabolic factors supplement the classification principle based on vessel size. Hypoperfusion, most likely of an episodic and repeated nature and due to heart failure or blood pressure drops, may cause dementing injury, often through collaboration with local cerebral vascular factors or regional hemodynamic conditions in border zones and white matter. This is a theme lately alluded to in an increasing number of publications. In addition, reduction in oxygen and/or glucose can produce brain lesions, either global (apallic or semiapallic syndromes) or focal due to special local metabolic demands (regional selective vulnerability). Venous occlusions may also cause large infarcts. A last group is formed by meningeal and brain hemorrhages. Against this background the pathophysiological classification of VaD, modified from Brun and Gustafson (1988), is used, as set out in Table 9.1.

Large vessel dementia

In the present classification large vessel dementia corresponds to MID. It is caused mainly by thromboembolism originating from atherosclerotic lesions in the heart and large vessels. A cardiac origin is also stressed, for example by the Cerebral Embolism Task Force (1989), as in cardiac dementia due to hypoperfusion of cardiac origin.

Occlusion of the larger vessels results in large infarcts involving the cortex plus the white matter and also central gray and brain stem structures. In an extensive neuropathological study of 175 cases of dementia (Brun, 1994) this was found to be the smallest group comprising about 15% of all VaD cases. This may explain the finding by Hulette et al (1997) who only investigated MID cases, that 'pure' VaD in general is rather uncommon. A significant part of the infarct pathology, especially in the white matter, is a perifocal incomplete infarct, often involving larger areas than the complete infarct. Here the tissue damage becomes less severe in a peripheral direction from the complete infarct center, in gray matter within a very narrow zone but in the white matter in wide areas. This is a penumbra zone (Astrup et al, 1981), which is probably not fully appreciated in its peripheral and less severely damaged areas on brain imaging, particularly computed tomography. It thus makes up an often undiscovered or poorly identified correlate to the functional brain deficit. This zone deserves attention in view of the possible benefits from treatment supporting and improving flow and metabolism, with the aim of preventing further growth of the penumbra zone or incorporation of the original penumbra zone in the complete infarct, as discussed by Back et al (1998). In the gray matter such incomplete infarcts are also named selective neuronal loss (Weiller et al, 1998); in the experience of the present author this (phenomenon!) is often best observed in hippocampal anoxic damage.

Table 9.1 Pathophysiological classification of VaD

1. Large vessel dementia
Multi-infarct dementia (MID)
Multiple large infarcts, cortical and subcortical, with perifocal incomplete infarcts, esp. in white matter
Strategic infarct dementia (SID)
Restricted, few infarcts in functionally important regions, often subcortical brain regions, e.g. striate body or thalamus, white matter key areas, basal forebrain, but also cortical, e.g. ACA and MCA territories incl. angular gyrus

2. Small vessel dementia
Subcortical infarct dementia
Multiple small lacunar infarcts with large perifocal incomplete infarcts, esp. in white matter
    lacunar state
    Binswanger's disease
    hereditary angiopathies
Cortical plus subcortical infarct dementia
Multiple, restricted small infarcts due to
    hypertensive and arteriolosclerotic angiopathy
    amyloid angiopathy, sometimes with hemorrhages
    collagen or inflammatory vascular disease
    hereditary forms

3. Hypoperfusive, hypoxic–ischemic dementia
    incomplete white matter infarcts
    borderzone infarcts
    diffuse hypoxic–ischemic encephalopathy or restricted according to regional selective vulnerability

4. Venous infarct dementia
Large hemorrhagic, congestive symmetric infarcts due to thrombosis of the sagittal sinuses or the great vein of Galen

5. Hemorrhagic dementia
    subdural hemorrhage
    subarachnoid hemorrhage
    intracerebral hemorrhage

Strategic infarct dementia

Strategic infarct dementia (SID) is a usually large vessel but sometimes a small vessel dementia, due to a single or few but topographically important infarcts, and in this sense it is the opposite to MID. This concept was introduced by Brun and Gustafson (1988) and has since been increasingly used to denote a dementia caused by few or single, often restricted, infarcts but with a strategic location in functionally important regions. One of the best known examples is bilateral anterior thalamic infarcts producing dementia of a frontal type. This places special emphasis on the role of brain imaging in dementia diagnostics as illustrated by a case clinically diagnosed as AD without CT lesions but with a thalamic strategic infarct shown on magnetic resonance, which prompted a revision of the diagnosis to strategic VaD (Wolf et al, 1997). Other strategic sites are the caudate nucleus and white matter key areas with important interconnecting loops but also cortical areas such as the angular gyrus.

Small vessel dementia

Small vessel dementia (SVD) is due to infarcts caused by obstruction of mainly intracerebral vessels of arteriolar size, subcortically represented by the long penetrants. The cause may be microemboli from heart valves or atheromatous large vessel lesions, particularly carotid stenosis or special vessel diseases such as collagen or inflammatory diseases (Lishman, 1997), amyloid angiopathy (especially the hemorrhagic familial forms), and other hereditary angiopathies. The major cause is, however, hypertensive angiopathy, which may assume two forms: cortical plus subcortical, and purely subcortical, referred to as Binswanger's disease (BD) or progressive subcortical vascular encephalopathy (PSVE); the lacunar state may be regarded as a milder form of the latter. The two varieties are basically similar, showing mostly small infarcts of lacunar size up to 10 to 15 mm in diameter. Esiri et al (1997) referred to small vessel dementia as microvascular disease and found it to be the most common variety in their neuropathological study. Small vessel dementia was also reported by Akiguchi et al (1997) to be the leading cause of VaD in Japan. This is in agreement with our finding that small vessel dementia accounts for 33% of cases of both pure and mixed AD/VaD. Further, the pure SVD group, with and without AD, was as big as the combination of the group composed of pure LVD and the group of LVD plus SVD, with and without AD (Brun, 1994).

Subcortical infarct dementia

Binswanger's disease, initially characterized pathologically by Alzheimer, is marked by lacunar infarcts usually measuring 5–10 mm in diameter and situated in the brain stem and central gray nuclei but above all in the frontal white matter, sparing the cortex and u-fibers. In the white matter the lacunes are surrounded by wide areas of incomplete infarcts with partial loss of axons, myelin and oligodendroglial cells accompanied by a mild astrocytic gliosis causing an extensive cortical undermining and disconnection. This change impresses as the main structural substrate for the functional deficit in BD explaining, for example, frontal symptoms, gait and incontinence problems. The small lacunes are probably of lesser importance. The loss of white matter is reflected in a widening of especially the frontal ventricular horns. Portions of less severe incomplete white matter infarcts may not be demonstrable on brain imaging, causing clinicopathological correlation difficulties. The incomplete infarcts can be assumed to evolve due to repeated episodes of ischemia in a penumbra zone around the lacunae which in combination with the relative discreteness of the damage may clinically simulate a progressive degenerative disorder with mild acute episodes. In contrast to some authors (Pantoni and Garcia, 1995), others (Roman, 1996; Caplan, 1995) consider BD to be a well-defined disorder and an important cause of VaD, particularly in the older age groups. Looking at all age groups, BD is common, in our study accounting for a quarter of pure small vessel dementia with and without AD (Brun, 1994).

Many of the BD cases suffer from hypertension. The absence of hypertension should raise the suspicion of cerebral autosomal dominant arteriopathy with subcortical infarcts and leukoencephalopathy (CADASIL) (Bowler and Hachinski, 1998). This condition is dominantly inherited, the gene localized to chromosome 19 notch 3 gene, as distinct from the ApoE gene (Tournier-Lasserve et al, 1993). In CADASIL the angiopathy is less florid than in BD, characterized by cerebral fibrohyaline arteriosclerosis with osmophilic material but also in other (e.g. skin) vessels (Kallimo et al, 2002). The resulting infarcts are mainly subcortical, complete and also incomplete in wide areas. It could be regarded as a presenile familial disorder in a PSVE or Binswanger spectrum but without hypertension (Hedera and Friedland, 1987).

Cortical plus subcortical infarct dementia

Cortical plus subcortical infarct dementia is usually associated with hypertension and arteriosclerosis. The vascular level and size involved is somewhat more varied than in BD and hence the infarcts show a greater variation in location, the lesions being less frontally accentuated than in BD and in size although they are mainly in the small to lacunar range. The complications of hypertensive angiopathy are mural and perivascular hemorrhages and microaneurysms. Other rarer causes of small vessel dementia are collagen/inflammatory vascular disease, hereditary angiopathies such as familial amyloid angiopathy, CADASIL with cortical infarcts, hereditary multi-infarct dementia and glycosaminoglycan angiopathy.

Hypoperfusive, hypoxic–ischemic dementia

Hypoperfusive, hypoxic–ischemic dementia is defined here as dementia due not to focal cessation of flow, as in preceding forms of VaD, but a temporary reduction of flow or substrate supply below the level necessary for neural structural integrity and for a period of time long enough to damage brain tissue. A chronic ischemic state causing brain damage appears unphysiologic, in agreement with Bowler and Hachinski (1998), in view of the existence of compensatory (e.g. autoregulatory) mechanisms and the possibility of variation in oxygen extraction. Hypoperfusion, hypoxia and ischemia are general rather than focal factors, and produce dementia through global anoxic encephalopathy, but also through focal lesions due to selective vulnerability or, based on hemodynamic principles, multifocal small or large borderzone (BZ) infarcts. It should be noted that BZ infarcts not only affect a cortical area but underneath there is a wedge of white matter where all kinds of connections become severed by the infarction. Such lesions are, however, less common causes of VaD. However, the large group here, roughly the size of small vessel VaD, is one with incomplete infarcts, particularly of white matter, called selective incomplete white matter infarcts (Brun and Englund, 1986), and treated in Chapter 10.

Venous infarct dementia

Venous occlusion infarcts rarely cause VaD due to the low survival rate after such incidents, which are in addition rare in themselves. The occlusion is a thrombosis often due to infection: a thrombophlebitis. The resulting infarcts are congestive, intensely hemorrhagic, usually bilaterally symmetrical, not following the arterial territories (and thus different from arterial infarcts), and may on gross inspection be mistaken for primary hemorrhages.

Hemorrhagic dementia

Dementia caused by hemorrhage is unusual but included here since it is clearly related to vascular disease and also causes secondary ischemic anoxic lesions, sometimes extensive due to brain swelling. It may be seen after sub-arachnoid, subdural and intracerebral hemorrhage, for example in familial congophilic angiopathy (CAA).

Overlap between VaD and AD

From a neuropathological point of view VaD can overlap with AD, either through a common etiology or pathogenesis of changes, or through colocal-ization of alterations, the distribution of vascular lesions more or less faith-fully imitating the basic AD topographic lesion pattern. Many facets of the interplay between the two disorders are covered in *Vascular Factors in Alzheimer's Disease* (Kalaria and Ince, 2000) and the clinical overlap together with small vessel subcortical dementia is reviewed by Roman et al (2002).

Of course, a common etiology remains speculative with an unknown cause for most cases of AD. AD and CADASIL might share a common genetic mechanism, the Notch 3 protein and amyloid precursor protein both being cleaved by γ-secretase (presenilin). Also Apo ε4 can be considered a link in view of its assumed role for both AD and VaD, perhaps converging on CAA.

Regarding pathogenesis, several authors have lately proposed a common pathway in terms of a variety of vascular mechanisms. A degenerative type of microangiopathy might cause not only VaD but also AD as claimed by de la Torre (2002). Further, CAA of AD could add a VaD of a hypoperfusive or SVD type, even with BZ infarcts (Suter et al, 2002) through stenosis, dis-turbed vascular autoregulation or through blood-brain barrier damage (Mueggler et al, 2002; Greenberg, 2002). Amyloid might also directly, or through induced reactive oxygen species and without CAA, affect autoregu-lation and perfusion (Niwa et al, 2001, 2002). In addition CAA causes hem-orrhages and then mainly in the familial forms. A reduction in AD of the blood pressure, from a previous hypertension or when dementia ensues, would be another mechanism behind hypoperfusive lesions in AD, particularly in cases of AD on medication for hypertension (Ruitenberg et al, 2001; Trenkwalder, 2002). Blood pressure may, however, long before the onset of dementia, decline from normal levels to a low and labile blood pressure, which together with failing heart function has been associated with cognitive decline, hypoperfusion and white matter lesions (Zuccala et al, 2001).

The second main mechanism, a structural and regional co-operation between the two disorders, may have mainly clinical implications. In contrast to the etiopathogenetic links discussed above one might view the concurrence of the two disorders as mainly coincidental in the majority of cases. The proportion of AD cases with vascular pathology, often minor, has been estimated to be 20–40% and in addition 3–5% AD with vascular lesions or mixed dementia (Jellinger, 2002). Counting all cases with any vascular lesion the figure rises to nearly 50%, those with a combined VaD and AD dementia amounting to 36%, with SVD as the dominating contributor (Brun, 1994). Even higher figures, 60–90%, have been quoted (Kalaria, 2000). Few and small vascular lesions may be of little or no clinical relevance in themselves. They do however add to the functional deficit in special, strategic positions. They are also a sign of a circulatory disturbance, which might not yet in all areas have reached a morphological level of expression demonstrable with presently available methods. An example of a small but important vascular lesion is a strategic complete or incomplete infarct within the AD pattern such as in the angular or supramarginal gyrus or underlying white matter. It would reinforce the regional dysfunction due to the AD degeneration here. Similarly a reinforcing effect, though through a different mechanism, would be exerted by a strategic type of infarct in the extreme capsule or its extension into the centrum semiovale, a common place for selective incomplete white matter infarcts in AD. Here lesions cut the distribution routes for acetylcholine (ACh) from the nucleus basalis of Meynert to neurones, but also to the vascular innervation, depriving it of the flow augmenting effect of ACh (Farkas and Luiten, 2001). With or without concurrent AD, symptoms based on such vascular lesions may therefore improve on Ach esterase inhibitor medication.

Another example of a strategic white matter infarct position is the capsular genu where incomplete or lacunar infarcts may interrupt thalamocortical frontal connections, adding confounding frontal cognitive symptoms in AD (Desmond, 2002). The more extensive white matter damage in selective white matter infarction (SIWI) and that accompanying BD undercuts large areas of the cortex, representing the presumably most common way of inter-action between vascular lesions and the cortical AD degeneration. These lesions develop insidiously much like the Alzheimer process and may therefore more or less silently augment the functional deficit due to the cor-tical AD pathology. With a frontal location such vascular lesions may in AD produce fluctuation and extrapyramidal symptoms as in the Lewy body variant of AD, or reinforce such symptoms in this variant of AD (Londos et al, 2002).

Summary

Vascular dementia comes in a large number of forms under a large variety of designations. They all have a common etiology, which is the more or less profound destruction of functionally important neuronal assemblies through vital substrate shortage or hemorrhage. They differ however with regard to pathogenic mechanism, which therefore lends itself for classification of VaD on a pathoanatomical basis. The translation of pathoanatomical to clinical forms meets with difficulties reflected in a bewildering variety of names, a problem that may in the future become solved to an increasing degree by imaging and other clinical methods of brain study. Interplay with other dis-eases and ageing adds to the confusion. Since VaD is the second commonest and one of the few dementing diseases where we know the cause and much of the pathogenic mechanisms, this is the group where intensified research should best pay off in terms of effective treatment strategies.

References

Akiguchi I, Tomimoto, H, Suenaga T et al, Alterations in glia and axons in the brains of Binswanger's disease patients, *Stroke* (1997) **28**:1423–9.

Amar K, Wilcock G, Vascular dementia, *BMJ* (1996) **312**:227–31.

Astrup J, Siesjö BK, Symon L, Thresholds in cerebral ischemia – the ischemic penumbra, Stroke (1981) **12**:723–5.

Back T, Nedergaard M, Ginsberg MD, The Ischemic Penumbra. Pathophysiology and relevance of spreading depression-like phenomena. In: Ginsberg MD, Bogous-slavsky J, eds, *Cerebrovascular Disease: Pathophysiology, Diagnosis and Management* (Blackwell Science: Berlin, 1998) 276–86.

Bowler J, Hachinski V, Vascular dementia. In: Ginsberg MD, Bogousslavsky J, eds, *Cere-brovascular Disease: Pathophysiology, Diagnosis and Management* (Blackwell Science: Berlin, 1998) 1126–44.

Brun A, Pathology and pathophysiology of cerebrovascular dementia: pure subgroups of obstructive and hypoperfusive etiology, *Dementia* (1994) **5**:145–7.

Brun A, Englund E, A white matter disorder in dementia of Alzheimer type: a pathoanatomical study, *Ann Neurol* (1986) **19**:253–62.

Brun A, Gustafson L, Zerebrovaskuläre Erkrankungen, In: Kisker KP, Lauter H, Meyer J-E, Muller C, Strömgren E, eds, *Psychiatrie der Gegenwart* (Springer: Berlin, 1988) 253–95.

Brun A, Gustafson L, Mårtensson SM, Ericsson C, Neuropathology of late life, *Dementia* (1992) **3**:125–30.

Caplan LR, Binswanger's disease: revisited, *Neurology* (1995) **45**:626–33.

Cerebral Embolism Task Force, Cardiogenic brain embolism. The second report of the Cerebral Embolism Task Force, *Arch Neurol* (1989) **46**:727–43.

De la Torre JC, Alzheimer's disease as a vascular disorder. Nosological evidence, *Stroke* (2002) **33**:1152–62.

Desmond DW, Cognition and white matter lesions, *Cerebrovasc Dis* (2002) **13** (Suppl 2):53–7.

Esiri MM, Wilcock GK, Morris JH, Neuropathological assessment of the lesions of significance in vascular dementia, *J Neurol Neurosurg Psychiatry* (1997) **63**:749–53.

Farkas E, Luiten PGM, Cerebral microvascular pathology in aging and Alzheimer's disease, *Progr Neurobiol* (2001) **64**:575–611.

Greenberg SM, Cerebral amyloid angiopathy and vessel dysfunction, *Cerebrovasc Dis* (2002) **13** (Suppl 2):42–7.

Hachinski V, Lassen NA, Marshall J, Multi-infarct dementia: a cause of mental deterioration in the elderly, *Lancet* (1974) **ii**:207–10.

Hedera P, Friedland R, Cerebral autosomal dominant arteriopathy with subcortical infarcts and leukoencephalopathy: study of two American families with predominant dementia, *J Neurol Sci* (1987) **146**:27–33.

Hulette C, Nochlin D, McKeel MD et al, Clinical-neuropathologic findings in multi-infarct dementia: a report of six autopsied cases, *Neurology* (1997) **48**:668–72.

Jellinger KA, Alzheimer's disease and cerebrovascular pathology: an update, *J Neural Transm* (2002) **109**:813–36.

Kalaria JN, The role of cerebral ischemia in Alzheimer's disease, *Neurobiol Aging* (2000) **21**:321–30.

Kalaria RN, Ince P, eds, *Vascular Factors in Alzheimer's Disease*, (Ann NY Acad Sci: New York, 2000).

Kallimo H, Ruchoux M-M, Viitanen M, Kalaria RN, CADASIL: a common form of hereditary arteriopathy causing brain infarcts and dementia, *Brain Pathol* (2002) **12**:371–84.

Lishman WA, Cerebrovascular disorders. In: Lishman WA, ed, *Organic Psychiatry. The Psychological Consequences of Cerebral Disorder*, 3rd edn (Blackwell Science: Oxford, 1997) 375–430.

Liu X, Ericsson C, Brun A, Cortical, synaptic changes and gliosis in normal ageing, Alzheimer's disease and frontal lobe degeneration, *Dementia* (1996) **7**:128–34.

Londos E, Passant U, Risberg J et al, Contributions of other brain pathologies in dementia with Lewy bodies, *Dement Geriatr Cogn Disord* (2002) **13**:130–48.

Mueggler T, Sturchler-Pierrat C, Baumann D et al, Compromised hemodynamic response in amyloid precursor protein transgenic mice, *J Neurosci* (2002) **22**:7218–24.

Nilsson K, Gustafson L, Hultberg B, Improvement of cognitive functions after cobalamin/folate supplementation in elderly patients with dementia and elevated plasma homocysteine, *Int J Geriatr Psychiatry* (2001) **16**:609–14.

Niwa K, Porter VA, Kazama K et al, A beta-peptides enhance vasoconstriction in cerebral circulation, *Am J Physiol Heart Circ Physiol* (2001) **281**:2417–24.

Niwa K, Kazama K, Younkin L et al, Cerebrovascular autoregulation is profoundly impaired in mice overexpressing amyloid precursor protein, *Am J Physiol Heart Circ Physiol* (2002) **283**:315–23.

O'Brien MD, How does cerebrovascular disease cause dementia? *Dementia* (1994) **5**:133–6.

Pantoni L, Garcia JH, The significance of cerebral white matter abnormalities 100 years after Binswanger's report. A review, *Stroke* (1995) **26**:1293–301.

Roman GC, From UBOs to Binswanger's disease. Impact of magnetic resonance imaging on vascular dementia research, *Stroke* (1996) **27**:1269–73.

Roman GC, Erkinjuntti T, Wallin A et al, Subcortical ischaemic vascular dementia, *Lancet Neurol* (2002) **1**:426–36.

Ruitenberg A, Skoog I, Ott A et al, Blood pressure and risk of dementia: results from the Rotterdam Study and the Gothenburg H-70 study, *Dement Geriatr Cogn Disord* (2001) **12**:33–9.

Suter O-C, Sunthorn T, Kraftsik R et al, Cerebral hypoperfusion generates cortical watershed microinfarcts in Alzheimer's disease, *Stroke* (2002) **33**:1986–92.

Tournier-Lasserve E, Joutel A, Melki J et al, Cerebral autosomal dominant arteriopathy with subcortical infarcts and leukoencephalopathy maps on chromosome 19q12, *Nat Genet* (1993) **3**:256–9.

Trenkwalder P, Potential for antihypertensive treatment with an AT(1)-receptor blocker to reduce dementia in the elderly, *J Hum Hypertens* (2002) **16** (Suppl 3):71–5.

Weiller C, Chollet F, Frackowiak RSJ, Physiologic aspects of functional recovery from stroke. In: Ginsberg MD, Bogousslavsky J, eds, *Cerebrovascular Disease: Pathophysiology, Diagnosis and Management* (Blackwell Science: Berlin, 1998) 2057–66.

Wolf R, Orszagh M, März W, Case study. Revision of an Alzheimer's diagnosis in a patient with an almost normal CT scan: why strategic vascular lesions may be overlooked, *Alzheimer's Research* (1997) **3**:73–6.

Zuccala G, Onder G, Pedone C et al, Hypotension and cognitive impairment. Selective association in patients with heart failure, *Neurology* (2001) **57**:1986–92.

chapter 10

White matter pathology of vascular dementia

Elisabet Englund

Introduction

In dementia associated with ischemic–vascular lesions, white matter damage occurs as a rule; it is only exceptionally that the white matter is unaffected in vascular dementia (VaD). However, the appearance of the white matter pathology varies from mild and regionally restricted to severe and extensive. The gray matter is different it does not always harbor lesions.

With regard to site, size and type of cerebrovascular lesions in VaD, distinct forms of either occlusive or hypoperfusive type are recognized. The forms of brain pathology reflect different pathogenetic principles and indicate several etiological factors which may work in co-operation. The prerequisite for diagnostic and pathogenetic considerations on a tissue level is an extensive neuropathological analysis, which allows a safe exclusion of all concurrent or confounding changes. It must necessarily, for all purpose of interpretation, be refered back to a thorough clinical work-up.

Against this background, the white matter lesions of hypoperfusive type due to intracranial vascular pathology and a general hemodynamic impairment are frequently seen, but may still be clinically difficult to recognize.

Comparing pathophysiological concepts with lesions, the ischemic penumbra remains the ideal description of a transient, often recurrent hypoxic condition, while the penumbra effect on the structural integrity of the white matter differs from that on the cortex and subcortical gray matter.

The high prevalence of histopathologically proven white matter pathology in VaD implies that damage to this part of the brain may be of major importance in the clinical expression of dementia, an impact that has been underestimated previously.

Firstly, as detailed below, the morphological white matter changes in aging are briefly described. The different forms of white matter changes in VaD are then presented and these changes are compared with those of mixed neurodegenerative and vascular dementia. Next, pathogenetic principles for the white matter pathology in VaD are discussed, with regard to vascular pathologies and cardiac/hemodynamic abnormalities, serving as potential risk factors in dementia. Lastly, some considerations on clinical and neuroradiological correlates to white matter changes are briefly discussed.

White matter changes in aging

The process of aging causes subtle-to-small structural changes in the white matter (Miller et al, 1980; Englund, 2000) with a subsequent enlargement of the ventricular system. Sometimes these alterations are more prominent, reaching the level at which a further minor accentuation would make them indistinguishable from the changes correlating with evident disease. A regionally nonspecific shrinkage of the brain also includes a mild decrease of myelinated tracts. The computed tomographic (CT) and magnetic resonance imaging (MRI) findings of white matter changes in aging are well known (Kobari et al, 1990; Wahlund et al, 2001) and the morphologic correlates include demyelination and gliosis (van Swieten et al, 1991; Grafton et al, 1991; Schmidt et al, 1993) especially around the lateral ventricles. A widespread arteriolosclerosis and dilated perivascular spaces are also well documented findings, which can be expected in the brains of mentally well-preserved elderly. Minor traumas may add subtle lesions with subsequent discrete degeneration of tracts.

Chronic edema and hypoxic acidosis can result in white matter demyelination and gliosis (Feigin et al, 1973) and may be the result of fluid transudation secondary to trauma and/or hypertension. Structurally the effects have similarities with incomplete white matter infarction (see below).

White matter changes in vascular dementia

The fundamental structural changes viewed macroscopically and through the microscope have already been described (Olsson et al, 1996) and comprehensibly covered in textbooks of neuropathology (Graham, 1992). The basic components of ischemic white matter pathology concern:

- loss of tissue components: axons, oligodendroglia and myelin, later astro-cytes and also vessels
- increase of reactive cells: astrocytes and microglial cell quantities
- tissue atrophy/attenuation and shrinkage
- necrosis: cavitation, sometimes scarring
- vascular changes: vessel wall degeneration, wall thickening, sclerosis and stenosis in gray and white matter.

Regionally, the pathologic components above form focal or diffuse changes, or both.

Focal lesions represent the complete infarct. In white matter only appearing exceptionally as isolated lesions in the form of minimal lacunes along the deeper parts of the large arterial supply borders. In the isolated appearance, they are minute lacunes of less than 1 mm in diameter.

Focal and diffuse changes together form a spectrum of relative proportions and represent the vast majority of white matter changes in VaD.

Diffuse changes alone comprise the morphological changes listed above, except necrosis. They appear isolated in a minority of cases – yet their preva-lence may be underestimated due to their sometimes subtle appearance in neuroimaging as in neuropathology.

The vascular alterations cover a number of vessel pathologies also beyond the white matter, from atherosclerosis and hypertensive alterations of large, medium-sized and small vessels, to amyloidosis of small and medium-sized vessels and to fibrohyalinosis/lipohyalinosis of the smallest arteries. In situations where diffuse lesions dominate, the smaller vessels are involved in the pathologic process.

The wide combination of these changes and the often simultaneous lesions in the gray matter are largely applicable to a classification of VaD and its modifications (Brun and Gustafson, 1988; Brun, 1994; Roman et al, 1993; Englund, 2000) based on pathophysiological principles, which are explained elsewhere in this book.

Focal changes: the complete infarct

The focal white matter lesions are either large cavitating, small or minor infarcts with cystic or lacunar (or slit-like) formation. In the recent infarct, necrotic material may be retained and progressively decomposed by activated macrophages, whereas the lacunar appearance provides evidence of older damage and the tissue is organized after both passage and clearing of macrophages and reactive astrocytes.

The large cystic infarcts may reach a diameter over 20 mm and the cyst lining is built by a mesh of fibrillary astrocytes and glial fibrillar detritus. Sometimes, a few remaining macrophages contain hemosiderin pigment, as evidence of a previous extravasation of blood. Traces of a minor, transient disruption of the blood–brain barrier can be found with immunohisto-chemical stainings for plasma proteins in the perivascular tissue. A localized microglial and astrocytic activation will also indicate a barrier disruption.

Edema is presumed to be transient with a settled, clear-cut lacunar infarct. Blood vessels of all calibers can be found altered by hypertensive changes, arteriosclerosis and other changes including vasculitis. The degree of vascular pathology varies and may be further focally accentuated.

Focal and diffuse changes: the complete and incomplete white matter infarction

These frequent coexisting pathologies would, by virtue of their high preva-lence, be the underlying substrate in the recognition of white matter disease (Goto et al, 1981; de Reuck, 2000; Garcia et al, 1996), leukoencephalopathy or leukoaraiosis (Hachinski et al, 1987) in general having been already described at the start of the 1900s (Alzheimer, 1902).

The model is that of the peri-infarct tissue in the white matter, namely the transitional zone between the glial scar or cavity of a complete infarct and the better preserved periphery at some distance from the infarct midpoint (Figure 10.1). The tissue within the incomplete infarction is partly atten-uated, exhibiting all grades except total devitalization. The diffuse changes generally cover a region many times larger than the central focal lesion and may dominate over the latter by 200 times the volume (Englund, 2002). The periphery merges with the surrounding normal white matter at a distance

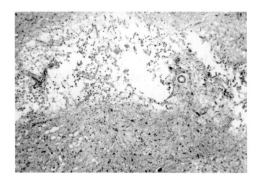

Figure 10.1 *Microphotograph of the border of a small complete (lacunar) white matter infarct surrounded by incomplete infarction.*

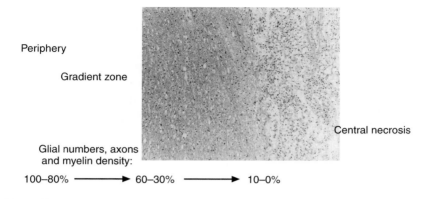

Periphery

Gradient zone

Central necrosis

Glial numbers, axons
and myelin density:

100–80% ———————▶ 60–30% ———————▶ 10–0%

Figure 10.2 *Schematic illustration of the perifocal infarct gradient, from the normal white matter (left) through the gradually impaired tissue, to the complete necrosis including a cavity (right). Percentage numbers represent the decreasing quantities of oligodendroglial cells and axons, paralleling lowered myelin density.*

from the infarct center that varies due to localization and specific preconditions in each situation. In between, the gradient shows increasing numbers of viable axons and myelin sheaths towards the periphery (Figure 10.2). The tissue gradient towards fully normal tissue was described by qualitative and quantitative neurochemical analyses of the white matter components (Gottfries et al, 1985; Englund et al, 1988). In these studies, the relative preservation of gangliosides versus decreased myelin lipids suggested a particular vulnerability of the myelin sheath, something also corroborated by correlative magnetic resonance and neuropathological studies of the very early stages of ischemia (Englund et al, 1987).

The diffuse damage may be functionally silent in an initial ischemic stage with an edema that later subsides, but may in a stabilized phase regain at least partial functioning.

Vascular changes are of various appearances and include thromboembolic occlusions, hemorrhage and luminal stenosis. The pattern of pathology complies with the general concepts of small vessel disease (Brun and Gustafson, 1988) and subcortical ischemic–vascular dementia (Roman et al, 2002), some of the so-called Binswanger type or lacunar state, others representing CADASIL (Ruchoux et al, 1995) or meningocortical amyloid angiopathy with multiple vascular lesions in cases not meeting the criteria for AD (Haglund and Englund, 2002).

The presentation of a broad transitional zone of incomplete infarction is a matter of conflicting opinion among morphologists, refuted by some (Neder-gaard et al, 1986) or at least in part contested by others (Torvik and Svind-land, 1986). It can be argued, however, that the pathophysiological and morphological differences between gray and white matter subjected to ischemic damage are far from fully explored.

A fundamental dissimilarity lies in the relatively dense vascularization of the gray matter, which ensures that the margins of the complete infarct are sharper and that the zone of partial devitalization, i.e. incomplete infarction, is often minimal or negligible.

Diffuse changes alone: the incomplete white matter infarction

Selective incomplete white matter infarction describes incomplete infarction without neighboring complete infarcts (Brun and Englund, 1986). In addition to its appearance as a component in Alzheimer's disease (AD), this is a finding in a number of brains from demented individuals in which there are no focal vascular or other pathologies, e.g. neurodegenerative pathologies found in either the gray or white matter (Englund, 2000). A central arteriolopathy is regularly present, often of a 'nonspecific', yet recognizable type, exhibiting an arteriolosclerosis with fibrohyaline degeneration confined to the attenuated, deep white matter areas. The vessels show a degeneration of the smooth muscle layer, which is replaced by collagen in a hyaline fibrosis, leading to a subtotal luminal occlusion. These arterioles share traits with nonhypertensive lipohyalinosis (Zhang et al, 1994), as well as with hypertensive arteriolosclerosis and may concur with hypertensive changes. There are, however, no microaneurysms or fibrinoid vessel wall necroses; there is also no marked association with large vessel arteriosclerosis.

Small vessel degeneration of nonspecific type is sometimes allegedly of diabetic type and the affected arterioles in such cases may appear particularly eosinophilic in routine hematoxylin–eosin staining.

In this situation, the entire pathology thus consists of diffuse white matter attenuation – a subtotal loss of all tissue elements, a mild reactive astrocytosis and macrophage reaction, and the named arteriolopathy. Macroscopically it can often not be detected, but severe cases may, on freshly cut sections, show a sunken surface and a mildly grayish discoloring.

In a series of 50 demented cases, neuropathologically verified as VaD, selective incomplete white matter infarction was the sole pathology found in 12 cases (Table 10.1).

Table 10.1 Neuropathological correlates in 50 consecutively studied cases of VaD, diagnosed clinically and neuropathologically

Cases (n)	Pathology	Target region
18	Medium-sized, small and large cortical–subcortical infarcts	Gray + white matter
19	Small subcortical infarcts (Binswanger type) and perifocal diffuse lesions	White >> gray matter*
12	Diffuse lesions alone, no complete infarcts	White matter
1	Focal perivascular lacunes**	White matter

* = subcortical gray > cortex
** = advanced cribriform state, not typical infarcts (Englund, 2000).

Wallerian degeneration

Any brain in which neurones in the cortex or subcortical nuclei are damaged, secondary or Wallerian degeneration occurs over time (Kreutzberg et al, 1997). It is a slow process of tissue and most prominently white matter regression, emanating from the damaged neuron through anterograde axonal breakdown and subsequent devitalization of myelin. It is readily discernible in cases with severe neuronal damage such as in AD or other neurodegenerative diseases, as well as following large hemorrhagic or ischemic–vascular lesions, as in VaD. This white matter degeneration may be differentiated from other pathological processes by its accentuation adjacent to the most pronounced cortical–neuronal damage (Englund 1998).

White matter changes in VaD and concurrent Alzheimer's disease

Alzheimer's disease

Alzheimer's disease of traditional type, as it presents in the brain, is often accompanied by selective incomplete white matter infarction (Brun and Englund, 1986). It seems to appear, in the course of AD, to be regionally accentuated in the frontal lobes and to be frequent and pathogenetically related but not unconditionally present (Englund, 2000).

Amyloid angiopathy, a recognized hallmark of AD, has for a long time been associated with cerebral white matter changes in dementia, including AD (Hollander and Strich, 1970; Heffner et al, 1976; Gray et al, 1985).

However, the amyloid angiopathy is highly variable in extent and is confined to the cortex and meninges. Quantitative analysis of the regional vascular amyloid load and white matter pathology in AD, in VaD and in VaD + AD revealed white matter pathology and an equal mean amount of amyloid vessels in all groups (Haglund and Englund, 2002). In the pure AD group, however, there was a statistically significant association between the amyloid load and the severity of white matter pathology.

This author's experience is that the high prevalence of diffuse white matter changes in Alzheimer's disease (approaching 60% in older individuals) underscores an association between AD and subcortical ischemic vascular lesions – one link may be vascular amyloidosis (Vinters 2001). The association however seems to be multifactorial and could easily be oversimplified. In other words, AD and its associated white matter pathology represent a form of 'mixed' or combined neurodegenerative and ischemic–vascular disease, albeit the latter rather appear as a complication of the former.

In addition to these diffuse white matter changes in AD, a Wallerian degeneration will appear, to be observed by the pathologist in the majority of investigated brains. It is accentuated, and hence first seen, in the basal temporal lobes, subjacent to the most intense cortical degeneration (Englund, 1998). These two white matter alterations are therefore dissimilar in terms of regional extent and local distance from the cortical degeneration, though seemingly co-operating in a progressive white matter atrophy.

Mixed AD and VaD

In AD and concurrent VaD, white matter pathology will be a mixture of all kinds: sometimes focal vascular lesions, perifocal diffuse or solely diffuse changes emanating from the two different diseases and furthermore from both, a secondary Wallerian degeneration. Of a presumably pathogenetic multitude, the repertoire of the tissue components is limited and the different morphological changes may not be discernible, even microscopically.

Pathogenetic principles

As a cause and contributory factor of dementia, vascular white matter lesions of a single, pure form may operate, whereas different types of vascular lesions may also be combined. Unmasking the subclinical effects of minimal or few ischemic lesions may be brought about by concurrent brain pathology of ischemic synergistic type. Furthermore vascular white matter lesions may add to primarily neurodegenerative changes such as those of Alzheimer's or Parkinson's disease and interact with these or aggravate the effects of otherwise subtle damage, whereas each on its own would not have triggered symptoms and signs of dementia.

The association between ischemic lesions and dementia is important in a more subtle form, which is when the damage is judged to minimize the reserve capacity of the brain and helps to precipitate a dementia or dementia-like clinical state under the influence of other types of impairment. Such impairment may be the presence of severe somatic illness, the negative effects or side-effects of drugs on the brain and low blood pressure levels.

The types of etiology and pathogenetic principles for white matter pathology in VaD may be divided in primary vascular and primary hemodynamic/hypoperfusive etiologies.

Being a rough simplification for a variety of etiologies and pathogenetic forms, the vascular etiology covers everything from the local vessel wall abnormalities (vasculitis, etc.) to the systemic vascular diseases that act on a general metabolic level, as in hypertension and diabetes.

The hemodynamic etiology covers several pathophysiological conditions, from local underperfusion to systemic hypotension.

Primary vascular etiology

Vascular pathology of local, regional or pancerebral type will exert its negative effects through endothelial and whole vessel wall damage, thickening and sclerosing. A number of events may follow in turn, such as a lowered transvascular passage and impaired vessel wall motility and hence a decreased capacity to compensate for perfusion-threatening flow changes. Late events may, according to the underlying cause, include microvascular hemorrhages, thrombotic stenosis and ultimately obliteration.

Systemic hypertension may intracranially result in large as well as small vessel disease, with contributions from both hypertension and atherosclerosis, as the former promotes the latter.

Diabetes mellitus results in small vessel hyalinosis (Zhang et al, 1994) and is supposedly an underestimated contributing etiologic factor in small vessel disease, but it is only occasionally dealt with in this aspect (Tatemichi et al, 1993). Here, an episodic hypoglycemia and proneness to develop ketoacidosis may further endanger the brain tissue under certain circumstances.

An age-related impairment of the vascular autoregulation (Wollner et al, 1979) due to impaired functioning of the autonomic nervous system (Kaijser and Sachs, 1985) can proposedly lead to symptom-producing blood pressure lability in the elderly. Additionally, age-related arteriolar changes, including endothelial changes (MacLennan et al, 1980), have been suggested to reduce the baroreflex activity and thereby predispose for deleterious blood pressure falls (Johnson, 1992). These mechanisms are proposedly often related and, against this background, even a minor impairment of the neural perivascular web may be sufficient to cause damage to the brain.

Primary hemodynamic etiology
Hypoperfusion

A primary hemodynamic etiology of vascular dementia concerns the cerebral hypoperfusion that affects either the whole brain, the deep central white matter (Ginsberg et al, 1976) or specific regions that are more susceptible to damage due to focal vascular pathology. In global hypoperfusion, a borderzone infarct often occurs in the most distal region of perfusion between the major intracerebral arteries (Romanul and Abramowicz, 1964). In milder insults, the white matter alone may show pathology with incomplete infarction, sometimes with small focal lesions along the major and deep borderzone lines.

The most common cause of hemodynamic disturbances with a drop in blood pressure is that of cardiovascular failure (Camm and Ward, 1984). Cardiac disease and cardiovascular failure contribute considerably to the development of VaD (Katzman, 1983), not only through cardiac embolism but also from the effects of hemodynamic insufficiency. The effects of arrythmia here will be a cerebral, notably episodic hypoperfusion (Harrison and Marshall, 1984), extended far along the penetrating arterioles and resulting in deep white matter damage (Mohr, 1977; Kawamura et al, 1991).

Longstanding ('chronic') hypoperfusion may lead to an ischemic penumbra (Astrup et al, 1981), a situation where the cerebral blood flow goes below the threshold for neuronal function and the energy supply is enough for most elements to survive on a structural level, but suboptimal for neuronal function. The penumbra concept is still alternatively used to describe a pathophysiological condition as well as morphology, with less clear distinctions regarding its application for gray compared to white (or all cerebral) matter.

Hypotension

Orthostatic and non-orthostatic hypotension cause symptoms of dementia due to CT scan detectable ischemic white matter lesions (Harrison and Marshall, 1984; Räihä et al, 1993). The clinical information on patients with 'primary orthostatic cerebral ischemia' (Stark and Wodak, 1983) indicates a partially reversible and probably incomplete white matter infarct pathology, with which the patients improved after extra- or intracerebral bypass surgery. Systemic hypotension is frequently found in dementia and is in many individuals not preceded by hypertension. The prevalence of orthostatic and non-orthostatic hypotension reached 50% in clinically evaluated VaD cases (Passant et al, 1996). It is probably an underestimated, important factor in the pathogenesis of white matter pathology. Thus not only *hypertension*, but also *hypotension* and in particular a *decline and recurrent drop of blood pressure* levels should deserve recognition as a potential pathogenetic factor in VaD.

Clinical and neuroradiological detection of white matter lesions in dementia

A problem of its own is the attribution of dementia to particular ischemic lesions in gray as well as white matter, as a stroke may be the cause of, as well as a contributing factor to dementia but it may also be of minor or no importance (Chui et al, 1992; Hennerici et al, 2000).

A defined number of infarcts required for the development of dementia (Chui et al, 1992) is to be considered, as well as infarct topography, but also a volume threshold of tissue damage (Hennerici et al, 2000). The volume of metabolically inactive tissue estimated by positron tomography may be critical for dementia severity (Mielke et al, 1992). This is applicable in situations of vast incomplete white matter infarction in individuals with marked dementia and signs of pathophysiological undercutting of important cortical regions that were only mildly damaged *per se* (Englund, 2000, 2002). Similarly, Tatemichi et al (1992), among others, illustrated how cognitive impairment followed from small lesions in critical white matter pathways that could functionally isolate larger cortical domains.

The volume of incomplete white matter infarction often by far dominates over the complete infarct's tissue loss, e.g. in Binswanger's disease (Brun et al, 1992; Englund, 2000). It is reasonable to believe that much of the symptomatology and also fluctuating somatic or neurological signs are due to this white matter impairment.

Considering its morphologically diffuse delineation and the difficulty in recognizing the full extent of white matter changes neuroradiologically, the perifocal incomplete white matter infarction should contribute considerably to the underestimation of the proportion of vascular dementia.

To advance the identification and accurate estimation of diffuse white matter changes, the use of new MRI techniques will be further applied (Kappeler et al, 2000). Diffusion tensor imaging (DTI) is a recently proposed method with which white matter abnormalities can be detected in areas that have a normal appearance according to high-performance conventional MRI (Jones et al, 1999; Rose et al, 2000; O'Sullivan et al, 2001). In this author's experience, it is possible not only to perform these investigations on post-mortem brains but also to assess the severity of white matter pathology, enabling a grading of white matter pathology on DTI which parallels that of the neuropathology, though in a less detailed fashion. DTI investigations thus appear to be promising for both detection and treatment monitoring of very subtle white matter changes. They may therefore be of particular interest in the mild forms or early phases of white matter disease, in which some of the tissue may still be saved.

References

Alzheimer A, Die seelen Störungen auf arteriosklerotischer Grundlage, *Z Psychiatr* (Berlin) (1902) **59**:695–711.

Astrup J, Siesjö B, Symon L, Thresholds in cerebral ischaemia – the ischaemic penumbra, *Stroke* (1981) **12**:723–5.

Brun A, Vascular dementia: pathological findings. In: Burns A, Levy R, eds. *Dementia* (Chapman & Hall: London, 1994) 653–63.

Brun A, Englund E, A white matter disorder in dementia of the Alzheimer type: a pathoanatomical study, *Ann Neurol* (1986) **19**:253–62.

Brun A, Gustafson L, Zerebrovaskuläre Erkrankungen. In: Kisker KP, Lauter H, Meyer J-E, Muller E, eds, *Organische Psychosen, Psychiatrie der Gegenwart*, Vol 6 (Springer-Verlag: Berlin, 1988) 253–97.

Brun A, Fredriksson K, Gustafson L, Pure subcortical arteriosclerotic encephalopathy (Binswanger's disease): a clinico-pathologic study. Part 2. Pathologic features, *Cerebrovasc Dis* (1992) **2**:87–92.

Camm AJ, Ward DE, Clinical electrocardiography. In: Martin A, Camm AJ, eds, *Heart Disease in the Elderly* (John Wiley: Chichester, 1984) 149–86.

Chui HC, Victoroff JI, Margolin D et al, Criteria for the diagnosis of ischemic vascular dementia proposed by the State of California Alzheimer's Disease Diagnostic and Treatment Centers, *Neurology* (1992) **42**:473–80.

De Reuck J, White matter disease: anatomical and physiological features in relation to modern cerebral blood flow techniques. In: Pantoni L, Inzitari D, Wallin A, eds,

The Matter of White Matter. Clinical and Pathophysiological Aspects of White Matter Disease Related to Cognitive Decline and Vascular Dementia. Current Issues in Neurodegenerative Diseases, Vol 10 (Academic Pharmaceutical Productions: Utrecht, 2000) 211–22.

Englund E, Neuropathology of white matter changes in Alzheimer's disease and vascular dementia, *Dement Geriatr Cogn Disord* (1998) **9** (Suppl 1):6–12.

Englund E, Neuropathology of white matter disease: parenchymal changes. In: Pantoni L, Inzitari D, Wallin A, eds, *The Matter of White Matter. Clinical and Pathophysiological Aspects of White Matter Disease Related to Cognitive Decline and Vascular Dementia.* Current Issues in Neurodegenerative Diseases, Vol 10 (Academic Pharmaceutical Productions: Utrecht, 2000) 223–46.

Englund E, Neuropathology of white matter lesions in vascular cognitive impairment, *Cerebrovasc Dis* (2002) **13** (Suppl 2):11–15.

Englund E, Brun A, Persson B, Correlations between histopathologic white matter changes and proton MR relaxation times in dementia, *Alzheim Dis Assoc Disord* (1987) **1**:156–70.

Englund E, Brun A, Alling C, White matter changes in dementia of Alzheimer's type, *Brain* (1988) **111**:1425–39.

Feigin I, Budzilovich G, Weinberg S, Degeneration of white matter in hypoxia, acidosis and edema, *J Neuropathol Exp Neurol* (1973) **32**:125–41.

Garcia JH, Lassen NA, Weiller C et al, Ischemic stroke and incomplete infarction, *Stroke* (1996) **27**:761–5.

Ginsberg MD, Hedley-Whyte ET, Richardson EP, Hypoxic–ischemic leukoencephalopathy in man, *Arch Neurol* (1976) **33**:5–14.

Goto K, Ishii N, Fukasawa H, Diffuse white matter disease in the geriatric population. Clinical, neuropathological and CT study, *Radiology* (1981) **141**:687–95.

Gottfries CG, Karlsson I, Svennerholm L, Senile dementia – A 'white matter' disease? In: Gottfries CG, ed, *Normal Aging, Alzheimer's Disease and Senile Dementia* (Editions de l'Université de Bruxelles: Brussels, 1985) 111–18.

Grafton ST, Sumi SM, Stimac GK et al, Comparison of post-mortem magnetic resonance imaging and neuropathological findings in the cerebral white matter. *Arch Neurol* (1991) **48**:293–8.

Graham DI, Hypoxia and vascular disorders. In: Adams JH, Duchen LW, eds, *Greenfield's Neuropathology*, 5th edn (Arnold: London, 1992) 153–268.

Gray F, Dubas F, Roullet E, Escourolle R, Leukoencephalopathy in diffuse hemorrhagic cerebral amyloid angiopathy, *Ann Neurol* (1985) **18**:54–9.

Hachinski VC, Potter P, Merskey H, Leukoaraiosis, *Arch Neurol* (1987) **44**:21–3.

Haglund M, Englund E, Cerebral amyloid angiopathy, white matter lesions and Alzheimer encephalopathy – a histopathological assessment, *Dement Geriatr Cogn Disord* (2002) **14**:161–6.

Harrison MJG, Marshall J, Hypoperfusion in the aetiology of subcortical arteriosclerotic encephalopathy (Binswanger type), *J Neurol Neurosurg Psychiatry* (1984) **47**:754–5.

Heffner RR, Porro RS, Olson ME, Earle KM, A demyelinating disorder associated with cerebrovascular amyloid angiopathy, *Arch Neurol* (1976) **33**:501–6.

Hennerici M, Bäzner H, Daffertshofer M, White matter changes: symptoms and signs. In: Pantoni L, Inzitari D, Wallin A, eds, *The Matter of White Matter. Clinical and Pathophysiological Aspects of White Matter Disease Related to Cognitive Decline and Vascular Dementia.* Current Issues in Neurodegenerative Diseases, Vol 10 (Academic Pharmaceutical Productions: Utrecht, 2000) 55–80.

Hollander D, Strich SJ, Atypical Alzheimer's disease with congophilic angiopathy presenting with dementia of acute onset. In: Wolstenholme GBW, O'Connor, eds,

Alzheimer's Disease and Related Conditions. A CIBA Foundation symposium (J&A Churchill: London, 1970) 105–24.

Johnson RH, Ageing and the autonomic nervous system. In: Bannister R, Mathias CJ, eds, *Autonomic Failure. A Textbook of Clinical Disorders of the Autonomic Nervous System* (Oxford University Press: Oxford, 1992) 882–903.

Jones DK, Lythgoe D, Horsfield MA et al, Characterization of white matter damage in ischemic leukoaraiosis with diffusion tensor MRI, *Stroke* (1999) **30**:393–7.

Kaijser L, Sachs C, Autonomic cardiovascular responses in old age, *Clin Physiol* (1985) **5**:347–57.

Kappeler P, Ropele S, Fazekas F, White matter imaging: technical considerations including histopathological correlation. In: Pantoni L, Inzitari D, Wallin A, eds, *The Matter of White Matter. Clinical and Pathophysiological Aspects of White Matter Disease Related to Cognitive Decline and Vascular Dementia*. Current Issues in Neurodegenerative Diseases, Vol 10 (Academic Pharmaceutical Productions: Utrecht, 2000) 123–39.

Katzman R, Vascular disease and dementia. In: Yahr MD, ed, *H. Houston Merrit Memorial Volume* (Raven Press, New York, 1983) 153–76.

Kawamura J, Meyer JS, Terayama Y, Weathers S, Cerebral hypoperfusion correlates with mild and parenchymal loss with severe multi-infarct dementia, *J Neurol Sci* (1991) **102**:32–8.

Kobari M, Meyer JS, Ichijo M, Oravez WT, Leukoaraiosis: correlation of MR and CT findings with blood flow, atrophy and cognition, *Am J Neuroradiol* (1990) **11**:273–81.

Kreutzberg GW, Blakemore WF, Graeber MB, Cellular pathology of the central nervous system, In: Graham DI, Lantos PL, eds, *Greenfield's Neuropathology*, 6th edn (Arnold: London, 1997) 85–156.

MacLennan WJ, Hall MRP, Timothy JI, Postural hypotension in old age: is it a disorder of the nervous system or the vessels? *Age Ageing* (1980) **9**:25–32.

Mielke R, Herholz K, Grond M et al, Severity of vascular dementia is related to volume of metabolically impaired tissue, *Arch Neurol* (1992) **49**:909–13.

Miller AKH, Alston RL, Corsellis JAN, Variation with age in the volumes of grey and white matter in the cerebral hemispheres of man: measurements with an image analyser. *Neuropath Appl Neurobiol* (1980) **6**:119–32.

Mohr JP, Neurologic complications of cardiac valvular disease and cardiac surgery including systemic hypotension. In: Vinken PJ, Bruyn GW, eds, *Handbook of Clinical Neurology, Vol 38* (Elsevier Science: Amsterdam, 1977) 143–71.

Nedergaard M, Vorstrup S, Astrup J, Cell density in the border zones around old small human brain infarcts, *Stroke* (1986) **6**:1129–37.

Olsson Y, Brun A, Englund E, Fundamental pathological lesions in vascular dementia, *Acta Neurol Scand* (1996) (Suppl) **168**:31–8.

O'Sullivan M, Summers PE, Jones DK et al, Normal-appearing white matter in ischemic leukoaraiosis: a diffusion tensor MRI study, *Neurology* (2001) **57**:2307–10.

Passant U, Warkentin S, Karlsson S et al, Orthostatic hypotension in organic dementia. Relationship between blood pressure, cortical blood flow and symptoms, *Clin Auton Res* (1996) **6**:1–8.

Räihä I, Tarvonen S, Kurki T et al, Relationship between vascular factors and white matter low attenuation of the brain, *Acta Neurol Scand* (1993) **87**:286–9.

Roman GC, Tatemichi TK, Erkinjuntti T et al, Vascular dementia: diagnostic criteria for research studies. Report of the NINDS-AIREN international work group, *Neurology* (1993) **43**:250–60.

Roman GC, Erkinjuntti T, Wallin A et al, Subcortical ischemic vascular dementia, *Lancet Neurol* (2002) **1**:421–36.

Romanul FCA, Abramowicz A, Changes in brain and pial vessels in arterial border zones: a study of 13 cases, *Arch Neurol* (1964) **11**:40–65.

Rose SE, Chen F, Chalk JB et al, Loss of connectivity in Alzheimer's disease: an evaluation of white matter tract integrity with colour coded MR diffusion tensor imaging, *J Neurol Neurosurg Psychiatry* (2000) **69**:528–30.

Ruchoux MM, Guerouaou D, Vandenhaute B et al, Systemic vascular smooth muscle impairment in cerebral autosomal dominant arteriopathy with subcortical infarcts and leukoencephalopathy, *Acta Neuropathol* (1995) **89**:500–12.

Schmidt R, Fazekas F, Offenbacher H et al, Neuropsychologic correlates of MRI white matter hyperintensities: a study of 150 normal volunteers, *Neurology* (1993) **43**:2490–4.

Stark RJ, Wodak J, Primary orthostatic cerebral ischaemia, *J Neurol Neurosurg Psych* (1983) **46**:883–91.

Tatemichi TK, Desmond DW, Prohovnik I et al, Confusion and memory loss from capsular genu infarction: a thalamocortical disconnection syndrome, *Neurology* (1992) **42**:1966–79.

Tatemichi TK, Desmond DW, Paik M et al, Clinical determinants of dementia related to stroke, *Ann Neurol* (1993) **33**:568–75.

Torvik A, Svindland A, Is there a transitional zone between brain infarcts and the surrounding brain? A histological study, *Acta Neurol Scand* (1986) **74**:365–70.

van Swieten JC, van der Hout JHW, van Ketel BA et al, Periventricular lesions in the white matter on magnetic resonance imaging in the elderly. A morphometric correlation with arteriolosclerosis and dilated perivascular spaces, *Brain* (1991) **114**:761–74.

Vinters HV, Cerebral amyloid angiopathy: a microvascular link between parenchymal and vascular dementia? *Ann Neurol* (2001) **49**:691–3.

Wahlund LO, Barkhof F, Fazekas F et al, A new rating scale for age-related white matter changes applicable to MRI and CT, *Stroke* (2001) **32**:1318–22.

Wollner L, McCarthy ST, Soper NDW, Macy DJ, Failure of cerebral autoregulation as a cause of brain dysfunction in the elderly, *BMJ* (1979) **1**:1117–18.

Zhang WW, Badonic T, Höög A et al, Structural and vasoactive factors influencing intracerebral arterioles in cases of vascular dementia and other cerebrovascular disease: a review, *Dementia* (1994) **5**:153–62.

chapter 11

Neurotransmitter changes in vascular dementia

Jennifer A Court, Elaine K Perry and Raj N Kalaria

Abstract

The occurrence of brain neurotransmitter deficits in vascular dementia (VaD) is indicated by autopsy and cerebrospinal fluid (CSF) investigations, and *in vivo* positron emission tomography (PET) studies. Changes in the cholinergic system have been the most frequently reported, although there are also indications of involvement of the serotonergic and dopaminergic systems and possibly changes in central nervous system glutamate and GABA and the hypothalamic–pituitary–adrenocortical axis in VaD. Deficits may in part be the result of mixed vascular and neurodegenerative pathology (e.g. vascular pathology in combination with Alzheimer's disease), but investigations using animal models are consistent with vascular disruption being associated with reduced cholinergic innervation. Since neurotransmitters modulate cerebral blood flow it is possible that neurotransmitter deficits in VaD not only contribute to behavioral and cognitive symptoms, but also further compromise cerebral perfusion and blood–brain barrier control. Clinical trials indicate potential benefits of cholinergic therapy in VaD and mixed dementia with vascular pathology.

Introduction

Brain neurotransmitter deficits are not only a feature of neurodegenerative disorders such as Alzheimer's disease (AD) and Lewy body pathologies, but also occur in vascular dementia (VaD). In AD, Parkinson's disease (PD) and dementia with Lewy bodies (DLB) extensive and detailed investigations of neurotransmitter changes have been carried out and attempts have been made to relate these to structural pathology and clinical features by the use of autopsy and *in vivo* techniques (e.g. Piggott et al, 1999; Ballard et al, 2000; Walker et al, 2002). Far fewer investigations have been undertaken in relation to VaD. However the findings reviewed below indicate neurotransmitter changes in VaD, which may in part be distinct from those of neurodegenerative disorders such as AD. These are likely to contribute to cognitive decline and behavioral symptoms, notably the movement disorder and depression frequently associated with this disorder (O'Brien et al, 2003).

There is convincing evidence that the innervation of blood vessels by both peripheral and central neurones plays a role in the regulation of regional brain blood flow and perfusion (Edvinsson et al, 1993). Several brain nuclei, including those of the basal forebrain (cholinergic), brain stem (noradrenergic and serotonergic) and midbrain (dopaminergic), innervate cerebral blood vessels and appear to participate in complex interactions involving ion flux, generation of second messengers and release of nitric oxide (NO) perivascular to or within arterioles and capillaries (Kummer and Haberberger, 1999; Saito et al, 1985; Vaucher and Hamel, 1995; Elhusseiny and Hamel, 2000; Elhusseiny et al, 1999; Zhang et al, 1995: Chataigneau et al, 1999; Cohen et al, 1997; Paspalas et al, 1998; Dieguez et al, 1998; Nobler et al, 1999; Krimer et al, 1998). Hence, transmitter deficits in VaD could potentially accentuate already compromised cerebral perfusion and blood–brain barrier control.

Evidence of cholinergic changes in VaD

A number of studies have demonstrated that presynaptic cholinergic indices including acetylcholine (ACh) and choline acetyltransferase (ChAT), the enzyme involved in the synthesis of ACh, are affected to a variable degree in dementias diagnosed as multi-infarct dementia (MID) and mixed dementia (Perry et al, 1977; Waller et al, 1986; Wallin et al, 1989; Gottfries et al, 1994; Bowen et al, 1982; Sakurada et al, 1990). For example, some studies reported that ChAT activity at autopsy was reduced by more than 40% in VaD or MID compared to controls (Table 11.1). The temporal cortex, hippocampus and basal ganglia were reported to be the most consistently affected (Perry et al. 1977; Gottfries et al 1994) although some of the studies examined relatively few cases. ^{3}H-hemicholiniun-3 binding to high-affinity choline uptake sites has also been found to be significantly reduced in the hippocampus and frontal cortex in MID, but not in AD (Krištofiková et al, 1995). However, no

Table 11.1 Cholinergic markers in cerebrovascular disease with dementia

Disorder(s)	Marker(s)	Change	Brain region	Remarks	References
MID	ChAT	↓ 30–45%	TC, HC, CP	More severe changes in SDAT	Perry et al, 1977
MID, Mixed	ChAT	↓ 30%	FC, TC, HC	↑ mAChR HC	Waller et al, 1986
VaD	ChAT	↓ 30%	FC, TC, CP	Infarction <15ml;	Wallin et al, 1989
					Gottfries et al, 1994
MID	ChAT	↔	TC	2 cases	Bowen et al 1982
MID, Mixed	ChAT	↓ 50–60%	HC	↓ mAChR, ↓ SP	Sakurada et al, 1990
MID	HCh-3 (ChT)	↓ 40%	HC, FC	↔ Cerebellum	Krištofiková et al, 1995
VDBT, MID	ACh	↓ 40%	CSF	Increased Ch, low vol infarctions	Tohgi et al, 1996
MID, AD	ChAT	↓	NbM	↓ DBH	Nakamura et al, 1984
MID	Cell count	↔	NbM	Some cellular pathology	Mann et al, 1986

Other studies showed ChAT (Rinne et al, 1988) and AChE (Perry et al, 1978) activities were not altered in MID patients compared to cognitively intact controls ↓, decrease; ↔, no change; AD, Alzheimer's disease; Ch, choline; ChAT, choline acetyltransferase; ChT, choline transporter; HCh-3, hemicholinium-3; CP, caudate-putamen; CSF, cerebrospinal fluid; DBH, dopamine β-hydroxylase; FC, frontal cortex; HC, hippocampus; mAChR, muscarinic ACh receptor; MID, multi-infarct dementia; Mixed, AD/VaD; nbM, nucleus basalis of Meynert; SDAT, senile dementia of Alzheimer type; SP, substance P; VaDBT, VaD of the Binswanger type.

significant changes in acetyl- or butyryl-cholinesterase activities in temporal cortex or hippocampus were observed in VaD, in marked contrast to AD (Perry et al 1978). Decreased concentrations of ACh in the cerebrospinal fluid in the 'Binswanger' and multiple small infarct variants of VaD (Tohgi et al, 1996) add further support for cholinergic deficits in VaD. These studies also indicate that cholinergic deficits are particularly seen in cases with long illness duration and disease involving small volume of infarction rather than lobar infarcts (Perry et al, 1977; Waller et al, 1986; Wallin et al, 1989; Gottfries et al, 1994; Bowen et al, 1982; Sakurada et al, 1990; Rinne et al, 1988; Krištofiková et al, 1995; Perry et al, 1978; Tohgi et al, 1996).

While deficits in ChAT activity could occur in focal regions such as the nucleus basalis of Meynert (nbM) due to retrograde changes from projection areas (Nakamura et al 1984), there appears no evidence that nbM cell size or cell number is changed in MID (Mann et al, 1986). Cortical cholinergic deficit in VaD could also occur due to interference in corticopetal cholinergic pathways (Selden et al, 1998) coursing through strategic sites affected by ischemic white matter damage. However, it is notable that reduced ChAT activity is evident in the striatum in VaD, an area with predominantly intrinsic cholinergic innervation (Gottfries et al, 1994).

There is little consistent evidence to date for changes in cholinergic receptors in VaD. Studies have reported that total muscarinic binding was both significantly decreased (Sakurada et al, 1990) and increased (Waller et al, 1986) in groups of patients including those with MID and MID/AD, and not changed in a small study ($n = 3$) of MID cases (Nordberg et al, 1992). In a group of patients who died with internal capsule stroke there was a reported increase in muscarinic binding in the frontal cortex (Bracco et al, 1982). These discrepant results could be due to differences in the stage of the disease process studied and/or heterogeneity in underlying pathology. Increases in muscarinic binding could be an adaptation to reduced cholinergic innervation at earlier stages of disease, whereas reduced density of binding could reflect more widespread pathology extending to postsynaptic elements which may occur later in the illness. In addition, since there are multiple subtypes of muscarinic receptors with differential distributions, and subtype specific ligands and antibodies are now available, there is a need to explore the possibility of selective muscarinic receptor subtype changes on different cell populations and brain regions in VaD. This is particularly important as muscarinic receptors appear to have a key role in the cholinergic control of cerebrovasculature and are also present on astrocytes which form an integral part of the blood–brain barrier (Luiten et al, 1996; Elhusseiny et al, 1999).

For high-affinity nicotinic acetylcholine receptors one small study ($n = 3$) demonstrated a 50% reduction in ^{3}H-ACh binding (Nordberg et al, 1992), whereas in larger series of cases no change in ^{3}H-epibatidine binding was observed when patients with a history of tobacco use were excluded (Martin-Ruiz et al, 2000). The latter is an important consideration since tobacco smoking is associated with a two-fold increase in high affinity nicotine binding in cortical areas (Benwell et al, 1988). The lack of change in ^{3}H-epibatidine binding in VaD was supported by the observation that there was also no change in α_4, α_7 or β_2 nicotinic receptor subunit proteins in the temporal cortex in VaD (Martin-Ruiz et al, 2000). In contrast, in AD, there have been consistent reports of reduced high-affinity nicotine receptors in the neocortex, including reductions observed in nicotinic receptor subunit proteins (reviewed in Court et al, 2001). In common with muscarinic receptors, nicotinic receptors are present on many neuronal (perikarya and terminals) and non-neuronal (blood vessels and glia) elements in the brain and are associated with a number of different transmitter systems, e.g. acetylcholine, serotonin, dopamine, glutamate and GABA (reviewed in Wonnacott, 1997; Court et al, 2000; Graham et al, 2002). It may be that the apparent lack of loss of nicotinic receptors in VaD in comparison to the deficit observed in AD is due to selective attrition and/or compensation of cell populations in these disorders. Impairments of the cholinergic neuronal markers including nicotinic receptors in cerebral vessels have been observed in AD (Kalaria, 1996) and recent findings indicate that α_7 nicotinic receptor subunits on astrocytes are upregulated in AD but not in DLB (Teaktong, 2003). To date no such investigations have been reported in VaD.

Neuronal changes subsequent to head injury have been described as similar to those in cerebral ischemic injury. Both tau-like pathology as well as accumulation of amyloid beta occurs in both conditions (Mann et al, 1986; Kalaria, 2000). Interestingly, ChAT activity was found to be reduced in the brains of subjects who suffered head injury but there was no evidence to suggest that other markers such as muscarinic or nicotinic receptors were affected (Dewar and Graham, 1996; Murdoch et al, 1998). Consistent with the cholinergic neuronal changes occurring in VaD cases with longer duration of illness, there was a greater reduction in enzyme activity in subjects surviving longer after injury.

Changes in cholinergic markers in animal models as a result of cerebral ischemia

Further evidence for the status of the cholinergic innervation during cerebrovascular disease may be derived from animal models of cerebral ischemia (Table 11.2). Several studies have reported brain ChAT activity and other neuronal markers such as glutamate decarboxylate to be impaired in rats and gerbils subjected to global brain ischemia. It is particularly relevant that cerebral ischemia induced by embolism to mimic MID was effective in demonstrating deficits in both ChAT activity and ACh concentrations in several brain regions with hippocampus and tempoparietal cortex being most affected (Narumi et al, 1986; Takagi et al, 1997). It is also interesting that the changes were consistently age dependent, with the most profound effects being observed in older animals irrespective of rodent strain or method used to induce cerebral ischemia (Nyberg and Waller, 1989; Narumi et al, 1986; Takagi et al, 1997; Ni et al, 1995; Ogawa et al, 1996; Tanaka et al, 1996; Egashira et al, 1996). For example, Narumi et al (1986) reported that ChAT activity was significantly reduced in neocortex and hippocampus by 30–60% at four weeks after four-vessel occlusion in 24-month-old Fischer 344 rats. In all these studies reductions in ChAT activities were also common in animals that survived longer than seven days after ischemic injury. As in VaD this could implicate retrograde axonal degeneration of cortical projection areas in the basal forebrain neurons. Further support for these observations is provided by the decreased basal concentrations and synthesis of ACh in cortical tissue from rats subjected to global cerebral ischemia produced by two or four vessel occlusion (Zaidan and Sims, 1990; Kumagae and Matsui, 1991; Ni et al, 1995). Focal models of ischemia involving middle cerebral artery occlusion were less effective in demonstrating deficits in ChAT and acetylcholinesterase activities (Kanemitsu et al, 1998). However, the stroke-prone spontaneously hypertensive rat (SP-SHR) appears an ideal model, revealing deficits in the neurotransmitter as well as in key components of nicotinic receptors (Saito et al, 1995; Togashi et al, 1996; Ferrari et al, 1999).

Additional support for the role for cholinergic innervation or influence of cortical microvessels has been derived from larger animals (Malatova et al, 1983) and non-human primates (Liberini et al, 1994). ChAT immunostained cholinergic neurons in basal forebrain were apparently not affected in animals subjected to occlusion of the pial artery that produced enzyme

numbers of dopamine uptake sites in the caudate nucleus in VaD, but with no change in dopamine D_2 receptors (Allard et al, 2002). The latter findings suggest that the D_2-bearing striatal GABAergic neurons associated with the indirect pathway to the globus pallidus may be intact in VaD.

Similarly to the loss of cholinergic neurons, previous studies have emphasized that loss of noradrenergic locus ceruleus cells also occur in AD and Parkinson's disease (German et al, 1992; Mann et al, 1982; Yang et al, 1999). It is plausible that morphological changes in the cortical or subcortical structures resulting from ischemic injury may induce retrograde effects in this nucleus, although a more recent report indicated no reduction in the number of locus ceruleus neurones in VaD in the absence of AD pathology (Yang et al, 1999).

The suggestions that both the dopaminergic and serotonergic system may be affected in VaD are consistent with slowing of motor performance, depression and loss of volition often associated with the disorder (O'Brien et al, 2003). Since it is also established that both these transmitter systems innervate the vasculature (Krimer et al, 1998; Nobler et al, 1999) and functional dopaminergic and serotonergic receptors are associated with cerebrovessels that affect vasoconstriction and/or dilation dependent on site and subtype, disruption of these pathways is likely to result in further impairments of the cerebrovasculature. In AD reduction in noradrenergic locus ceruleus neurons was associated with alterations of alpha and beta adrenergic receptors localized within cerebral microvessels (Kalaria, 1996; Kalaria and Harik, 1989). Much more work is required to explore the patterns of change in the monoaminergic systems in VaD at both a neuronal and microvascular level.

Changes in amino acids, neuropeptides and hormonal factors in VaD

Few studies have reported alterations in amino acids and neuropeptides in subtypes of VaD. The excitatory amino acids aspartate and glutamate as well as gamma-aminobutyric acid and many other amino acids were found to be decreased in the CSF in VaD of the Binswanger type, whereas aspartate and glutamate were selectively decreased in AD (Tohgi et al, 1992a). Among the neuropeptides, concentrations of neurotensin and somatostatin in several brain regions, including the caudate, were found to be increased in VaD.

One of the main regions being affected was the hypothalamus (Gottfries et al, 1994). Two different studies suggested decreased CSF concentrations of somatostatin (Molins et al, 1991; Heilig et al, 1995) along with beta-endorphine and corticotropin-releasing hormone (Higashi et al, 1994) in VaD compared to aged matched controls. However, similar peptide changes were also evident in AD (Heilig et al, 1995). Other studies have assessed pituitary function in dementia. Growth hormone and prolactin secretions were affected in both VaD and AD suggesting pituitary dysfunction is a feature of both disorders (Higashi et al, 1994). However, basal concentrations of growth hormone or thyroid-stimulating hormone (TSH) were not affected in dementia of vascular origin (Gomez et al, 1994). In contrast to AD there were also no changes in brain methionine- or leucine-enkephalin receptors in patients with VaD (Rinne et al, 1993). Basal levels of the adrenal neurosteroid GABA-agonist allopregnanolone were reduced in both VaD and AD (Bernardi et al, 2000). Cortisol secretion was sensitive to corticotropin releasing factor stimulation, with the cortisol response being higher in both AD and VaD compared to controls. These studies emphasize that the hypothalamic–pituitary–adrenocortical axis is disturbed in both VaD and AD (Suemaru et al, 1993).

Therapeutic strategies based on neurotransmitter pathology

(These are also discussed in detail in Chapters 23 and 24.) Over the last decade several different approaches involving neurotransmitter or messenger replacement therapy have been attempted in VaD and VaD-related animal models. Some of these have focused on cholinergic therapy using cholinesterase inhibitors (McLendon et al, 2000), which has been shown to be effective in AD. Donepezil in a small cohort of VaD patients with subcortical lesions and mild-to-moderate cognitive impairment stabilized cognitive measures and daily living activities including improved patient activity, engagement and self-care (Mendez et al, 1999). Rivastigmine, a joint acetyl- and butyrylcholinesterase inhibitor, also showed efficacy in patients diagnosed with probable VaD assessed by an open trial (Moretti et al, 2002); patients showed significant improvements in executive function and behavioral symptoms after 22 months of treatment as compared to the control group. The acetylcholinesterase inhibitor with additional nicotinic allosteric agonist properties, galantamine, has been shown in a randomized trial of patients with VaD and combined AD and VaD to be equally as effective as in AD (Erkinjuntti et al, 2002); values for ADAS-cog, disability assessment and the neuropsychiatric inventory were maintained at or above baseline over a six-month period.

Other potential therapeutic agents include posatirelin, a synthetic peptide having modulatory activity on monoaminergic and cholinergic systems as well as neurotropic effects. This drug significantly improved cognitive functions, attention and motivation assessed by several measures including the GBS rating scale (Parnetti et al, 1996). Interestingly, cholinergic deficits were ameliorated by bifemelane HCl, which prevented decreases in mAChR and receptor mRNA in a rat model of chronic cerebral hypoperfusion induced by bilateral carotid artery occlusion (Kondo et al, 1996). Selegiline, a selective monoamine oxidase-B inhibitor, administered two hours after carotid artery occlusion for five minutes in the gerbil, reduced hippocampal pyramidal cell damage (Lahtinen et al, 1997). Further, this drug appeared to be neuroprotective administered chronically prior to middle cerebral artery lesion in the mouse (Ünal et al, 2001), although the mode of action may be via mechanisms other than monoamine oxidase activity. It has been shown that risperidone, a benzisoxazole derivative efficacious against psychotic symptoms and active primarily against serotonin 5-HT2A and dopamine D_2 receptors, was effective in VaD as well as other dementias (Bhana and Spencer, 2000). Memantine, an uncompetitive N-methyl-D-aspartate (NMDA) antagonist has been shown to improve the clinical global impression of change (CGI-C) rating in dementia patients independent of etiology (Winblad and Poritis, 1999) and more recently, results of multicenter placebo-controlled trials have indicated the efficacy of memantine specifically for VaD (Wilcock et al, 2002; Orgogozo et al, 2002).

Summary

The most consistent transmitter alterations in VaD are associated with ACh-containing neurons. However, changes in cholinergic markers do not appear to occur to the same extent as in AD, with cholinergic terminal markers rather than receptors being affected. Recent trials indicate that strategies that ameliorate cholinergic deficits can be beneficial in VaD. In addition, partial blockade of NMDA channels appears efficacious in VaD. Other transmitter-based therapies, which would modulate neuronal and vascular function, may also be of benefit in VaD.

References

Allard P, Englund E, Marcusson JO, Reduced number of caudate nucleus dopamine uptake sites in vascular dementia, *Dementia* (1999) **10**:77–80.

Allard P, Englund E, Marcusson J, Caudate nucleus dopamine D2 receptors in vascular dementia, *Dement Geriatr Cogn Disord* (2002) **14**:22–7.

Araki T, Kato H, Fujiwara T et al, Alteration of [3H]hemicholinium-3 binding in the post-ischaemic gerbil brain, *Neuroreport* (1995) **6**:561–4.

Ballard C, Piggott M, Johnson M et al, Delusions associated with elevated muscarinic binding in dementia with Lewy bodies, *Ann Neurol* (2000) **48**:868–76.

Benwell ME, Balfour DJ, Anderson JM, Evidence that tobacco smoking increases the density of (-)-[3H]nicotine binding sites in human brain, *J Neurochem* (1988) **50**:1243–7

Bernardi F, Lanzone A, Cento RM et al, Allopregnanolone and dehydroepiandrosterone response to corticotropin-releasing factor in patients suffering from Alzheimer's disease and vascular dementia, *Eur J Endocrinol* (2000) **142**:466–71.

Bhana N, Spencer CM, Risperidone: a review of its use in the management of the behavioural and psychological symptoms of dementia, *Drugs Aging* (2000) **16**:451–71.

Blin J, Ivanoiu A, Coppens A et al, Cholinergic neurotransmission has different effects on cerebral glucose consumption and blood flow in young normals, aged normals, and Alzheimer's disease patients, *Neuroimage* (1997) **6**:335–43.

Bowen DM, Benton JS, Spillane JA et al, Choline acetyltransferase activity and histopathology of frontal neocortex from biopsies of demented patients, *J Neurol Sci* (1982) **57**:191–202.

Bracco L, Corradetti R, Amaducci L, Acute subcortical lesions modify cortical muscarinic receptors in human brain, *Neurosci Lett* (1982) **31**:227–31.

Chataigneau T, Feletou M, Huang PL et al, Acetylcholine-induced relaxation in blood vessels from endothelial nitric oxide synthase knockout mice, *Br J Pharmacol* (1999) **126**:219–26.

Cohen Z, Molinatti G, Hamel E, Astroglial and vascular interactions of noradrenaline terminals in the rat cerebral cortex, *J Cereb Blood Flow Metab* (1997) **17**:894–904.

Court JA, Martin-Ruiz C. Graham A, Perry E, Nicotinic receptors in human brain: topography and pathology, *J Chem Neuroanat* (2000) **20**:281–98.

Court J, Martin-Ruiz C, Piggott M et al, Nicotinic receptor abnormalities in Alzheimer's disease, *Biol Psychiatry* (2001) **49**:175–84.

Dauphin F, Lacombe P, Sercombe R et al, Hypercapnia and stimulation of the substantia innominata increase rat frontal cortical blood flow by different cholinergic mechanisms, *Brain Res* (1991) **553**:75–83.

Dauphin F, Linville DG, Hamel E, Cholinergic dilatation and constriction of feline cerebral blood vessels are mediated by stimulation of phosphoinositide metabolism via two different muscarinic receptor subtypes, *J Neurochem* (1994) **63**:544–51.

Dewar D, Graham DI, Depletion of choline acetyltransferase activity but preservation of M1 and M2 muscarinic receptor binding sites in temporal cortex following head injury: a preliminary human postmortem study, *J Neurotrauma* (1996) **13**:181–7.

Dieguez G, Fernandez N, Sanchez MA et al, Adrenergic reactivity after inhibition of nitric oxide synthesis in the cerebral circulation of awake goats, *Brain Res* (1998) **813**:381–9.

Edvinsson L, MacKenzie ET, McCulloch J, *Cerebral Blood Flow and Metabolism* (Raven Press: New York, 1993).

Egashira T, Takayama F, Yamanaka Y, Effects of bifemelane on muscarinic receptors and choline acetyltransferase in the brains of aged rats following chronic cerebral hypoperfusion induced by permanent occlusion of bilateral carotid arteries, *Jpn J Pharmacol* (1996) **72**:57–65.

Elhusseiny A, Hamel E, Muscarinic – but not nicotinic – acetylcholine receptors mediate a nitric oxide-dependent dilation in brain cortical arterioles: a possible role for the M5 receptor subtype, *J Cereb Blood Flow Metab* (2000) **20**:298–305.

Elhusseiny A, Cohen Z, Olivier A et al, Functional acetylcholine muscarinic receptor subtypes in human brain microcirculation: identification and cellular localization, *J Cereb Blood Flow Metab* (1999) **19**:794–802.

Erkinjuntti T, Kurtz A, Gauthier S et al, Efficacy of galantamine in probable vascular dementia and Alzheimer's disease combined with cerebrovascular disease: a randomised trial, *Lancet* (2002) **359**:1283–90.

Farkas E, Luiten PG, Cerebral microvascular pathology in aging and Alzheimer's disease, *Prog Neurobiol* (2001) **64**:575–611.

Ferrari R, Frasoldati A, Leo G et al, Changes in nicotinic acetylcholine receptor subunit mRNAs and nicotinic binding in spontaneously hypertensive stroke prone rats, *Neurosci Lett* (1999) **277**:169–72.

Francis A, Pulsinelli W, The response of GABAergic and cholinergic neurons to transient cerebral ischemia, *Brain Res* (1982) **243**:271–8.

Geaney DP, Soper N, Shepstone BJ, Cowen PJ, Effect of central cholinergic stimulation on regional cerebral blood flow in Alzheimer disease, *Lancet* (1990) **335**:1484–7.

German DG, Manaye KF, Smith WK et al, Disease-specific patterns of locus coeruleus cell loss, *Ann Neurol* (1992) **32**:667–76.

Gomez JM, Aguilar M, Navarro MA et al, Secretion of growth hormone and thyroid-stimulating hormone in patients with dementia, *Clin Investig* (1994) **72**:489–93.

Gottfries CG, Blennow K, Karlsson I, Wallin A, The neurochemistry of vascular dementia, *Dementia* (1994) **5**:163–7.

Graham AJ, Martin-Ruiz CM, Teaktong T et al, Human brain nicotinic receptors, their distribution and participation in neuropsychiatric disorders, *Current Drug Targets – CNS Neurolog Disord* (2002) **1**:387–97.

Gsell W, Strein I, Riederer P, The neurochemistry of Alzheimer type, vascular type and mixed type dementias compared, *J Neural Transm Suppl* (1996) **47**:73–101.

Hansson G, Alafuzoff I, Winblad B, Marcusson J, Intact brain serotonin system in vascular dementia, *Dementia* (1996) **7**:196–200.

Harkany T, Penke B, Luiten PG, beta-Amyloid excitotoxicity in rat magnocellular nucleus basalis. Effect of cortical deafferentation on cerebral blood flow regulation and implications for Alzheimer's disease. *Ann NY Acad Sci* (2000) **903**:374–86.

Heilig M, Sjogren M, Blennow K et al, Cerebrospinal fluid neuropeptides in Alzheimer's disease and vascular dementia, *Biol Psychiatry* (1995) **38**:210–16.

Higashi S, Fujita M, Nishimoto Y et al, Neuroendocrine studies in dementia patients: reponses of plasma GH and PRL following bromocriptine administration, *Acta Neurol Scand* (1994) **90**:39–44.

Itoh M, Meguro K, Fujiwara T et al, Assessment of dopamine metabolism in brain of patients with dementia by means of 18F-fluorodopa and PET, *Ann Nucl Med* (1994) **8**:245–51.

Kalaria RN, Cerebral vessels in ageing and Alzheimer's disease, *Pharm Therap* (1996) **72**:193–214.

Kalaria RN, The role of cerebral ischemia in Alzheimer's disease, *Neurobiol Aging* (2000) **21**:321–30.

Kalaria RN, Harik SI, Increased α_2- and β_2-adrenergic receptors in cerebral microvessels in Alzheimer disease, *Neurosci Lett* (1989) **106**: 233–8.

Kanemitsu H, Suematsu M, Ishii T et al, Changes in acetylcholine level and its related enzyme activities in rat brain following focal ischemia, *No To Shinkei* (1998) **50**:39–44.

Kawakami M, Itoh T, Effects of idebenone on monoamine metabolites in cerebrospinal fluid of patients with cerebrovascular dementia, *Arch Gerontol Geriatr* (1989) **8**:343–53.

Kondo Y, Ogawa N, Asanuma M et al, Preventive effects of bifemelane hydrochloride on decreased levels of muscarinic acetylcholine receptor and its mRNA in a rat model of chronic cerebral hypoperfusion, *Neurosci Res* (1996) **24**:409–14.

Krimer LS, Muly CE, Williams GV, Goldman-Rakic PS, Dopaminergic regulation of cerebral cortical microcirculation, *Nature Neurosci* (1998) **1**:286.

Krištofiková Z, Fales E, Majer E, Klaschka J, (^{3}H)Hemicholunium-3 binding sites in postmortem brains of human patients with Alzheimer's disease and multi-infarct dementia, *Exp Gerontol* (1995) **30**:125–36.

Kumagae Y, Matsui Y, Output, tissue levels, and synthesis of acetylcholine during and after transient forebrain ischemia in the rat, *J Neurochem* (1991) **56**:1169–73.

Kummer W, Haberberger R, Extrinsic and intrinsic cholinergic systems of the vascular wall, *Eur J Morphol* (1999) **37**:223–6.

Lacombe P, Sercombe R, Verrecchia C et al, Cortical blood flow increases induced by stimulation of the substantia innominata in the unanesthetized rat, *Brain Res* (1989) **491**:1–14.

Lahtinen H, Koitinaho J, Kauppinen R et al, Selegiline treatment after global ischemia in gerbils enhances the survival of CA1 pyramidal neurons in the hippocampus, *Brain Res* (1997) **757**:260–7.

Le Mestric C, Chavoix C, Chapon F et al, Effects of damage to the basal forebrain on brain glucose utilization: a re-evaluation using positron emission tomography in baboons with extensive unilateral excitotoxic lesion, *J Cereb Blood Flow Metab* (1998) **18**:476–90.

Liberini P, Pioro EP, Maysinger D, Cuello AC, Neocortical infarction in subhuman primates leads to restricted morphological damage of the cholinergic neurons in the nucleus basalis of Meynert, *Brain Res* (1994) **648**:1–8.

Luiten PGM, de Jong GI, van der Zee EA et al, Ultrastructural localization of cholinergic muscarinic receptors in rat brain cortical capillaries, *Brain Res* (1996) **720**:225–9.

Malatova Z, Pomfy M, Marsala J, Cholinergic enzyme activity during partial brain ischemia in the dog, *Act Nerv Super (Praha)* (1983) **25**:43–8.

Mann DMA, Yates PO, Hawkes J, The noradrenergic system in Alzheimer and multi-infarct dementias, *J Neurol Neurosurg Psychiatry* (1982) **45**:113–19.

Mann DMA, Yates PO, Marcyniuk B, The nucleus basalis of Meynert in multi-infarct (vascular) dementia, *Acta Neuropathol* (1986) **71**:332–7.

Martin-Ruiz C, Court J, Lee M et al, Nicotinic receptors in dementia of Alzheimer, Lewy body and vascular types, *Acta Neurol Scand Suppl* (2000) **176**:34–41.

McLendon BM, Chen GG, Doraiswamy PM, Current and future treatments for cognitive deficits in dementia, *Curr Psychiatry Rep* (2000) **2**:20–3.

Mehlhorn G, Loffler T, Apelt J et al, Glucose metabolism in cholinoceptive cortical rat brain regions after basal forebrain cholinergic lesion, *Int J Dev Neurosci* (1998) **16**:675–90.

Mendez MF, Younesi FL, Perryman KM, Use of donepezil for vascular dementia: preliminary clinical experience, *J Neurosci Clin Neurosci* (1999) **11**:268–70.

Molins A, Catalan R, Sahuquillo J et al, Somatostatin cerebrospinal fluid levels in dementia, *J Neurol* (1991) **238**:168–70.

Moretti R, Torre P, Antonello RM et al, Rivastigmine in subcortical vascular dementia: an open 22-month study, *J Neurol Sci* (2002) **203–4**:141–6

Murdoch I, Perry EK, Court JA et al, Cortical cholinergic dysfunction after human head injury, *J Neurotrauma* (1998) **15**:295–305.

Nakamura S, Koshimura K, Kato T et al, Neurotransmitters in dementia, *Clin Ther* (1984) **7**:18–34.

Narumi S, Kiyota Y, Nagaoka A, Cerebral embolization impairs memory function and reduces cholinergic marker enzyme activities in various brain regions in rats, *Pharmacol Biochem Behav* (1986) **24**:1729–31.

Ni JW, Matsumoto K, Li HB et al, Neuronal damage and decrease of central acetylcholine level following permanent occlusion of bilateral common carotid arteries in rat, *Brain Res* (1995) **673**:290–6.

Nobler MS, Mann JJ, Sackeim HA, Serotonin, cerebral blood flow, and cerebral metabolic rate in geriatric major depression and normal aging, *Brain Res Rev* (1999) **30**:250–63.

Nordberg A, Alafuzoff I, Winblad B, Nicotinic and muscarinic subtypes in the human brain: changes with aging and dementia, *J Neurosci Res* (1992) **31**:103–11.

Nyberg P, Waller S, Age-dependent vulnerability of brain choline acetyltransferase activity to transient cerebral ischemia in rats, *Stroke* (1989) **20**:495–500.

O'Brien JT, Erkinjuntti T, Reisberg B et al, Vascular cognitive impairment, *Lancet Neurology* (2003) **2**:11–20.

Ogawa N, Asanuma M, Tanaka K et al, Long-term time course of regional changes in cholinergic indices following transient ischemia in the spontaneously hypertensive rat brain, *Brain Res* (1996) **712**:60–8.

Oishi M, Mochizuki Y, Yoshihashi H et al, Laboratory examinations correlated with severity of dementia, *Ann Clin Lab Sci* (1996) **26**:340–5.

Orgogozo JM, Rigaud AS, Stoffler A et al, Efficacy and safety of memantine in patients with mild to moderate vascular dementia: a randomised, placebo controlled trial (MMM 300), *Stroke* (2002) **33**:1834–9.

Parnetti L, Ambrosoli L, Agliati G et al, Posatirelin in the treatment of vascular dementia: a double-blind multi-centre study vs placebo, *Acta Neurol Scand* (1996) **93**:456–63.

Paspalas CD, Papadopoulos GC, Ultrastructural evidence for combined action of noradrenaline and vasoactive intestinal polypeptide upon neurons, astrocytes and blood vessels of the rat cerebral cortex, *Brain Res* (1998) **45**:247–59.

Perry EK, Perry RH, Blessed G, Tomlinson BE, Changes in brain cholinesterases in senile dementia of the Alzheimer type, *Neuropathol Appl Neurobiol* (1978) **4**:273–7.

Perry EK, Gibson PH, Blessed G et al, Neurotransmitter enzyme abnormalities in senile dementia. Choline acetyltransferase and glutamic acid decarboxylase activities in necropsy brain tissue, *J Neurol Sci* (1977) **34**:247–65.

Peruzzi P, von Euw D, Lacombe P, Differentiated cerebrovascular effects of physostigmine and tacrine in cortical areas deafferented from the nucleus basalis magnocellularis suggest involvement of basalocortical projections to microvessels, *Ann N Y Acad Sci* (2000) **903**:394–406.

Peruzzi P, Lacombe P, Moro V et al, The cerebrovascular effects of physostigmine are not mediated through the substantia innominata, *Exp Neurol* (1993) **122**:319–26.

Piggott MA, Marshall EF, Thomas N et al, Striatal dopaminergic markers in dementia with Lewy bodies, Alzheimer's and Parkinson's diseases: rostracaudal distribution, *Brain* (1999) **122**:1440–68.

Rinne JO, Sako E, Paljarvi L et al, A comparison of brain choline acetyltransferase activity in Alzheimer's disease, multi-infarct dementia, and combined dementia, *J Neural Transm* (1988) **73**:121–8.

Rinne JO, Lonnberg P, Marjamaki P et al, Brain methionine- and leucine-enkephalin receptors in patients with dementia, *Neurosci Lett* (1993) **161**:77–80.

Roher AE, Kuo YM, Potter PE et al, Cortical cholinergic denervation elicits vascular A beta deposition, *Ann NY Acad Sci* (2000) **903**:366–73.

Sadoshima S, Ibayashi S, Fujii K et al, Inhibition of acetylcholinesterase modulates the autoregulation of cerebral blood flow and attenuates the ischemic brain metabolism in hypertensive rats, *J Cereb Blood Flow Metab* (1995) **15**:845–51.

Saito A, Wu JY, Lee TJ, Evidence for the presence of cholinergic nerves in cerebral arteries: an immunohistochemical demonstration of choline acetyltransferase, *J Cereb Blood Flow Metab* (1985) **5**:327–34.

Saito H, Togashi H, Yoshioka M et al, Animal models of vascular dementia with emphasis on stroke-prone spontaneously hypertensive rats, *Clin Exp Pharmacol Physiol* (1995) **22** (Suppl 1):S257–S259.

Sakurada T, Alufuzoff I, Winblad B, Nordberg A, Substance P-like immunoreactivity, choline acetyltransferase activity and cholinergic muscarinic receptors in Alzheimer's disease and multi-infarct dementia, *Brain Res* (1990) 52:329–32.

Scremin OU, Jenden DJ, Time-dependent changes in cerebral choline and acetylcholine induced by transient global ischemia in rats, *Stroke* (1991) **22**:643–7.

Scremin OU, Jenden DJ, Cholinergic control of cerebral blood flow in stroke, trauma and aging, *Life Sci* (1996) **58**:2011–18.

Scremin OU, Li MG, Jenden DJ, Cholinergic modulation of cerebral cortical blood flow changes induced by trauma, *J Neurotrauma* (1997) **14**:573–86.

Scremin OU, Scremin AM, Heuser D et al, Prolonged effects of cholinesterase inhibition with eptastigmine on the cerebral blood flow-metabolism ratio of normal rats. *J Cereb Blood Flow Metab* (1993) **13**:702–11.

Selden NR, Gitelman DR, Salamon-Murayama N et al, Trajectories of cholinergic pathways within the cerebral hemispheres of the human brain, *Brain* (1998) **121**:2249–57.

Sercombe R, Lacombe P, Springhetti V et al, Basal forebrain control of cortical blood flow and tissue gases in conscious aged rats, *Brain Res* (1994) **662**:155–64.

Suemaru S, Suemaru K, Hashimoto K et al, Cerebrospinal fluid corticotropin-releasing hormone and ACTH, and peripherally circulating choline-containing phospholipid in senile dementia, *Life Sci* (1993) **53**:697–706.

Takagi N, Miyake K, Taguchi T et al, Changes in cholinergic neurons and failure in learning function after microsphere embolism-induced cerebral ischemia. *Brain Res Bull* (1997) **43**:87–92.

Tanaka K, Ogawa N, Asanuma M et al, Relationship between cholinergic dysfunction and discrimination learning disabilities in Wistar rats following chronic cerebral hypoperfusion, *Brain Res* (1996) **729**:55–65.

Teaktong T, Graham A, Court J et al, Alzheimer's disease is associated with a selective increase in α7 nicotinic acetylcholine receptor immunoreactivity on astrocytes, *Glia* (2003) **41**:207–11.

Togashi H, Kimura S, Matsumoto M et al, Cholinergic changes in the hippocampus of stroke-prone spontaneously hypertensive rats, *Stroke* (1996) **27**:520–5.

Tohgi H, Abe T, Takahashi S et al, Indoleamine concentrations in cerebrospinal fluid from patients with Alzheimer type and Binswanger type dementias before and after administration of citalopram, a synthetic seratonin uptake inhibitor. *J Neurol Transm Park Dis Dement Sect* (1995) 9:121–31.

Tohgi H, Abe T, Takahashi S, Kimura M, A selective reduction of excitatory amino acids in cerebrospinal fluid of patients with Alzheimer type dementia compared with vascular dementia of the Binswanger type, *Neurosci Lett* (1992a) **141**:5–8.

Tohgi H, Ueno M, Abe T et al, Concentrations of monoamines and their metabolites in the cerebrospinal fluid from patients with senile dementia of the Alzheimer type and vascular dementia of the Binswanger type, *J Neural Transm* (1992b) 4:69–77.

Tohgi H, Abe T, Kimura M et al, Cerebrospinal fluid acetylcholine and choline in vascular dementia of Binswanger and multiple small infarct types as compared with Alzheimer-type dementia, *J Neural Transm* (1996) **103**:1211–20.

Tohgi H, Yonezawa H, Takahashi S et al, Cerebral blood flow and oxygen metabolism in senile dementia of Alzheimer's type and vascular dementia with deep white matter changes, *Neuroradiology* (1998) **40**:131–7.

Tsukada H, Sato K, Kakiuchi T, Nishiyama S, Age-related impairment of coupling mechanism between neuronal activation and functional cerebral blood flow response was restored by cholinesterase inhibition: PET study with microdialysis in the awake monkey brain, *Brain Res* (2000) **857**:158–64.

Ünal I, Gûrsoy-Õzdemir Y, Bolay H et al, Chronic daily administration of selegiline and EGb 761 increases brain's resistance to ischemia in mice, *Brain Res* (2001) **917**:174–81.

Van Dyck CH, Lin CH, Robinson R et al, The acetylcholine releaser linopirdine increases parietal regional cerebral blood flow in Alzheimer's disease, *Psychopharmacol (Berl)* (1997) **132**:217–26.

Vaucher E, Hamel E, Cholinergic basal forebrain neurons project to cortical microvessels in the rat: electron microscopic study with antrograde transported Phaseolus vulgaris leucoagglutinin and choline acetyltransferase immunocytochemistry, *J Neurosci* (1995) **15**:1727–41.

Vaucher E, Dauphin F, Seylaz J, Lacombe P, Autoradiographic study of the cerebrovascular effects of stimulation of the substantia innominata: convenient stimulation paradigm, *J Auton Nerv Syst* (1994) **49** (Suppl):S43–S47.

Waite JJ, Holschneider DP, Scremin OU, Selective immunotoxin-induced cholinergic deafferentation alters blood flow distribution in the cerebral cortex, *Brain Res* (1999) **818**:1–11.

Walker Z, Costa DC, Walker RW et al, Differentiation of dementia with Lewy bodies from Alzheimer's disease using a dopaminergic presynaptic ligand, *J Neurol Neurosurg Psychiatry* (2002) **73**:134–40.

Waller SB, Ball MJ, Reynolds MA, London ED, Muscarinic binding and choline acetyltransferase in postmortem brains of demented patients, *Can J Neurol Sci* (1986) **13** (Suppl 4):528–32.

Wallin A, Alafuzoff I, Carlsson A et al, Neurotransmitter deficits in a non-multi-infarct category of vascular dementia, *Acta Neurol Scand* (1989) **79**:397–406.

Wilcock G, Mobius HJ, Stoffler A, A double-blind, placebo-controlled multicentre study of memantine in mild to moderate vascular dementia (MMM500), *Int Clin Psychopharmacol* (2002) **17**:297–305.

Wilson K, Bowen D, Francis P, Tyrrell P, Effect of central cholinergic stimulation on regional cerebral blood flow in Alzheimer's disease, *Br J Psychiatry* (1991) **158**:558–62.

Winblad B, Poritis N, Memantine in severe dementia: results of the 9M-Best Study (Benefit and efficacy in severely demented patients during treatment with memantine), *Int J Geriatr Psych* (1999) **14**:135–46.

Wonnacott S, Presynaptic nicotinic Ach receptors, *Trends Neurosci* (1997) **20**: 92–8.

Yang Y, Beyreuther K, Schmitt HP, Spatial analysis of the neuronal density of aminergic brainstem nuclei in primary neurodegenerative and vascular dementia: a comparative immunocytochemical and quantitative study using a graph method. *Anal Cell Pathol* (1999) **19**:125–38.

Zaidan E, Sims NR, Alterations in the production of $^{14}CO_2$ and [^{14}C] acetylcholine from [U-^{14}C]glucose in brain subregions following transient forebrain ischemia in the rat, *J Neurochem* (1990) **55**:1882–9.

Zhang F, Xu S, Iadecola C, Role of nitric oxide and acetylcholine in neocortical hyperemia elicited by basal forebrain stimulation: evidence for an involvement of endothelial nitric oxide, *Neuroscience* (1995) **69**:1195–204.

chapter 12

Hereditary forms of vascular dementia

Martin Dichgans

Introduction

Monogenic conditions are responsible for only a minority of cases of dementia. However, they may provide important insights into the more common sporadic forms. Thus, for example, cloning of the genes for familial Alzheimer's disease and cerebral autosomal dominant arteriopathy with sub-cortical infarcts and leukoencephalopathy (CADASIL) has revealed pathways involved in the degeneration of neurons and vascular smooth muscle cells (VSMC), respectively (Sisodia and George-Hyslop, 2002; Wang et al, 2002a). Studies with transgenic animals and cells overexpressing the mutant proteins have led to new therapeutic strategies (Fassbender et al, 2001; Schenk, 2002; Wang et al, 2002a). Some of these strategies are currently tested in sporadic disease (Simons et al, 2002).

Vascular dementia is closely connected to strokes. Table 12.1 gives an overview on monogenic conditions associated with stroke. In principle, each of these conditions may cause vascular dementia (VaD) (see, for example, Mendez et al, 1997; DeBaun et al, 1998; Schatz et al, 2001). However, in many cases information regarding the prevalence and profile of cognitive deficits is limited. This chapter focuses on CADASIL and hereditary forms of cerebral amyloid angiopathy (CAA). CADASIL has recently been recognized as an important cause of subcortical VaD (Dichgans, 2002). Similarly, hered-itary forms of CAA may provide important clues on CAA-related dementia (Natte et al, 2001).

Table 12.1 Monogenic causes of stroke

Small vessel disease
  CADASIL
  CARASIL
  Cerebroretinal vasculopathy and HERNS

Large artery disease
  Moyamoya disease
  Ehlers–Danlos syndrome type IV
  Marfan's syndrome
  Pseudoxanthoma elasticum
  Neurofibromatosis type I

Disorders affecting both small *and* large arteries
  Fabry's disease
  Homocystinuria
  Sickle cell disease

Embolic causes of stroke
  Hereditary hemorrhagic telangiectasia
  Familial cardiomyopathies and dysrhythmias

Hemorrhagic stroke
  Cerebral amyloid angiopathies
  Cavernous angiomas
  Other types of vascular malformations

Prothrombotic disorders

Mitochondrial disorders

CADASIL

CADASIL is an autosomal dominantly inherited non-amyloid angiopathy caused by mutations in *Notch3* (Joutel et al, 1996; Dichgans et al, 1998). Previous descriptions of families with 'hereditary multi-infarct dementia', 'familial subcortical dementia' and 'chronic familial vascular encephalopathy' represent early reports of the same condition. In 1993, Tournier-Lasserve et al (1993) mapped the gene to chromosome 19 and coined the acronym CADASIL. Since then several hundred families have been reported from all over the world – more than 180 families in Germany (Dichgans et al, 2000 and unpublished data).

Clinical phenotype

The phenotypic spectrum of CADASIL has been delineated by two large studies from Europe (Chabriat et al, 1995a; Dichgans et al, 1998) as well as multiple reports on single patients or families (Desmond et al, 1999).

Migraine with aura

Migraine with aura is an early manifestations of CADASIL and is found in about 30% of the cases (Dichgans et al, 1998; Chabriat et al, 1995a). Aura symptoms tend to involve the visual and sensory system. However, in a considerable number of cases, symptoms are those of hemiplegic migraine, basilar migraine or isolated aura, which may be difficult to differentiate from ischemic episodes. Migraine may account for some unusual presentations such as prolonged coma and confusion (Le Ber et al, 2002). In an individual patient the type of aura may vary or be invariantly the same. In most patients who develop migraine, it is the first symptom (onset usually before age 40 years). The frequency of migraine attacks seems to decrease after the first stroke (Dichgans et al, 1998).

TIA and stroke

Transient ischemic attacks (TIA) and stroke are the most frequent presentations found in about 85% of symptomatic individuals (Chabriat et al, 1995a; Desmond et al, 1999). Mean age at onset for ischemic episodes is 46 years (range of 30–70 years). In many cases they present as a classic lacunar syndrome (pure motor stroke; ataxic hemiparesis/dysarthria or clumsy hand syndrome, pure sensory stroke; sensorimotor stroke) but other lacunar syndromes (brainstem or hemispheric) are also observed. They are often recurrent leading to severe disability with gait disturbance, urinary incontinence and pseudobulbar palsy. Strokes involving the territory of a large artery have occasionally been reported (Rubio et al, 1997). However, those observations may be coincidental. Strokes related to small vessel pathology are clearly the main manifestation of the disease.

Dementia

Cognitive deficits are found in about 60% of symptomatic individuals and by the age of 65-two thirds of the cases have become demented (Dichgans et al, 1998). Dementia in CADASIL is characterized by a dysexecutive syndrome (frontal lobe impairment), memory deficits, behavioral disturbance and mood disturbance (see below) (Taillia et al, 1998; Trojano et al, 1998, Hedera and Friedland, 1997; Filley et al, 1999). Frontal lobe signs that are frequently observed in CADASIL patients include apathy and abulia, cognitive slowing and difficulties with the following capacities: goal formulation, initiation, planning, decision making and set shifting. These symptoms are often accompanied by psychomotor slowing and a narrowing of the field of interest. Memory deficits in CADASIL are characterized by impaired recall whereas recognition is relatively preserved. Behavioral abnormalities include agitation, social withdrawal and personality change. Some patients exhibit visuospatial impairment and difficulties with calculation or language. However, most often language is relatively spared.

Cognitive deficits may evolve in a stepwise or slowly progressive fashion (Dichgans et al, 1998; Chabriat et al, 1995a). They are associated with gait disturbance (unprovoked falls), urinary incontinence and pseudobulbar palsy.

Psychiatric manifestations

Mood disorders are the most frequent psychiatric manifestations and occur in about 30% of cases. Many patients develop an adjustment disorder or moderate depression. Severe major depression is seen in only a few cases (Dichgans et al, 1998). Psychiatric manifestations further include manic depressive disorder, panic disorder, hallucinatory syndromes and delusional episodes (Dichgans et al, 1998; Chabriat et al, 1995a). Rarely, CADASIL may present with a picture of schizophrenia (Lagas and Juvonen, 2001).

Other manifestations

Like other patients with stroke CADASIL patients may develop epileptic seizures (up to 10% of cases) which may require treatment. There have been single reports on spinal cord signs (Hutchinson et al, 1995) or infarcts (Sourander and Walinder, 1977; Gutierrez-Molina et al, 1994), intracerebral hemorrhages (Sourander and Walinder, 1977) and episodes of raised intracranial pressure (Baudrimont et al, 1993, Feuerhake et al, 2002). Also, there have been single reports on early myocardial infarction (Wielaard et al,

1995; Filley et al, 1999). However, it is still unclear whether the latter are related to the underlying angiopathy of small blood vessels in CADASIL.

Overall course

The overall course of CADASIL is highly variable even within single families. Some patients remain asymptomatic until their seventies whereas others are severely disabled at an early age. Early onset does not necessarily predict rapid progression. In a large group of patients the duration from onset to death varied between three and 43 years (mean 23 years) (Dichgans et al, 1998). Advanced stages correspond to the clinical syndrome of severe Binswanger's encephalopathy (Caplan, 1995). Mean age at death is about 60 years (Dichgans et al, 1998; Chabriat et al, 1995a; Desmond et al, 1999).

Autopsy findings

Macroscopic examination of the brains from advanced cases reveals a pronounced rarefication of the subcortical white matter with periventricular preference (Figure 12.1a) (Ruchoux and Maurage, 1997). Another regular finding is lacunar infarcts which are predominantly located within the basal ganglia, thalamus and brainstem (in particular the pons). Histopathological examination shows various degress of demyelination, axonal loss, enlargement of the extracellular space and mild astrocytic gliosis compatible with chronic ischemia. The underlying vascular lesion is a unique non-arteriosclerotic, amyloid-negative angiopathy involving small arteries (100–400 μm) and capillaries primarily in the brain but also in other organs. The diagnosis may therefore be established by a simple skin biopsy (Ruchoux et al, 1994; Mayer et al, 1999; Joutel et al, 2001). Ultrastructural examination reveals characteristic granular osmiophilic deposits within the vascular basal lamina which are considered diagnostic (Figure 12.1b). These deposits are often seen in close contact with vascular smooth muscle cells which degenerate and eventually disappear. Yet they have not been characterized biochemically and their origin remains unresolved. Even though CADASIL is a generalized angiopathy, vascular complications appear to be limited to the brain. This discrepancy might in part be related to the predominant involvement of leptomeningeal and long penetrating arteries of the brain. However, additional factors such as properties of the blood–brain barrier may be suspected (Ruchoux and Maurage, 1997; Dichgans et al, 1999a).

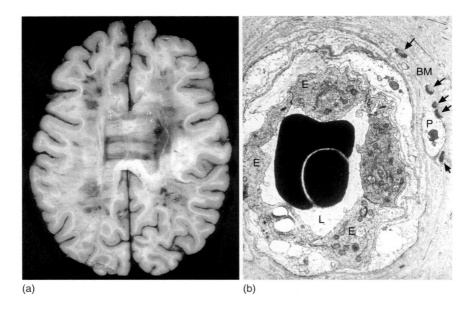

(a)   (b)

Figure 12.1 *Pathological findings in CADASIL. (a) Numerous small infarcts and diffuse white matter changes in an axial slice from a 64-year-old male CADASIL patient with spastic tetraparesis, dementia, and urinary incontinence (autopsy material; photographs kindly provided by R. Meyermann, Tübingen). Note the relative sparing of the subcortical u-fibers. (b) Granular osmiophilic material (GOM) in a patient with CADASIL. GOM can only be detected on electron microscopy. Granular deposits (arrows) within the basilar membrane (BM) of a skin capillary (skin biopsy sample, kindly processed by PD Dr M Bergmann, Bremen). L, lumen of blood vessel; E, endothelial cells; P, pericyte.*

Neuroimaging

MRI shows two major types of abnormalities (Figure 12.2) (Chabriat et al, 1998; Auer et al, 2001a): Firstly, there are small circumscribed regions that are isointense to free CSF on T1- and T2-weighted images. Many of these lesions are suggestive of lacunar infarcts regarding size, shape and location. Secondly, there are less well demarcated T2-hyperintensities of variable size which may show different degrees of hypointensity on T1-weighted images but are clearly distinct from free CSF. The majority of these lesions are located in the subcortical white matter but similar lesions may be seen in other brain regions including the subcortical gray matter (Chabriat et al, 1998; Auer et al, 2001a). Small irregular T2-hyperintensities of the periventricular and deep white matter are usually the first sign seen in younger indi-

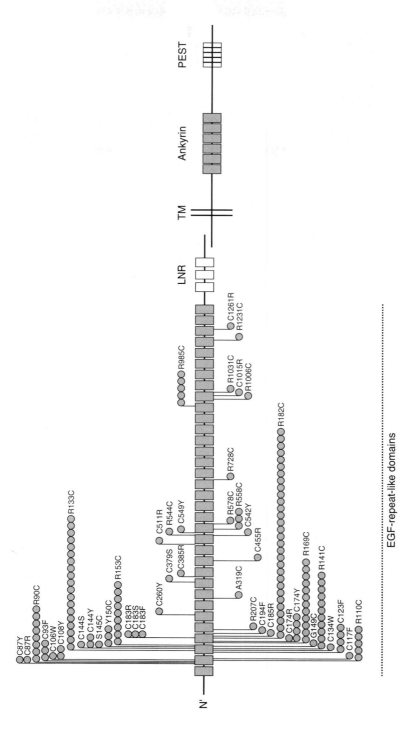

Figure 12.5 Graphical illustration of the human Notch3 receptor and spectrum of mutations (pooled data from Joutel et al, 1997; Dichgans et al, 2000; Oberstein et al, 1999; Arboleda-Velasquez et al, 2002; Dichgans et al. unpublished data). CADASIL mutations are located in epidermal growth factor (EGF)-like repeat domains of the Notch3 receptor with a strong cluster at the N-terminus.

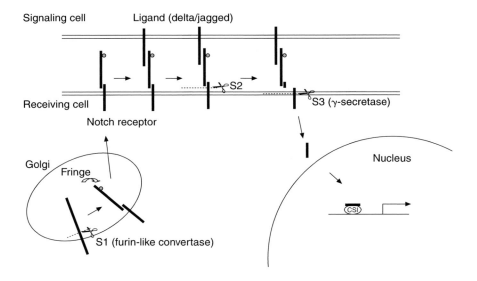

Figure 12.6 *Maturation and proteolytic processing of Notch receptor. Maturation of Notch receptors involves a constitutive cleavage in the trans-Golgi network as the receptor traffics toward the plasma membrane. Cleavage at the S1 site results in a larger extracellular fragment containing all the EGF-repeat like domains and a smaller intracellular fragment which contains the transmembrane region. Only the heterodimeric proteins are present at the cell surface. The next step is binding of the ligand. Ligands of Notch are presented by neighboring cells. Binding of the ligand facilitates cleavage within the extracellular juxtamembrane region (S2 site). S2 cleavage induces a third intracellular cleavage within the transmembrane region (S3 site). S3 cleavage results in the release of the intracellular portion of Notch. Upon release, the intracellular domain translocates to the nucleus where it modifies transcription of target genes.*

Mutations in CADASIL show a highly stereotyped nature – they all involve highly conserved cysteine residues (Joutel et al, 1997; Dichgans et al, 2000, 2001) thus changing the regular number of six cysteine residues within wild-type EGF-like repeat domains toward an odd number. It has been suggested that the unpaired cysteine residue generated by the mutations could cause aberrant interactions of Notch3 with other Notch3 molecules or other proteins and, in fact, recent data have provided evidence for multimerization of mutant Notch3 (Joutel et al, 2000b).

Expression of the human Notch3 receptor is restricted to vascular smooth muscle cells (VSMC) and pericytes. In CADASIL there is an excessive accumulation of the ectodomain of the Notch3 receptor within blood vessels (Joutel et al, 2000b). Accumulation takes place at the cytoplasmic membrane of VSMC and pericytes, in close vicinity to (but not within) the deposits that characterize the disease. Notch3 immunostaining of dermal blood vessels derived from skin biopsies has been shown to be diagnostic (Joutel et al, 2001).

Recent data suggest that the Notch3 receptor may have a role in promoting vascular smooth muscle cell survival. Rat embryonic aorta cells, which have been transfected with the constitutively active intracellular form of the Notch3 receptor, show enhanced resistance to apoptosis (Wang et al, 2002b). Moreover, in an *in vivo* model of arterial injury expression of Notch3 was shown to be upregulated in neointimal tissue (Wang et al, 2002b). Taken together these data suggest a critical role for Notch3 in vascular remodeling.

Cerebral amyloid angiopathies

CAA and dementia

Cerebral amyloid angiopathy (CAA) is the deposition of congophilic material in the walls of small and medium-sized blood vessels in the cortex and leptomeninges (Vinters, 1987). The arteriolar media, including its smooth muscle cell component, is gradually replaced by fibrillar amyloid. As a result vessels undergo various degenerative changes such as concentric cracking (vessel-within-vessel configuration), microaneurysm formation and fibrinoid necrosis.

CAA is widely recognized as an important cause of intracerebral hemorrhage (ICH). CAA may further cause ischemic infarction (Cadavid et al, 2000) mediated by stenotic changes and functional disturbances of cerebral blood vessels (Greenberg, 2002a; Mueggler et al, 2002; Zhang et al, 1997). In the typical case MRI reveals a lobar hemorrhage together with hemosiderin deposits evidencing past hemorrhages (Knudsen et al, 2001). Other findings include diffuse white matter signal hyperintensities (Gray et al, 1985; Greenberg, 2002a) and ischemic infarcts.

CAA commonly overlaps with Alzheimer's disease because of a closely related biology of the two conditions. Consequently, the relationship between CAA and cognitive impairment has been difficult to assess. However, recent data from the Honolulu–Asia Aging Study (Pfeifer et al, 2002) suggest that CAA represents an independent risk factor for dementia (Greenberg, 2002b). Also, studies in hereditary cerebral hemorrhage with amyloidosis–Dutch type (HCHWA-D) show that CAA in the absence of parenchymal Alzheimer's disease-like pathology (neuritic plaques and neurofibrillary tangles) is sufficient to cause dementia (Natte et al, 2001).

Hereditary forms of CAA

There are several hereditary forms of CAA, which may be differentiated based on clinical, pathological, biochemical and genetic findings (Revesz et al, 2002). These disorders are inherited in an autosomal dominant fashion.

Amyloid precursor protein (APP)-related CAA

Several point mutations within the amyloid precursor protein (APP) gene are associated with enhanced deposition of beta amyloid (Aβ), a 39–43 amino-acid fragment of APP. As a general rule, mutations associated with severe CAA are located within the Aβ region, while mutations associated primarily with senile plaques (Alzheimer's disease type pathology) flank the Aβ region (Figure 12.7). 'CAA mutations' affect three neighboring codons close to the α-cleavage site (Figure 12.7, Table 12.2).

The most thoroughly characterized form of familial CAA is the Dutch type. Affected individuals generally present with recurrent strokes with onset between the ages of 40 and 65 years (mean 50 years) (Wattendorff et al, 1995; Bornebroek et al, 1997). In at least 80% of the cases strokes are hemorrhagic and almost one-third of the patients die within a year following their first hemorrhage. Another prominent feature is dementia which may develop in the absence of clinically overt stroke (Wattendorff et al, 1995; Haan et al, 1990, 1992; Bornebroek et al, 1996a; Natte et al, 2001). Cognitive deficits may evolve in a stepwise fashion related to strokes, as in VaD, or slowly progressive suggesting a more chronic type of tissue damage. The profile of neuropsychological abnormalities in HCHWA-D seems to be variable and includes deficits in memory, language, calculation, and constructional abilities (Haan et al, 1990; Bornebroek et al, 1996a).

The mechanisms by which CAA may cause dementia are partly unknown. In an autopsy study of 19 patients dementia was associated with cerebral amyloid angiopathy (CAA-load and vessel wall thickening) but was independent of plaques and neurofibrillary tangles, i.e. AD-like pathological changes (Natte et al, 2001) (Figure 12.8). In another study, semiquantitative measures of CAA were shown to be associated with the number of cerebrovascular lesions. Taken together these data suggest that dementia in HCHWA-D is largely mediated by (small) hemorrhages and infarcts. However, other factors are likely to play a role (Bornebroek et al, 1996b). The impact of diffuse white matter changes (WMC) on cognition is still a matter of debate (Gray et al, 1985; Bornebroek et al, 1996b). They are a frequent finding – even in presymptomatic individuals (Bornebroek et al, 1996a) –

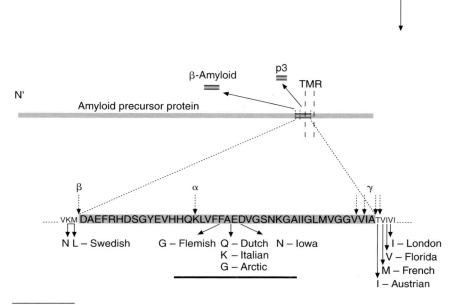

Figure 12.7 *Amyloid precursor protein (APP) is a transmembrane receptor that is cleaved proteolytically in two alternative ways depending on cleavage at the alpha or beta site. Cleavage by the alpha secretase causes release of the p3 peptide which is not amyloidogenic whereas cleavage by the beta-secretase releases the Aβ peptide. Aggregates of Aβ are found as a major component of two different pathologies: neuritic plaques and vascular amyloid deposition. Mutations associated with familial CAA (Flemish, Dutch, Italian, Arctic, Iowa) are located within the Aβ sequence close to the alpha site whereas those associated with familial AD are located at the beta site (Swedish) or gamma site (London, Florida, French, Australian). All CAA mutations result in enhanced amyloid deposition within blood vessels whereas they have differential effects on the extent of Alzheimer-type pathology.*

and are likely to contribute. However, most studies have failed to find correlations between WMC and cognitive parameters (Bornebroek et al., 1996a, b).

Whereas the dementia in HCHWA-D may be classified as VaD, dementia in the Flemish and Arctic type of CAA is compatible with AD both clinically and neuropathologically (see Table 12.2) (Roks et al, 2000; Nilsberth et al, 2001). Gradual worsening of cognitive functions has further been reported for carriers of the Iowa mutation who typically present with progressive aphasic dementia (Grabowski et al, 2001). Compared with the Dutch type intracerebral hemorrhage is less frequent in the Flemish variant and it has not been mentioned in the Arctic and Iowa types. The mechanisms by which these mutations cause distinct clinical and neuropathological phenotypes

Table 12.2 Hereditary forms of cerebral amyloid angiopathy

	Gene (Chromosome)	Precursor protein	Mutation(s)	Amyloid component	Cerebral hemorrhage	Ishemic white matter lesions (MRI)	Dementia	Brain parenchymal changes other than CAA
Amyloidois–Flemish	APP (21)	Amyloid Precursor Protein (APP)	A692G	Aβ (4kDa)	+	+	++ (AD-like)	Neuritic plaques (++), NFT (++)
HCHWA–Dutch			E693Q		++	++	+ (VaD-like)	Diffuse plaques rare: NP and NFT
Amyloidosis–Arctic			E693G		-	-	++ (AD-like)	Neuritic plaques (++), NFT (++)
Amyloidosis–Italian			E693K		++	?	+	'Amyloid' plaques, NFT (+)
Amyloidosis–Iowa			D694N		(-) microhemorrhages	++ posterior calcifications	++ aphasic dementia	Neuritic plaques (+) NFT (++)
HCHWA–Icelandic	CYST C (20)	Cystatin C (Cys C)	L68Q	Acys (20 kDa)	++	+	+	-
FBD	BRI2 (13)	Abri precursor protein (ABriPP)	STOP267R	ABri (4kDa)	relatively rare (+)	++	++	Amyloid plaques, NF degeneration
FDD			Decamer duplication	ADan (4kDa)				
FAP/MVA	TTR (18)	Transthyretin (TTR)	D18G V30G	ATTR (10kDa)	-	-	++	Subependymal TTR-immunoreactive amyloid deposits, subpial calcifications
FAF	GEL (9)	Gelsolin (Gel)	D187N	AGel (7kDa)	-	++	cognitive impairment	-
PrP-CAA	PRNP (20)	Prion protein (PrP)	Y145STOP	APrP (7.5kDa)				

HCHWA, hereditary cerebral hemorrhage with amyloidosis; FBD, familial British dementia; FDD, familial Danish dementia; FAP/MVA, familial amyloid polyneuropathy/meningovascular amyloidosis; FAF, familial amyloidosis Flemish type; PrP-CAA, prion protein-related cerebral amyloid angiopathy; NFT, neurofibrillary tangles; NP, neuritic plaques.

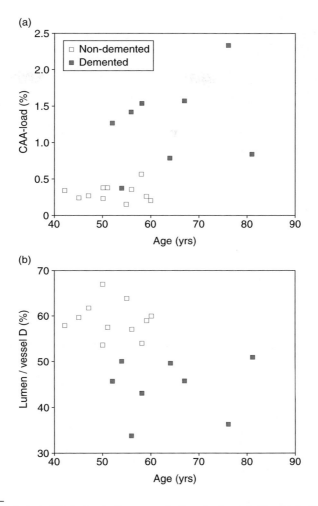

Figure 12.8 *Association between the amount of cerebral amyloid angiopathy (CAA) and age as well as dementia in HCHWA–Dutch type. (a) CAA load is the area of cortical vessel wall Aβ immunoreactivity as a percentage of the area of cortex. (b) Lumen/vessel D = lumen diameter as a percentage of vessel diameter, (reproduced with kind permission from Natte et al, 2001).*

are not fully understood. However, several studies suggest that the various mutations have differential effects on Aβ secretion, fibrillogenesis, and toxicity (Table 12.3) (Miravalle et al, 2000; Nilsberth et al, 2001; Van Nostrand et al, 2001; Murakami et al, 2002).

Table 12.3 Biochemical and biological properties of mutated Aβ fragments in familial CAA

	Effects on *Aβ secretion*	*Effects on* *Aβ fibrillogenesis*	*Aβ toxicitiy*
Flemish (A692G)	↑	↓	↔
Dutch (E693Q)	(↓)	↑	↑
Arctic (E693G)	(↓)	↑	↑
Iowa (D694N)	↔	↑	↑

For further details see text.

Cystatin C-related CAA

Hereditary cerebral hemorrhage with amyloidosis–Iceland (HCHWA-I) has been described in several families from Western Iceland (Gudmundsson et al, 1972; Jensson et al, 1987; Olafsson et al, 1996). The condition is characterized by severe amyloid deposition within small arteries and arterioles of the leptomeninges, cortex, basal ganglia, cerebellum and brain stem.

Affected individuals usually present with recurrent intracerebral hemorrhage (ICH) starting between age 20 and 40 years (mean 27.3 years). Cognitive deficits are frequent and may develop in a stepwise or slowly progressive fashion (Jensson et al, 1987; Sveinbjornsdottir et al, 1996). Single patients present with dementia as the sole manifestation (Sveinbjornsdottir et al, 1996). However, there is little detailed information on the profile of neuropsychological deficits in patients with HCHWA-I.

Pathological and MRI examination of the brain show single or multiple hemorrhages, diffuse white matter changes and occasional ischemic infarctions. The main amyloid component in HCHWA-I is cystatin C (CYS C), a type II cysteine protease inhibitor (Table 12.2). Affected individuals carry a mis-sense mutation at position 68 of the *CYS C* gene. A role for Cys C in the pathogenesis of other amyloidoses is further suggested by the fact that Cys C colocalizes with amyloid deposits in Aβ-, TTR- and gelsolin-related amyloidosis (Vinters et al, 1990; Vidal et al, 1996; Kiuru et al, 1999).

Transthyretin (TTR)-related CAA

Transthyretin (TTR) amyloidoses are a large group of late-onset autosomal dominant conditions characterized by the deposition of TTR – a carrier protein for thyroid hormone and retinol binding protein – in the extracellular space of several organs (Benson, 1996). Meanwhile, more than 60 different mutations have been described (http://archive.uwcm.ac.uk/uwcm/mg/search/119471.html).

By far the most common phenotype is sensorimotor polyneuropathy, usually associated with autonomic neuropathy. Additional manifestations include cardiomyopathy and renal insuffiency. Amyloid deposition may also occur in the leptomeninges and meningeal vessels (Benson, 1996). Meningocerebrovascular amyloidosis (Vidal et al, 1996; Garzuly et al, 1996) and oculoleptomeningeal amyloidosis (Petersen et al, 1997), in which amyloid deposition also takes place in the vitreous, are associated with distinct point mutations (see Table 12.2). Patients with the D18G mutation present with progressive cognitive deficits, ataxia, and spasticity (Garzuly et al, 1996; Vidal et al, 1996). Some patients develop episodic confusion, hallucinations, hearing loss or migraine, which seem to be related to the involvement of leptomeningeal blood vessels. MRI shows prominent meningeal enhancement but no obvious parenchymal lesions (Garzuly et al, 1996).

Patients with the V30G mutation develop progressive dementia, seizures and ataxia together with hemiparesis and decreased vision (Petersen et al, 1997). At autopsy the brains exhibit some degree of diffuse atrophy. Upon histopathological examination Petersen et al found widespread cortical neuronal loss as well as remote and recent cystic infarcts which may explain the neuropsychological deficits. However, there was no apparent involvement of the subcortical white matter on neuroimaging.

Intracranial manifestations of TTR amyloidoses further include subarachnoid hemorrhage (Ellie et al, 2001; Mascalchi et al, 1999) and intracerebral hemorrhages (Sakashita et al, 2001) which have been associated with distinct mutations.

ABri precursor protein (ABriPP)-related CAA

Familial British dementia (FBD) and familial Danish dementia (FDD) are the new terms for two conditions associated with mutations in the *BRI2* gene.

FBD has been described in a few pedigrees from Great Britain (Plant et al, 1990; Vidal et al, 1999; Mead et al, 2000). Clinically, the disorder is characterized by progressive memory loss or dementia (>95%), spastic tetraparesis (>90%) and cerebellar ataxia (75%) (Mead et al, 2000). Additional manifestations include stroke-like episodes (30%) and headache (20%), whereas intracerebral hemorrhages or epileptic seizures are rather uncommon (<10%).

Mean age of onset is 48 years with a mean disease duration of nine years (mean age at death 56 years).

Mead et al. (2000) studied the neuropsychological profile in early affected cases. They found memory loss to be the most consistent finding. However, MRI white matter changes in those patients were not severe enough to explain the neuropsychological deficits satisfactorily. Also, there were no frontal or executive abnormalities as would be expected if ischemic white matter changes were contributing to the neuropsychological findings. Thus, the authors concluded, that the memory loss in early affected cases results largely from the loss of hippocampal neurons. Interestingly, many of the early cases had a history of depression, anxiety or sleep disturbance which occurred early on.

FDD was initially described in a large family from Denmark under the term 'heredopathia ophtalmo-oto-encephalica' (Stromgren et al, 1970). Affected individuals may present with cataracts and other ocular disorders including ocular hemorrhages in the third decade followed by severe hearing loss. Cerebellar ataxia usually occurs shortly after the age of 40. Paranoid psychosis develops in the sixth decade and is followed by dementia in the majority of cases. Some patients show temporal disturbance of consciousness. Most patients die in their fifth to sixth decade (Holton et al, 2002; Stromgren et al, 1970; Vidal et al, 2000).

Neuropathologically, FBD and FDD are characterized by a diffuse atrophy of the brain (including the cerebellum), cranial nerves and spinal cord. Another prominent feature is the presence of ischemic white matter changes and lacunar infarcts (Holton et al, 2001; Mead et al, 2000; Holton et al, 2002; Stromgren et al, 1970) (Figure 12.9), whereas cerebral hemorrhages are relatively rare. Ischemic lesions are connected with extensive CAA, which involves leptomeningeal vessels as well as blood vessels of the cortex, white matter (see Figure 12.9), and spinal cord (Holton et al, 2002; Revesz et al, 2002). Histopathological findings further include parenchymal (pre-amyloid) plaques and neurofibrillary tangles. Thus, the pathology in FBD and FDD comprises both vascular (predominantly ischemic) and neurodegenerative alterations. Most likely, both components contribute to the development of dementia in ABriPP-related CAAs.

The wild-type ABri precursor protein is a 266-amino-acid (AA)-long type II, single-pass transmembrane protein (see Table 12.2). FBD is associated with a point mutation in the stop codon of the *BRI2* gene resulting in an extended precursor protein (Vidal et al, 1999). FDD is due to a decamer duplication

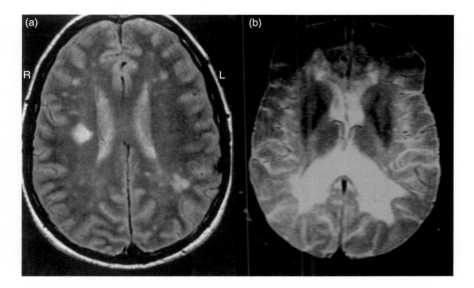

Figure 12.9 MRIs from patients with familial British dementia (FBD) showing (a) early and (b) confluent white matter lesions (kindly provided by Prof G Plant).

(TTTAATTTGT) which occurs between codons 265 and 266 and leads to a frame-shift (Vidal et al, 2000). Both the FBD and FDD mutation result in 277 AA-long extended precursor proteins. Cleavage of 34 amino-acids at the C-terminus by a furin-like protease results in the release of the amyloidogenic peptides (ABri and ADan, respectively). The two peptides share a common *N*-terminal 22 AA-long sequence but have distinct *C*-termini. ABri and ADan are deposited as amyloid in leptomeningeal vessels and in blood vessels of the cortex, white matter and spinal cord (Holton et al, 2001, 2002).

Summary and future perspectives

Hereditary angiopathies have provided important insights into the mechanisms underlying vascular dementia. Carefully designed studies combining detailed neuropsychological testing and advanced neuroimaging protocols such as fiber-tracking diffusion tensor imaging, voxel-based morphometry, statistical parametric mapping and functional imaging are now required to further elucidate the morphological and functional correlates of VaD. Hereditary angiopathies are particularly suited for such studies because the underlying vascular lesion is clearly defined with a low rate of combined pathologies. Functional and interventional studies in animal models for CAA and CADASIL (Ruchoux et al, 2003) may assist in exploring new therapeutic strategies for hereditary and sporadic forms of VaD.

References

Arboleda-Velasquez JF, Lopera F, Lopez E et al, C455R notch 3 mutation in a Colombian CADASIL kindred with early onset of stroke, *Neurology* (2002) 59:277–9.

Artavanis-Tsakonas S, Rand MD, Lake, RJ, Notch signaling: cell fate control and signal integration in development, *Science* (1999) 284:770–6.

Auer DP, Putz B, Gossl C et al, Differential lesion patterns in CADASIL and sporadic subcortical arteriosclerotic encephalopathy: MR imaging study with statistical parametric group comparison. *Radiology* (2001a) 218:443–51.

Auer D, Schirmer T, Heidenreich JO et al, Altered white and gray matter metabolism in CADASIL as detected by chemical shift imaging and single voxel ^{1}H-MRS, *Neurology* (2001b) 56:635–42.

Baudrimont M, Dubas F, Joutel A et al, Autosomal dominant leukoencephalopathy and subcortical ischemic stroke. A clinicopathological study, *Stroke* (1993) 24:122–5.

Benson MD, Leptomeningeal amyloid and variant transthyretins, *Am J Pathol* (1996) 148:351–4.

Bornebroek M, Haan J, van Buchem, MA et al, White matter lesions and cognitive deterioration in presymptomatic carriers of the amyloid precursor protein gene codon 693 mutation, *Arch Neurol* (1996a) 53:43–8.

Bornebroek M, van Buchem MA, Haan J et al, Hereditary cerebral hemorrhage with amyloidosis–Dutch type: better correlation of cognitive deterioration with advancing age than with number of focal lesions or white matter hyperintensities, *Alzheimer Dis Assoc Disord* (1996b) 10:224–31.

Bornebroek M, Westendorp RG, Haan J et al, Mortality from hereditary cerebral haemorrhage with amyloidosis–Dutch type. The impact of sex, parental transmission and year of birth, *Brain* (1997) 120:2243–9.

Brüning R, Dichgans M, Berchtenbreiter C et al, CADASIL: decrease in regional cerebral blood volume in hyperintense subcortical lesions inversely correlates with disability and cognitive performance, *Am J Neuroradiol* (2001) 22:1268–74.

Cadavid D, Mena H, Koeller K, Frommelt RA, Cerebral beta amyloid angiopathy is a risk factor for cerebral ischemic infarction. A case control study in human brain biopsies, *J Neuropathol Exp Neurol* (2000) 59:768–73.

Caplan LR, Binswanger's disease–revisited, *Neurology* (1995) 45:626–33.

Chabriat H, Bousser MG, Pappata S, Cerebral autosomal dominant arteriopathy with subcortical infarcts and leukoencephalopathy: a positron emission tomography study in two affected family members, *Stroke* (1995b) 26:1729–30.

Chabriat H, Levy C, Taillia H et al, Patterns of MRI lesions in CADASIL, *Neurology* (1998) 51:452–7.

Chabriat H, Pappata S, Ostergaard L et al, Cerebral hemodynamics in CADASIL before and after acetazolamide challenge assessed with MRI bolus tracking, *Stroke* (2000) 31:1904–12.

Chabriat H, Pappata S, Poupon C et al, Clinical severity in CADASIL related to ultra-structural damage in white matter: *in vivo* study with diffusion tensor MRI, *Stroke* (1999) 30:2637–43.

Chabriat H, Vahedi K, Iba-Zizen MT et al, Clinical spectrum of CADASIL: a study of 7 families. Cerebral autosomal dominant arteriopathy with subcortical infarcts and leukoencephalopathy, *Lancet* (1995a) **346**:934–9.

DeBaun MR, Schatz J, Siegel MJ et al, Cognitive screening examinations for silent cerebral infarcts in sickle cell disease, *Neurology* (1998) **50**:1678–82.

Desmond DW, Moroney JT, Lynch T et al, The natural history of CADASIL: a pooled analysis of previously published cases, *Stroke* (1999) **30**:1230–3.

Dichgans M, CADASIL: a monogenic condition causing stroke and subcortical vascular dementia, *Cerebrovasc Dis* (2002) **13** (Suppl 2):37–41.

Dichgans M, Filippi M, Bruning R et al, Quantitative MRI in CADASIL: correlation with disability and cognitive performance, *Neurology* (1999b) **52**:1361–7.

Dichgans M, Herzog J, Gasser T, *Notch 3* in-frame deletion involving three cysteine residues causes typical CADASIL, *Neurology* (2001) **57**:1714–17.

Dichgans M, Holtmannspötter K, Herzog J et al, Cerebral microbleeds in CADASIL: a gradient-echo MRI and autopsy study, *Stroke* (2002) **33**:67–71.

Dichgans M, Ludwig H, Müller-Höcker J et al, Small in-frame deletions and missense mutations in CADASIL: 3D models predict misfolding of Notch 3 EGF-like repeat domains, *Eur J Hum Genet* (2000) **8**:280–5.

Dichgans M, Mayer M, Uttner I et al, The phenotypic spectrum of CADASIL: clinical findings in 102 cases, *Ann Neurol* (1998) **44**:731–9.

Dichgans M, Petersen D, Angiographic complications in CADASIL. *Lancet* (1997) **349**:776–7.

Dichgans M, Wick M, Gasser T, Cerebrospinal fluid findings in CADASIL. *Neurology* (1999a) **53**:233.

Ellie E, Camou F, Vital A et al, Recurrent subarachnoid hemorrhage associated with a new transthyretin variant (Gly53Glu), *Neurology* (2001) **57**:135–7.

Fassbender K, Simons M, Bergmann C et al, Simvastatin strongly reduces levels of Alzheimer's disease beta-amyloid peptides Abeta 42 and Abeta 40 *in vitro* and *in vivo*, *Proc Natl Acad Sci USA* (2001) **98**:5856–61.

Feuerhake F, Volk B, Ostertag B et al, Reversible coma with raised intracranial pressure: an unusual clinical manifestation of CADASIL, *Acta Neuropathol (Berl)* (2002) **103**:188–92.

Filley CM, Thompson LL, Sze CI et al, White matter dementia in CADASIL, *J Neurol Sci* (1999) **163**:163–7.

Forteza AM, Brozman B, Rabinstein AA et al, Acetazolamide for the treatment of migraine with aura in CADASIL, *Neurology* (2001) **57**:2144–5.

Garzuly F, Vidal R, Wisniewski T et al, Familial meningocerebrovascular amyloidosis, Hungarian type, with mutant transthyretin (TTR Asp18Gly), *Neurology* (1996) **47**:1562–7.

Grabowski TJ, Cho HS, Vonsattel JP et al, Novel amyloid precursor protein mutation in an Iowa family with dementia and severe cerebral amyloid angiopathy, *Ann Neurol* (1996) **49**:697–705.

Gray F, Dubas F, Roullet E, Escourolle, R et al, Leukoencephalopathy in diffuse hemorrhagic cerebral amyloid angiopathy, *Ann Neurol* (1985) **18**:54–9.

Greenberg SM, Cerebral amyloid angiopathy and vessel dysfunction, *Cerebrovasc Dis* (2002a) **13** (Suppl 2):42–7.

Greenberg SM, Cerebral amyloid angiopathy and dementia: two amyloids are worse than one, *Neurology* (2002b) **58**:1587–8.

Gudmundsson G, Hallgrimsson J, Jonasson TA, Bjarnason O, Hereditary cerebral haemorrhage with amyloidosis, *Brain* (1972) **95**:387–404.

Gutierrez-Molina M, Caminero RA, Martinez GC et al, Small arterial granular degeneration in familial Binswanger's syndrome, *Acta Neuropathol (Berl)* (1984) **87**:98–105.

Haan J, Bakker E, Jennekens-Schinkel A, Roos RA, Progressive dementia, without cerebral hemorrhage, in a patient with hereditary cerebral amyloid angiopathy, *Clin Neurol Neurosurg* (1992) **94**:317–18.

Haan J, Lanser JB, Zijderveld I et al, Dementia in hereditary cerebral hemorrhage with amyloidosis–Dutch type, *Arch Neurol* (1990) **47**:965–7.

Hedera P, Friedland RP, Cerebral autosomal dominant arteriopathy with subcortical infarcts and leukoencephalopathy: study of two American families with predominant dementia, *J Neurol Sci* (1997) **146**:27–33.

Holton JL, Ghiso J, Lashley T et al, Regional distribution of amyloid-Bri deposition and its association with neurofibrillary degeneration in familial British dementia, *Am J Pathol* (2001) **158**:515–26.

Holton JL, Lashley T, Ghiso J et al, Familial Danish dementia: a novel form of cerebral amyloidosis associated with deposition of both amyloid-Dan and amyloid-beta, *J Neuropathol Exp Neurol* (2002) **61**:254–67.

Hutchinson M, O'Riordan J, Javed M et al, Familial hemiplegic migraine and autosomal dominant arteriopathy with leukoencephalopathy (CADASIL). *Ann Neurol* (1995) **38**:817–24.

Iannucci G, Dichgans M, Rovaris M et al, Correlations between clinical findings and magnetization transfer imaging metrics of tissue damage in individuals with cerebral autosomal dominant arteriopathy with subcortical infarcts and leukoencephalopathy, *Stroke* (2001) **32**:643–8.

Jensson O, Gudmundsson G, Arnason A et al, Hereditary cystatin C (gamma-trace) amyloid angiopathy of the CNS causing cerebral hemorrhage, *Acta Neurol Scand* (1987) **76**:102–14.

Joutel A, Andreux F, Gaulis S et al, The ectodomain of Notch3 receptor accumulates within the cerebrovasculature of CADASIL patients, *J Clin Invest* (2000b) **105**:597–605.

Joutel A, Chabriat H, Vahedi K et al, Splice site mutation causing a 7 amino-acids Notch3 in-frame deletion in CADASIL, *Neurology* (2000a) **54**:1874–5.

Joutel A, Corpechot C, Ducros A et al, Notch3 mutations in CADASIL, a hereditary adult-onset condition causing stroke and dementia, *Nature* (1996) **383**:707–10.

Joutel A, Favrole P, Labauge P et al, Skin biopsy immunostaining with a Notch3 monoclonal antibody for CADASIL diagnosis, *Lancet* (2001) **358**:2049–51.

Joutel A, Vahedi K, Corpechot C et al, Strong clustering and stereotyped nature of Notch3 mutations in CADASIL patients, *Lancet* (1997) **350**:1511–15.

Kiuru S, Salonen O, Haltia M, Gelsolin-related spinal and cerebral amyloid angiopathy, *Ann Neurol* (1999) **45**:305–11.

Knudsen KA, Rosand J, Karluk D, Greenberg SM, Clinical diagnosis of cerebral amyloid angiopathy: validation of the Boston criteria, *Neurology* (2001) **56**:537–9.

Lagas PA, Juvonen V, Schizophrenia in a patient with cerebral autosomally dominant arteriopathy with subcortical infarcts and leucoencephalopathy (CADASIL disease), *Nord J Psychiatry* (2001) **55**:41–2.

Le Ber I, Carluer L, Derache N et al, Unusual presentation of CADASIL with reversible coma and confusion, *Neurology* (2002) **59**:1115–16.

Liebetrau M, Herzog J, Hamann G, Dichgans M, Prolonged cerebral transit time in CADASIL: a transcranial ultrasound study, *Stroke* (2002) **33**:509–12.

Mascalchi M, Salvi F, Pirini MG et al, Transthyretin amyloidosis and superficial siderosis of the CNS, *Neurology* (1999) **53**:1498–503.

Mayer M, Straube A, Bruening R et al, Muscle and skin biopsies are a sensitive diagnostic tool in the diagnosis of CADASIL, *J Neurol* (1999) **246**:526–32.

Mead S, James-Galton M, Revesz T et al, Familial British dementia with amyloid angiopathy: early clinical, neuropsychological and imaging findings, *Brain* (2000) **123**:975–91.

Mellies JK, Baumer T, Muller JA et al, SPECT study of a German CADASIL family: a phenotype with migraine and progressive dementia only, *Neurology* (1998) **50**:1715–21.

Mendez MF, Stanley TM, Medel NM et al, The vascular dementia of Fabry's disease, *Dement Geriatr Cogn Disord* (1997) **8**:252–7.

Miravalle L, Tokuda T, Chiarle R et al, Substitutions at codon 22 of Alzheimer's abeta peptide induce diverse conformational changes and apoptotic effects in human cerebral endothelial cells, *J Biol Chem* (2000) **275**:27110–16.

Molina C, Sabin JA, Montaner J et al, Impaired cerebrovascular reactivity as a risk marker for first-ever lacunar infarction: a case-control study, *Stroke* (1999) **30**:2296–301.

Mueggler T, Sturchler-Pierrat C, Baumann D et al, Compromised hemodynamic response in amyloid precursor protein transgenic mice, *J Neurosci* (2002) **22**:7218–24.

Murakami K, Irie K, Morimoto A et al, Synthesis, aggregation, neurotoxicity, and secondary structure of various A beta 1-42 mutants of familial Alzheimer's disease at positions 21–23, *Biochem Biophys Res Commun* (2002) **294**:5–10.

Natte R, Maat-Schieman ML, Haan J et al, Dementia in hereditary cerebral hemorrhage with amyloidosis-Dutch type is associated with cerebral amyloid angiopathy but is independent of plaques and neurofibrillary tangles, *Ann Neurol* (2001) **50**:765–72.

Nilsberth C, Westlind-Danielsson A, Eckman CB et al, The 'Arctic' APP mutation (E693G) causes Alzheimer's disease by enhanced Abeta protofibril formation, *Nat Neurosci* (2001) **4**:887–93.

Oberstein SA, Ferrari MD, Bakker E et al, Diagnostic Notch3 sequence analysis in CADASIL: three new mutations in Dutch patients. Dutch CADASIL Research Group, *Neurology* (1999) **52**:1913–15.

Olafsson I, Thorsteinsson L, Jensson O, The molecular pathology of hereditary cystatin C amyloid angiopathy causing brain hemorrhage, *Brain Pathol* (1996) **6**:121–6.

O'Sullivan M, Jarosz JM, Martin RJ et al, MRI hyperintensities of the temporal lobe and external capsule in patients with CADASIL, *Neurology* (2001) **56**:628–34.

Petersen RB, Goren H, Cohen M et al, Transthyretin amyloidosis: a new mutation associated with dementia, *Ann Neurol* (1997) **41**:307–13.

Pfefferkorn T, von Stuckrat-Barre S, Herzog J et al, Reduced cerebrovascular C02 reactivity in CADASIL: a transcranial doppler sonography study, *Stroke* (2001) **32**:17–21.

Pfeifer LA, White LR, Ross GW et al, Cerebral amyloid angiopathy and cognitive function: the HAAS autopsy study, *Neurology* (2002) **58**:1629–34.

Plant GT, Revesz T, Barnard RO et al, Familial cerebral amyloid angiopathy with non-neuritic amyloid plaque formation, *Brain* (1990) **113**:721–47.

Revesz T, Holton JL, Lashley T et al, Sporadic and familial cerebral amyloid angiopathies, *Brain Pathol* (2002) **12**:343–57.

Roks G, van Harskamp F, De Koning I et al, Presentation of amyloidosis in carriers of the codon 692 mutation in the amyloid precursor protein gene (APP692), *Brain* (2000) **123**:2130–40.

Rubio A, Rifkin D, Powers JM et al, Phenotypic variability of CADASIL and novel morphologic findings, *Acta Neuropathol (Berl)* (1997) **94**:247–54.

Ruchoux MM, Chabriat H, Bousser MG et al, Presence of ultrastructural arterial lesions in muscle and skin vessels of patients with CADASIL, *Stroke* (1994) **25**:2291–2.

Ruchoux MM, Guerouaou D, Vandenhaute B et al, Systemic vascular smooth muscle cell impairment in cerebral autosomal dominant arteriopathy with subcortical infarcts and leukoencephalopathy, *Acta Neuropathol (Berl)* (1995) **89**:500–12.

Ruchoux MM, Maurage CA, CADASIL: cerebral autosomal dominant arteriopathy with subcortical infarcts and leukoencephalopathy, *J Neuropathol Exp Neurol* (1997) **56**:947–64.

Ruchoux MM, Domenga V, Brulin P et al, Transgenic mice expressing mutant notch3 develop vascular alterations characteristic of cerebral autosomal dominant arteriopathy with subcortical infarcts and leukoencephalopathy, *Am J Pathol* (2003) **162**:329–42.

Sakashita N, Ando Y, Jinnouchi K et al, Familial amyloidotic polyneuropathy (ATTR Val30Met) with widespread cerebral amyloid angiopathy and lethal cerebral hemorrhage, *Pathol Int* (2001) **51**:476–80.

Schatz J, Brown RT, Pascual JM et al, Poor school and cognitive functioning with silent cerebral infarcts and sickle cell disease, *Neurology* (2001) **56**:1109–11.

Schenk D, Opinion: amyloid-beta immunotherapy for Alzheimer's disease: the end of the beginning, *Nat Rev Neurosci* (2002) **3**:824–8.

Simons M, Schwarzler F, Lutjohann D et al, Treatment with simvastatin in normocholesterolemic patients with Alzheimer's disease: a 26-week randomized, placebo-controlled, double-blind trial, *Ann Neurol* (2002) **52**:346–50.

Sisodia SS, George-Hyslop PH, gamma-Secretase, Notch, Abeta and Alzheimer's disease: where do the presenilins fit in? *Nat Rev Neurosci* (2002) **3**:281–90.

Sourander P, Walinder J, Hereditary multi-infarct dementia. Morphological and clinical studies of a new disease, *Acta Neuropathol (Berl)* (1979) **39**:247–54.

Stromgren E, Dalby A, Dalby MA, Ranheim, B, Cataract, deafness, cerebellar ataxia, psychosis and dementia – a new syndrome, *Acta Neurol Scand* (1970) **46** (Suppl 43):261.

Sveinbjornsdottir S, Blondal H, Gudmundsson G et al, Progressive dementia and leucoencephalopathy as the initial presentation of late onset hereditary cystatin-C amyloidosis. Clinicopathological presentation of two cases, *J Neurol Sci* (1996) **140**:101–8.

Taillia H, Chabriat H, Kurtz A et al, Cognitive alterations in non-demented CADASIL patients, *Cerebrovasc Dis* (1998) **8**:97–101.

Terborg C, Gora F, Weiller C, Rother J, Reduced vasomotor reactivity in cerebral microangiopathy: a study with near-infrared spectroscopy and transcranial Doppler sonography, *Stroke* (2000) **31**:924–9.

Tournier-Lasserve E, Joutel A, Melki J et al, Cerebral autosomal dominant arteriopathy with subcortical infarcts and leukoencephalopathy maps to chromosome 19q12, *Nat Genet* (1993) **3**:256–9.

Trojano L, Ragno M, Manca A, Caruso G, A kindred affected by cerebral autosomal dominant arteriopathy with subcortical infarcts and leukoencephalopathy (CADASIL). A 2-year neuropsychological follow-up, *J Neurol* (1998) **245**:217–22.

Tuominen S, Juvonen V, Amberla K et al, Phenotype of a homozygous CADASIL patient in comparison to 9 age-matched heterozygous patients with the same R133C Notch3 mutation, *Stroke* (2001) **32**:1767–74.

Van Nostrand WE, Melchor JP, Cho HS et al, Pathogenic effects of D23N Iowa mutant amyloid beta-protein, *J Biol Chem* (2001) **276**:32860–6.

Vidal R, Frangione B, Rostagno A et al, A stop-codon mutation in the BRI gene associated with familial British dementia, *Nature* (1999) **399**:776–81.

Vidal R, Garzuly F, Budka H et al, Meningocerebrovascular amyloidosis associated with a novel transthyretin mis-sense mutation at codon 18 (TTRD 18G), *Am J Pathol* (1996) **148**:361–6.

Vidal R, Revesz T, Rostagno A et al, A decamer duplication in the 3' region of the BRI gene originates an amyloid peptide that is associated with dementia in a Danish kindred, *Proc Natl Acad Sci USA* (2000) **97**:4920–5.

Vinters HV, Cerebral amyloid angiopathy. A critical review, *Stroke* (1987) **18**:311–24.

Vinters HV, Nishimura GS, Secor DL, Pardridge WM, Immunoreactive A4 and gamma-trace peptide colocalization in amyloidotic arteriolar lesions in brains of patients with Alzheimer's disease, *Am J Pathol* (1990) **137**:233–40.

Wang W, Campos AH, Prince CZ et al, Coordinate Notch3-hairy-related transcription factor pathway regulation in response to arterial injury. Mediator role of platelet-derived growth factor and ERK, *J Biol Chem* (2002a) **277**:23165–71.

Wang W, Prince C, Mou Y, Pollman MJ, Notch3 signaling in vascular smooth muscle cells induces c-FLIP expression via ERK/MAPK activation: resistance to FasL-induced apoptosis, *J Biol Chem* (2002b) **277**:21723–9..

Wattendorff AR, Frangione B, Luyendijk W, Bots GT, Hereditary cerebral haemorrhage with amyloidosis, Dutch type (HCHWA-D): clinicopathological studies, *J Neurol Neurosurg Psychiatry* (1995) **58**:699–705.

Wielaard R, Bornebroek M, Ophoff RA et al, A four-generation Dutch family with cerebral autosomal dominant arteriopathy with subcortical infarcts and leukoencephalopathy (CADASIL), linked to chromosome 19p13, *Clin Neurol Neurosurg* (1995) **97**:307–13.

Yousry TA, Seelos K, Mayer M et al, Characteristic MR lesion pattern and correlation of T1 and T2 lesion volume with neurologic and neuropsychological findings in cerebral autosomal dominant arteriopathy with subcortical infarcts and leukoencephalopathy (CADASIL), *Am J Neuroradiol* (1999) **20**:91–100.

Zhang F, Eckman C, Younkin S et al, Increased susceptibility to ischemic brain damage in transgenic mice overexpressing the amyloid precursor protein, *J Neurosci* (1997) **17**:7655–61.

chapter 13

Homocysteine, cerebrovascular disease, cognitive function and aging

Katherine L Tucker, Tammy M Scott and Marshal Folstein

Introduction

Memory deficit and dementia are common among elderly individuals. Prevention of most types of cognitive impairment is not possible because we do not understand the pathogenesis of the diseases, such as Alzheimer's disease (AD), that cause impairment. It has long been known that deficiency of vitamins such as niacin, vitamin B_{12} and thiamine cause cognitive impairment, and that replacement of deficient nutrients can prevent or ameliorate those forms of cognitive impairment that are caused by deficiency. However, new studies suggest that even moderately low or subclinically deficient levels of B vitamins are associated with cognitive impairment and other psychiatric disorders. In this chapter, we review the possible link between homocysteine and associated B vitamins as a contributing causal pathway to cognitive decline and dementia.

Homocysteine is a known risk factor for cardiovascular disease, and elevated homocysteine concentrations have been shown to result in atherosclerosis and stroke in many studies. A meta-analysis of 27 studies calculated a summary odds ratio of 1.9 for every 5 μmol/l of homocysteine (Boushey et al, 1995). Subsequent prospective studies have shown a mixture of positive risk associations with myocardial infarction and stroke (Perry et al, 1995; Ridker et al, 1999; Bostom et al, 1999; Bots et al, 1999; Maxwell et al, 2002) and null findings (Evans et al, 1997; Folsom et al, 1998; Fallon et al, 2001). Because the effects on the vasculature that contribute to heart disease and stroke are also likely to increase risk of vascular dementia (VaD), it has more recently been hypothesized that inadequate B vitamin status and high homocysteine may also contribute to cognitive decline through silent brain infarction (Matsui et al, 2001).

While severe vitamin deficiencies or congenital defects are not common, milder sub-clinical B vitamin deficiencies are prevalent in the elderly. The importance of these deficiencies to cognitive function in later years of life is not yet known. There is considerable evidence that subclinical vitamin deficiencies are prevalent (Tucker et al, 2000; van Asselt et al, 1998; Lindenbaum et al, 1994; Joosten et al, 1993). Should these inadequacies of B vitamins contribute to cognitive decline, it is possible that intervention could significantly reduce the public health costs of dementia.

Associative studies on B vitamins, homocysteine and cognitive function

An accumulating number of studies have linked nutritional deficiencies to poor cognitive function and dementia. Healthy, independently living elderly individuals with 'subclinical' malnutrition, as measured by relatively low B vitamin concentrations, have been shown to score lower than average on tests of verbal memory and nonverbal abstract reasoning compared to their nondeficient peers. The Mini-Mental State Examination (MMSE) (Folstein et al, 1975) and other tests have shown cognitive impairment associated with poor B vitamin status in geriatric patients (Bell et al, 1990; Franchi et al, 2001), AD patients and free-living elderly subjects (Bernard et al, 1998). Studies using more extensive neuropsychological batteries have found significant associations of levels of B vitamins, homocysteine and antioxidants with scores obtained on tests of executive functioning (Robins Wahlin et al, 2001), visuospatial skills and short term memory.

In addition, studies have found that patients with dementia, especially AD, have lower serum concentrations of B vitamins (Karnaze and Carmel, 1987; Ikeda et al, 1990; Clarke et al, 1998; Serot et al, 2001; McIlroy et al, 2002) and serum concentrations of these micronutrients have also been related to the severity of the disease (Snowdon et al, 2000; Sommer and Wolkowitz, 1988). Several have also found that patients with AD had significantly higher concentrations of serum total homocysteine than did age-matched hospitalized controls (Joosten et al, 1997) and healthy community-dwelling elderly individuals. In a small study by Leblhuber et al (2001) consisting of 19 AD patients, 12 VaD patients and 19 control subjects, homocysteine concentrations were significantly higher in both dementia groups as compared to controls. Approximately 40% of AD patients have been found to have elevated homocysteine concentrations (Clarke et al, 1998; Gottfries et al, 1998). Combining AD patients with controls, however, Miller et al (2002) found that high homocysteine was associated with VaD, but not with AD diagnosis. Rather, they found that low vitamin B_6 status was associated with AD, and suggested that this vitamin, which is an essential cofactor for enzymes involved in neurotransmitter synthesis, may be of greater importance to prevention of AD than is homocysteine, acknowledging that further research is needed in this area.

Recent reports have also been highly suggestive of an association between homocysteine and brain morphology. In community dwelling elderly subjects without clinical memory problems, hippocampal width was inversely associated with homocysteine concentration, suggesting that homocysteine may damage the hippocampus (Williams et al, 2002). Hippocampal atrophy on magnetic resonance imaging (MRI) has been associated with impaired memory performance in healthy elderly people (O'Brien et al, 1997) and patient populations (Lencz et al, 1992; Bremner et al, 1993; Scott, 1993).

MRI analysis is also useful in measuring brain infarcts and white matter damage. In the Rotterdam study, silent brain infarcts were seen to be 2.5 times as frequent, and white matter lesions more than twice as likely, in the highest versus lowest quintile of homocysteine concentration (Vermeer et al, 2002). Using computed tomographic (CT) scanning, Hogervorst et al (2002) found an odds ratio for moderate-to-severe cerebral white matter changes (leukoaraiosis) of 1.4 for each 5 µmol/l of homocysteine in a combined sample of AD patients and age-matched controls (adjusted for diagnosis). Moderate to severe leukoaraiosis was three times more common in AD cases than in age-matched controls and was associated with homocysteine with an odds ratio of 2.0 per 5 µmol/l in cases alone.

Longitudinal studies of B vitamins, homocysteine and cognitive decline

The growing number of cross-sectional studies is highly suggestive but leads to the question of whether the associated poor B vitamin status and elevated homocysteine are a product of the disease (possibly secondary to decreased dietary intake) or whether these micronutrient inadequacies are responsible for some of the cognitive impairments that are evident in these patients. In autosomal recessive disorders of methionine metabolism leading to high homocysteine (the variations of homocystinuria), young individuals develop cognitive impairment and cerebrovascular disease (McCully, 1969). This suggests that cognitive impairment and brain disease can be *caused* by elevated homocysteine and related compounds and that in these cases the elevation is not secondary to the dementia. Other examples of disorders in which micronutrient deficiencies have been demonstrated to *cause* cognitive impairment include Wernicke–Korsakoff syndrome (thiamine) (Victor and Adams, 1953; Butters, 1981), pernicious anemia (B_{12}) (Hector and Burton, 1988), pellagra (niacin) and neural tube defects (maternal folate deficiency) (Allen, 1996).

Longitudinal studies generally support the hypothesis that low B vitamin status and high homocysteine are causal contributors to cognitive decline and dementia. In studies by La Rue et al (1997) and Ebly et al (1998), past micronutrient intakes were predictive of current cognitive performance. McCaddon et al (2001) found that higher baseline homocysteine predicted greater five-year declines in MMSE scores. Most recently, the Epidemiology of Vascular Ageing (EVA) Study from France found consistent positive associations between homocysteine and cognitive decline (Dufouil et al, 2003). Comparing people with baseline homocysteine greater than 15 µmol/l versus <10 µmol/l, two-year declines differed significantly for the MMSE ($p < 0.05$), for measures of attention (digit symbol substitution; $p < 0.004$) and psychomotor speed (finger tapping; $p < 0.0001$).

One large prospective study, the Rotterdam Study, did not find an association between homocysteine levels and cognitive decline, as measured by the MMSE, over a 2.7-year follow-up (Kalmijn et al, 1999). However, a more recent cross-sectional analysis from the same Rotterdam Study, using more sensitive cognitive tests, found that elevated homocysteine was associated with significantly poorer psychomotor speed (Prins et al, 2002). The authors suggest that the earlier reported lack of association was likely due to the limited sensitivity of the MMSE to measure the relatively small average decline noted over the observed period in that population.

B vitamins and homocysteine have also been associated prospectively with incident cases of dementia and AD (Wang et al, 2001). In Sweden, a three-year follow-up study determined that subjects with low baseline concentrations of folate or vitamin B_{12} were twice as likely to develop AD. Results from the Framingham Heart Study showed clear associations with the incidence of dementia and AD over an eight-year follow-up period (Seshadri et al, 2002).

New imaging techniques are also contributing to understanding these associations. Higher concentrations of homocysteine in AD patients were associated with greater progression of hippocampal atrophy as measured by medial temporal lobe thickness, as well as with a similar (although non-significant) trend in MMSE score decline over a 2.7-year follow-up period (Clarke et al, 1998). In a study by Snowdon et al (2000), neuropathological examinations of the brains of deceased participants of the Nun Study, for whom earlier blood measures were available, were conducted. They found that cerebral atrophy was significantly related to earlier serum folate levels in those individuals with a significant number of AD lesions. In contrast, the EVA study in France found only a nonsignificant ($p = 0.09$) trend for the association between homocysteine concentration and presence of moderate or severe white matter hyperintensities on MRI two years later (Dufouil et al, 2003). Furthermore, this study found that adjustment for these white matter hyperintensities did not weaken the association between homocysteine and cognitive decline, suggesting that these brain lesions may not provide an explanation for the observed association.

Intervention studies

Cognitive recovery following replacement of low B_{12} is related to duration of symptoms, suggesting that early periods of micronutrient deficiency can cause structural damage. Patients with subsequent restoration of vitamin status might present the normal micronutrient concentrations but with vitamin-induced brain damage. The effectiveness of vitamin therapy appears to depend on the duration of cognitive symptoms. In a study by Martin et al (1992), patients who were symptomatic for less than 12 months gained an average of 20 points on the Dementia Rating Scale (DRS) (paired t test $p = 0.0076$) after vitamin therapy. However, patients who were symptomatic for greater than 12 months lost an average of three points (paired t test

$p = 0.34$), regardless of therapy. Another study of elderly dementia patients also found that patients with moderate dementia and elevated homocysteine improved with supplementation of vitamin B_{12} and folic acid. However, those who were severely demented did not improve (Nilsson et al, 2001). Conversely, in a study of relatively healthy elderly subjects with low plasma vitamin B_{12} status and no obvious cognitive impairment, cobalamin supplementation led to reductions in plasma homocysteine and significant improvements on tests of verbal learning and verbal fluency as well as to electrographic signs of improved cerebral function (van Asselt et al, 2001). Together, these studies suggest that early vitamin intervention, preferably before symptoms become obvious, may be effective in preventing cognitive decline in deficient individuals, but that after symptoms have been apparent for some time, impairment may not be reversed with vitamins.

Hypothesized mechanisms

An inverse correlation of serum homocysteine concentration with folate, vitamin B_{12} and vitamin B_6 status is well established. Homocysteine is an intermediate metabolite resulting from the demethylation of methionine, an essential amino acid that is found in protein in foods. Homocysteine is metabolized by two main pathways (Figure 13.1). First, it may be remethylated to methionine, catalyzed by methionine synthase with vitamin B_{12} as a cofactor, and requiring methyltetrahydrofolate as a methyl donor. In the absence of sufficient folate or vitamin B_{12}, homocysteine accumulates and leads to lower concentrations of s-adenosylmethionine (SAM), an important methyl donor, essential for normal methylation of DNA, RNA and neurotransmitters among numerous other molecules essential for normal cell function. A second pathway for homocysteine metabolism is the trans-sulfuration pathway in which homocysteine is converted to cystathionine and then to cysteine by enzymes dependent on vitamin B_6 as a cofactor. Therefore, low vitamin B_6 may also be associated with accumulation of homocysteine (Selhub et al, 2000).

Elevated homocysteine concentrations are typically a function of poor dietary intake and/or poor absorption of B vitamins (Basun et al, 1994; Selhub et al, 1993; Brussaard et al, 1997a,b). Elevated homocysteine is also, but less frequently, found in autosomal recessive disorders (such as homocystinuria) and end-stage renal disease patients (McCully, 1969; Bostom et al, 1996). In these cases, high homocysteine most likely reflects a disruption in the metabolism of folate, vitamin B_{12}, or vitamin B_6 rather than poor intake

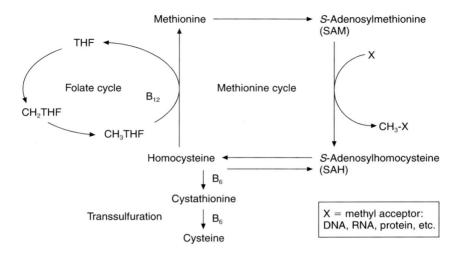

Figure 13.1 *Metabolic pathways associated with homocysteine*

(Selhub et al, 2000). Elevated homocysteine appears to result in atherosclerosis, vasotoxic and excitotoxic effects, leading to small vessel disease cerebral infarcts, and cerebral atrophy (Beal et al, 1990; 1991; Clarke et al, 1998; Fassbender et al, 1999; Lipton et al, 1997; Yoo et al, 1998).

High homocysteine concentrations have been clearly associated with vascular disease (Boushey et al, 1995) and homocysteine has been shown to promote damage to the vascular endothelium and to enhance platelet aggregation. These effects are thought to contribute to the observed association between high plasma homocysteine and occlusion of large vessels in heart disease (Voutilainen et al, 1998). Recent evidence suggests that even moderate hyperhomocystinemia may be an independent risk factor for cerebral infarction and may predict the severity of cerebral atherosclerosis for patients with cerebral infarction (Yoo et al, 1998). Hyperhomocystinemia has also been identified in more than 40% of survivors with stroke and was seen not only in carotid artery disease or lacunar stroke but also in hemorrhagic and embolic strokes (Brattstrom, 1992). In a multiracial, nationally representative sample of US adults, homocysteine concentration was independently associated with an increased likelihood of nonfatal stroke (Giles et al, 1998). In addition to effects on clinically diagnosed stroke, it is possible that these effects of homocysteine also contribute to cognitive decline through repeated 'silent' brain infarcts.

A second mechanism, which is receiving considerable attention, concerns the effects of hypomethylation, resulting from the lower availability of methyl donors when homocysteine is elevated. In addition to reduced SAM under these conditions, there is an accumulation of *s*-adenosylhomocysteine, which is thought to further inhibit methylation through its high-affinity binding to the catalytic region of most SAM-dependent methyltransferases (James et al, 2002). Hypomethylation interferes with protein synthesis and affects neurotransmitter metabolism (Bottiglieri et al, 1995; Alpert and Fava, 1997; Bailey and Gregory, 1999). It may, therefore, lead directly to cognitive impairment through the accumulation of neuronal DNA damage (Mischoulon, 1996; Rosenberg and Miller, 1992). A study using hippocampal cultures in a folic acid-deficient medium or with homocysteine noted that methyl donor deficiency in these conditions caused DNA damage that potentiated Aβ toxicity (Kruman et al, 2002). In a study treating cultured murine cortical neurons with homocysteine, increases in cytosolic calcium, reactive oxygen species, phospho-tau immunoreactivity and other indicators of apoptosis were observed (Ho et al, 2002). These authors noted that the homocysteine mediated apoptosis was reduced by co-treatment with SAM, suggesting that inhibition of methylation reactions mediated the homocysteine induced apoptosis. Homocysteine is thought to have a neurotoxic effect by activating the *N*-methyl-D-aspartate (NMDA) receptor, leading to cell death (Lipton et al, 1997; Parnetti et al, 1997). However, Ho et al (2001) did not find that addition of an NMDA channel antagonist to their cultured cortical neurons reduced apoptosis after homocysteine treatment, although it did reduce tau phosphorylation.

Interactions with other proponents of oxidative stress may have a role in the association between homocysteine and cognitive decline. In a study of mouse neuronal cultures, homocysteine was shown to potentiate toxicity from copper. Homocysteine was also found to generate high levels of hydrogen peroxide in the presence of copper and to promote neurotoxicity, suggesting that the combination of high copper and homocysteine may promote oxidant damage to neurons that may lead to AD (White et al, 2001).

Summary

The evidence that poor B vitamin status and resulting high homocysteine concentrations contribute to cognitive decline is increasing rapidly. There are several potential mechanisms and it is likely that the causal pathways are complex. Despite this complexity, the majority of epidemiologic studies find consistent associations between low concentrations of B vitamins, high homocysteine and cognitive function. Despite continuing concern that initially observed cross-sectional associations may be measuring a response to the cognitive decline or dementia rather than a causal process, more recent longitudinal studies and detailed mechanistic work with cell culture suggest that a causal connection is likely. Further studies to confirm and refine the observed associations are needed along with long-term randomized trials to demonstrate the effect of vitamin supplementation in the general population. Should the provision of these vitamins prove to reduce cognitive decline, it could have a major impact on the health and well-being of our aging population.

References

Allen WP, Folic acid in the prevention of birth defects, *Curr Opin Pediatr* (1996) **8**:630–4.

Alpert JE, Fava M, Nutrition and depression: the role of folate, *Nutr Rev* (1997) **55**:145–9.

Bailey LB, Gregory JF, Folate metabolism and requirements, *J Nutr* (1999) **129**:779–82.

Basun H, Fratiglioni L, Winblad B, Cobalamin levels are not reduced in Alzheimer's disease: results from a population-based study, *J Am Geriatr Soc* (1994) **42**:132–6.

Beal MF, Kowall NW, Swartz KJ, Ferrante RJ, Homocysteic acid lesions in rat striatum spare somatostatin-neuropeptide Y (NADPH-diaphorase) neurons, *Neurosci Lett* (1990) **108**:36–42.

Beal MF, Swartz KJ, Finn SF et al, Neurochemical characterization of excitotoxin lesions in the cerebral cortex, *J Neurosci* (1991) **11**:147–58.

Bell IR, Edman JS, Marby DW et al, Vitamin B_{12} and folate status in acute geropsychiatric inpatients: affective and cognitive characteristics of a vitamin nondeficient population, *Biol Psychiatry* (1990) **27**:125–37.

Bernard MA, Nakonezny PA, Kashner TM, The effect of vitamin B_{12} deficiency on older veterans and its relationship to health, *J Am Geriatr Soc* (1998) **46**:1199–206.

Bostom AG, Shemin D, Yoburn D et al, Lack of effect of oral N-acetylcysteine on the acute dialysis-related lowering of total plasma homocysteine in hemodialysis patients, *Atherosclerosis* (1996) **120**:241–4.

Bostom AG, Rosenberg IH, Silbershatz H et al, Nonfasting plasma total homocysteine levels and stroke incidence in elderly persons: the Framingham Study, *Ann Intern Med* (1999) **131**:352–5.

Bots ML, Launer LJ, Lindemans J et al, Homocysteine and short-term risk of myocardial infarction and stroke in the elderly: the Rotterdam Study, *Arch Intern Med* (1999) **159**:38–44.

Bottiglieri T, Crellin RF, Reynolds EH, Folate and neuropsychiatry. In: Bailey LB, ed, *Folate in Health and Disease* (Marcel Dekker: New York, 1995) 435–62.

Boushey CJ, Beresford SA, Omenn GS, Motulsky AG, A quantitative assessment of plasma homocysteine as a risk factor for vascular disease. Probable benefits of increasing folic acid intakes, *JAMA* (1995) **274**:1049–57.

Brattstrom L, Lindgren A, Israelsson B et al, Hyperhomocysteinaemia in stroke: prevalence, cause, and relationships to type of stroke and stroke risk factors, *Eur J Clin Invest* (1992) **22**:214–21.

Bremner JD, Scott TM, Delaney RC et al, Deficits in short-term memory in posttraumatic stress disorder, *Am J Psychiatry* (1993) **150**:1015–19.

Brussaard JH, Lowik MR, van den Berg H et al, Folate intake and status among adults in the Netherlands, *Eur J Clin Nutr* (1997a) **51** (Suppl 3):S46–S50.

Brussaard JH, Lowik MR, van den Berg H et al, Dietary and other determinants of vitamin B_6 parameters, *Eur J Clin Nutr* (1997b) **51** (Suppl 3):S39–S45.

Butters N, The Wernicke–Korsakoff syndrome: a review of psychological, neuropathological and etiological factors, *Curr Alcohol* (1981) **8**:205–32.

Clarke R, Smith AD, Jobst KA et al, Folate, vitamin B_{12}, and serum total homocysteine levels in confirmed Alzheimer disease, *Arch Neurol* (1998) **55**:1449–55.

Dufouil C, Alperovitch A, Ducros V, Tzourio C, Homocysteine, white matter hyperintensities, and cognition in healthy elderly people, *Ann Neurol* (2003) **53**:214–21.

Ebly EM, Schaefer JP, Campbell NR, Hogan DB, Folate status, vascular disease and cognition in elderly Canadians, *Age Ageing* (1998) **27**:485–91.

Evans RW, Shaten BJ, Hempel JD et al, Homocysteine and risk of cardiovascular disease in the Multiple Risk Factor Intervention Trial, *Arterioscler Thromb Vasc Biol* (1997) **17**:1947–53.

Fallon UB, Elwood P, Ben-Shlomo Y et al, Homocysteine and ischaemic stroke in men: the Caerphilly study, *J Epidemiol Comm Health* (2001) **55**:91–6.

Fassbender K, Mielke O, Bertsch T et al, Homocysteine in cerebral macroangiography and microangiopathy, *Lancet* (1999) **353**:1586–7.

Folsom AR, Nieto FJ, McGovern PG et al, Prospective study of coronary heart disease incidence in relation to fasting total homocysteine, related genetic polymorphisms, and B vitamins: the Atherosclerosis Risk in Communities (ARIC) Study *Circulation* (1998) **98**:204–10.

Folstein MF, Folstein SE, McHugh PR, 'Mini-Mental State'. a practical method for grading the cognitive state of patients for the clinician, *J Psychiat Res* (1975) **12**:189–98.

Franchi F, Baio G, Bolognesi AG et al, Deficient folate nutritional status and cognitive performances: results from a retrospective study in male elderly inpatients in a geriatric department, *Arch Gerontol Geriatr* (2001) **33** (Suppl 1):145–50.

Giles WH, Croft JB, Greenlund KJ et al, Total homocysteine concentration and the likelihood of nonfatal stroke: results from the Third National Health and Nutrition Examination Survey, 1988–1994, *Stroke* (1998) **29**:2473–7.

Gottfries CG, Lehmann W, Regland B, Early diagnosis of cognitive impairment in the elderly with the focus on Alzheimer's disease, *J Neural Transm* (1998) **105**:773–86.

Hector M, Burton JR, What are the psychiatric manifestations of vitamin B_{12} deficiency? *J Am Geriatr Soc* (1988) **36**:1105–12.

Ho PI, Ortiz D, Rogers E, Shea TB, Multiple aspects of homocysteine neurotoxicity: glutamate excitotoxicity, kinase hyperactivation and DNA damage, *J Neurosci Res* (2002) **70**:694–702.

Ho PI, Collins SC, Dhitavat S et al, Homocysteine potentiates beta-amyloid neurotoxicity: role of oxidative stress, *J Neurochem* (2001) **78**:249–53.

Hogervorst E, Ribeiro HM, Molyneux A et al, Plasma homocysteine levels, cerebrovascular risk factors, and cerebral white matter changes (leukoaraiosis) in patients with Alzheimer disease, *Arch Neurol* (2002) **59**:787–93.

Ikeda T, Furukawa Y, Mashimoto S et al, Vitamin B_{12} levels in serum and cerebrospinal fluid of people with Alzheimer's disease, *Acta Psychiatr Scand* (1990) **82**:327–9.

James SJ, Melnyk S, Pogribna M et al, Elevation in S-adenosylhomocysteine and DNA hypomethylation: potential epigenetic mechanism for homocysteine-related pathology, *J Nutr* (2002) **132**:2361S–2366S.

Joosten E, van den Berg A, Riezler R et al, Metabolic evidence that deficiencies of vitamin B-12 (cobalamin), folate, and vitamin B-6 occur commonly in elderly people, *Am J Clin Nutr* (1993) **58**:468–76.

Joosten E, Lesaffre E, Riezler R et al, Is metabolic evidence for vitamin B-12 and folate deficiency more frequent in elderly patients with Alzheimer's disease? *J Gerontol* (1997) **52A**:M76–M79.

Kalmijn S, Launer LJ, Lindemans J et al, Total homocysteine and cognitive decline in a community-based sample of elderly subjects, *Am J Epidemiol* (1999) **150**:283–9.

Karnaze DS, Carmel R, Low serum cobalamin levels in primary degenerative dementia: do some patients harbor atypical cobalamin deficiency states? *Arch Intern Med* (1987) **147**:429–31.

Kruman II, Kumaravel TS, Lohani A et al, Folic acid deficiency and homocysteine impair DNA repair in hippocampal neurons and sensitize them to amyloid toxicity in experimental models of Alzheimer's disease, *J Neurosci* (2002) **22**: 1752–62.

La Rue A, Koehler KM, Wayne SJ et al, Nutritional status and cognitive functioning in a normally aging sample: a 6-year reassessment, *Am J Clin Nutr* (1997) **65**:20–9.

Leblhuber F, Walli J, Widner B et al, Homocysteine and B vitamins in dementia, *Am J Clin Nutr* (2001) **73**:127–8.

Lencz T, McCarthy G, Bronen RA et al, Quantitative MR imaging studies in temporal lobe epilepsy: relationship to neuropathology and neuropsychological function, *Ann Neurol* (1992) **31**:629–37.

Lindenbaum J, Rosenberg IH, Wilson PW et al, Prevalence of cobalamin deficiency in the Framingham elderly population, *Am J Clin Nutr* (1994) **60**:2–11.

Lipton SA, Kim WK, Choi YB et al, Neurotoxicity associated with dual actions of homocysteine at the N-methyl-D-aspartate receptor, *Proc Natl Acad Sci USA* (1997) **94**:5923–8.

Martin DC, Francis J, Protetch J, Huff FJ, Time dependency of cognitive recovery with cobalamin replacement: report of a pilot study, *J Am Geriatr Soc* (1992) **40**:168–72.

Matsui T, Arai H, Yuzuriha T et al, Elevated plasma homocysteine levels and risk of silent brain infarction in elderly people, *Stroke* (2001) **32**:1116–19.

Maxwell CJ, Hogan DB, Ebly EM, Serum folate levels and subsequent adverse cerebrovascular outcomes in elderly persons, *Dement Geriatr Cogn Disord* (2002) **13**:225–34.

McCaddon A, Hudson P, Davies G et al, Homocysteine and cognitive decline in healthy elderly, *Dement Geriatr Cogn Disord* (2001) **12**:309–13.

McCully KS, Vascular pathology of homocysteinemia: implications for the pathogenesis of arteriosclerosis, *Am J Pathol* (1969) **56**:111–28.

McIlroy SP, Dynan KB, Lawson JT et al, Moderately elevated plasma homocysteine, methylenetetrahydrofolate reductase genotype, and risk for stroke, vascular dementia, and Alzheimer disease in Northern Ireland, *Stroke* (2002) **33**:2351–6.

Miller JW, Green R, Mungas DM et al, Homocysteine, vitamin B$_6$, and vascular disease in AD patients, *Neurology* (2002) **58**:1471–5.

Mischoulon D, The role of folate in major depression: mechanisms and clinical implications, *Am Soc Clin Psychopharmacol Prog Notes* (1996) **7**:4–5.

Nilsson K, Gustafson L, Hultberg B, Improvement of cognitive functions after cobalamin/folate supplementation in elderly patients with dementia and elevated plasma homocysteine, *Int J Geriatr Psychiatry* (2001) **16**:609–14.

O'Brien JT, Desmond P, Ames D et al, Magnetic resonance imaging correlates of memory impairment in the healthy elderly: association with medial temporal lobe atrophy but not white matter lesions, *Int J Geriatr Psychiatry* (1997) **12**:369–74.

Parnetti L, Bottiglieri T, Lowenthal D, Role of homocysteine in age-related vascular and non-vascular diseases, *Aging (Milano)* (1997) **9**:241–57.

Perry IJ, Refsum H, Morris RW et al, Prospective study of serum total homocysteine concentration and risk of stroke in middle-aged British men, *Lancet* (1995) **346**:1395–8.

Prins ND, Den Heijer T, Hofman A et al, Homocysteine and cognitive function in the elderly: the Rotterdam Scan Study, *Neurology* (2002) **59**:1375–80.

Ridker PM, Manson JE, Buring JE et al, Homocysteine and risk of cardiovascular disease among postmenopausal women, *JAMA* (1999) **281**:1817–21.

Robins Wahlin TB, Wahlin A, Winblad B, Backman L, The influence of serum vitamin B_{12} and folate status on cognitive functioning in very old age, *Biol Psychol* (2001) **56**:247–65.

Rosenberg IH, Miller JW, Nutritional factors in physical and cognitive functions of elderly people, *Am J Clin Nutr* (1992) **55**:1237S–1243S.

Scott T, Hippocampal and Temporal Lobe Magnetic Resonance Volume Measurements as an Index of Memory Impairment in Patients with Temporal Lobe Epilepsy, Doctoral Dissertation (Department of Psychology, Yale University, 1993).

Selhub J, Jacques PF, Wilson PW et al, Vitamin status and intake as primary determinants of homocysteinemia in an elderly population, *JAMA* (1993) **270**:2693–8.

Selhub J, Jacques PF, Bostom AG et al, Relationship between plasma homocysteine and vitamin status in the Framingham Study population. Impact of folic acid fortification, *Public Health Rev* (2000) **28**:117–45.

Serot JM, Christmann D, Dubost T et al, CSF-folate levels are decreased in late-onset AD patients, *J Neural Transm* (2001) **108**:93–9.

Seshadri S, Beiser A, Selhub J et al, Plasma homocysteine as a risk factor for dementia and Alzheimer's disease, *N Engl J Med* (2002) **346**:476–83.

Snowdon DA, Tully CL, Smith CD et al, Serum folate and the severity of atrophy of the neocortex in Alzheimer disease: findings from the Nun Study, *Am J Clin Nutr* (2000) **71**:993–8.

Sommer BR, Wolkowitz OM, RBC folic acid levels and cognitive performance in elderly patients: a preliminary report, *Biol Psychiatry* (1988) **24**:352–4.

Tucker KL, Rich S, Rosenberg I et al, Plasma vitamin B-12 concentrations relate to intake source in the Framingham Offspring Study, *Am J Clin Nutr* (2000) **71**:514–22.

van Asselt DZ, de Groot LC, van Staveren WA et al, Role of cobalamin intake and atrophic gastritis in mild cobalamin deficiency in older Dutch subjects, *Am J Clin Nutr* (1998) **68**:328–34.

Van Asselt DZ, Pasman JW, van Lier HJ et al, Cobalamin supplementation improves cognitive and cerebral function in older, cobalamin-deficient persons, *J Gerontol A Biol Sci Med Sci* (2001) **56**:M775–M779.

Vermeer SE, van Dijk EJ, Koudstaal PJ et al, Homocysteine, silent brain infarcts, and white matter lesions: the Rotterdam Scan Study, *Ann Neurol* (2002) **51**:285–9.

Victor M, Adams RD, The effects of alcohol on the nervous system, *Res Pub Assoc Res Nerv Ment Dis* (1953) **32**:526–73.

Voutilainen S, Alfthan G, Nyyssonen K et al, Association between elevated plasma total homocysteine and increased common carotid artery wall thickness, *Ann Med* (1998) **30**:300–6.

Wang HX, Wahlin A, Basun H et al, Vitamin B(12) and folate in relation to the development of Alzheimer's disease, *Neurology* (2001) **56**:1188–94.

White AR, Huang X, Jobling MF et al, Homocysteine potentiates copper- and amyloid beta peptide-mediated toxicity in primary neuronal cultures: possible risk factors in the Alzheimer's-type neurodegenerative pathways, *J Neurochem* (2001) **76**:1509–20.

always be paid to the mode of onset of the disorder, the duration of symptoms and the way they have progressed.

It is important that the investigation of the patient's symptomatology is comprehensive and well structured. This makes the work easier for the clinician and facilitates the documentation of silent symptoms in various phases of the disease process. It also facilitates the identification of various VaD subtypes. Destruction of even a minor part of the brain causes changes in a number of functions that are difficult to study objectively (Brodal, 1973). A comprehensive investigation enables the clinician to identify symptoms or groups of symptoms that frequently occur in the various dementing illnesses and to follow the intensities of the symptoms over time. A tool for identification of regional brain syndromes in dementia is the Stepwise Comparative Status Analysis (STEP). It is adapted to the physician's way of working and may be used by both specialists and relatively inexperienced physicians (Wallin et al, 1996).

Vascular cognitive impairment

The cognitive syndrome of VaD differs from that of AD. VaD is characterized by predominant executive, subcortical and frontal lobe dysfunction rather than deficits in memory and language function. By requiring impairment in activities of daily living for a diagnosis of dementia, many VaD cases are detected only when the brain damage has reached a degree where successful treatment is no longer possible. Thus, it has been suggested that the traditional concept of dementia should be substituted with a broader category including the whole spectrum of cognitive impairment related to cerebrovascular disease (Bowler and Hachinski, 1995).

Hypoperfusion due to congestive heart failure is a significant risk factor for cognitive decline in old people (Zuccala et al, 2001). The cognitive impairment is correlated with the degree of left-ventricular dysfunction and with systolic blood pressures below 130 mmHg (Pullicino et al, 2001). Other patients at risk include those after coronary-artery bypass graft and those recovering from major surgery, particularly hip fracture repair (Newman et al, 2001), and patients with diabetes and hypertension. Atrial fibrillation has also been associated with impaired cognitive function and dementia (Kilander et al, 1998; Ott et al, 1997). In subjects with atrial fibrillation a reduced cardiac output might be responsible for cerebral hypoperfusion. It has been shown that subjects with atrial fibrillation have twice the frequency of severe periventricular white matter lesions, but are at no increased risk of subcortical white matter lesions (de Leeuw et al, 2000). It has been suggested that periventricular white matter lesions are associated with impaired cognitive performance (de Groot et al, 2000). The periventricular white matter is a vulnerable area because of its terminal arterial supply in this watershed area.

Subtypes of VaD

Different forms of VaD produce clinical pictures that differ to some extent. One part of the clinical presentation consists of symptoms and behavior patterns directly related to the site of the brain damage. These are referred to as primary or deficit symptoms. The other part of the clinical presentation consists of what is called secondary, noncognitive or psychic and behavioral symptoms. These may be connected to the disease process, the patients' personalities, their efforts to compensate for difficulties, side-effects of drugs or an unfavorable psychosocial situation (Gustafson and Hagberg, 1975). Primary symptoms reflect disturbances in different parts of the brain (Table 15.1). These include impaired practical abilities, a lowered ability to interpret sensory impressions, reduced mental speed and motor activity, a reduced ability to take initiatives and personality changes. Primary symptoms also encompass a reduction of memory and abstract thinking.

In one study 31 consecutive patients with the clinical diagnosis of VaD – defined as dementia with pronounced vascular disease – were examined with regard to symptoms reflecting disturbances in various brain regions. Frontal (77%) and subcortical (68%) disturbances were the most common clinical patterns (Wallin et al, 1991); 91% of the VaD patients were characterized by dominance of frontal and/or subcortical symptomatology (Wallin and Blennow, 1996). Slowness in the rate of information processing has been described as a key component of the subcortical symptom complex. This complex also includes behavioral disturbances similar to those seen in patients with frontal damage. Although the patients were defined as VaD in general, most of them appeared to fit into the SVD category.

Multi-infarct dementia

Multiple large complete infarcts, usually from large-vessel occlusions involving cortical areas, may result in a clinical syndrome of dementia

Table 15.1 Symptoms and signs in some regional brain syndromes

Regional brain syndromes	Symptoms and signs
Parietal brain syndrome	Sensory aphasia (fluent aphasia; impaired ability to understand spoken language) Visual agnosia (impaired ability to interpret primary visual acuity or field deficits, e.g. difficulty in identifying a knife) Visuospatial dysfunction (perceptual spatial dysfunction) Body agnosia (inability to orient the body spatially) Apraxia (impaired ability to perform purposeful movements)
Frontal brain syndrome	Emotional bluntness (apathy; indifference; stereotypy; aspontaneity; lack of initiative) Impaired control and modulation of emotions and behavior (disinhibition; tearfulness; inadequate smiling; indolent euphoria) Lack of insight and judgment (loss of tact) Change of oral/dietary/sexual behavior Perseveration Poverty of language
Subcortical brain syndrome	Mental slowness Psychomotor retardation Bilateral pyramidal signs (spasticity; increased tendon reflexes; Babinski's sign; subclonus; paraparetic gait; marche à petits pas) Bilateral extrapyramidal signs (limb rigidity; cogwheel phenomenon; limb tremor; hypokinesia) Pseudobulbar symptoms (positive masseter reflex; compulsive crying; dysarthria; dysphagia)
Global brain syndrome	Memory impairment Disorientation Reduced problem-solving ability Anomia Concentration difficulties Visuospatial disturbances

(Roman et al, 1993). Multi-infarct dementia (MID) is characterized by TIAs or stroke episodes in close time relation to the development of dementia. Stepwise deterioration is considered a hallmark of MID but this is sometimes difficult to identify. The history of illness usually comprises various types of vascular disease. Clinical examination reveals asymmetric neurological signs, such as field of vision deficits, hemiparesis and reflex abnormalities. Erkinjuntti (1987) found the four most common symptoms after stroke in patients with MID to be motor-sensory hemiparesis (22.6%), aphasia (19.5%), vertigo with dysequilibrium (12.3%) and apractic–atactic gait (9.9%). Erkinjuntti also found that patients with MID more often tended to have abrupt onset of cognitive failure, nocturnal confusion and atrial fibrillation than those with SVD.

Strategic infarct dementia

The symptomatology of SID varies with the infarct location (Brun et al, 1988). Certain small deep infarcts may result in significant cognitive impairment or dementia, particularly when the thalamus or the anterior limb or genu of the internal capsule are involved. Some patients may exhibit progressive cognitive decline due to recurrent stroke, whether clinically evident or silent. In addition to infarct volume and location, cerebral atrophy may be another important correlate of dementia in patients with cerebrovascular disorder. Focal, often small, ischemic lesions involving specific regions important for higher cortical functions may cause symptoms. The angular gyrus is one example of the cortical sites. The subcortical sites include the deep gray matter nuclei, white matter pathways between association areas and frontolimbic connections. Other subcortical sites include hippocampal infarcts, thalamic lesions, bifrontal infarcts, bilateral infarcts of the fornix or of the cingulate gyrus, basal forebrain lesions, caudate lesions, lesions in globus pallidus and genu of anterior capsule. Bilateral hippocampal infarcts are mainly characterized by amnesia.

The visual disturbances of cortical stroke often affect the visual pathways coming from the lateral geniculate bodies and next to the occipital cortex. Damage to this part of the visual pathways causes defects of the visual field. Damage after the visual impulses leave the occipital cortex disturb the awareness and translation of what patients see. The stroke may cause optic ataxia and visuospatial disturbances, with difficulty in tasks such as drawing. Other lesions result in disturbances of object recognition, with manifesta-

Table 15.2 Syndromes of misidentification.

Capgras' syndrome	The delusion that significant people have been replaced by identical imposters
Fregoli's syndrome	The patient identifies his persecutor in several persons, the persecutor being accused of changing faces, like an actor
Intermetamorphosis syndrome	The delusion that people have taken on the physical appearance of others
De Clerambault's syndrome	Erotomania or the delusional belief that one is secretly loved by another person

tions such as prosopagnosia and an inability to read written symbols. Prosopagnosia is an inability (not due to eye problems) to recognize faces, visual field defects or dementia. The combination of defects in the left or right visual field and loss of sensation from the same side of the body can cause the patient to behave as if what is on the same side does not exist (hemineglect). An infarct in the posterior part of the brain can cause functional blindness. A stroke may cause complete blindness by lesions to the occipital cortex on both sides. When this cortical blindness is denied, this is Anton's syndrome. A lesion in the left parieto-occipital area of the cortex may cause visual agnosia (Birkett, 1996). Tagawa et al (1990) found that lesions of the right occipital cortex cause spatial agnosia in the left visual field; lesions of the left occipital cortex cause pure alexia and color agnosia; and bilateral lesions in both occipital cortices cause prosopagnosia, color blindness and object agnosia. Difficulty with visual recognition combined with impaired reasoning and memory sometimes produce false recognitions and faulty orientation in place. Unfamiliar things and people tend to be mistaken for familiar things and people may be interpreted as hostile or persecutory. Thus, the patient may misidentify the doctor as an old friend or enemy or a nurse as a relative, the hospital ward may be mistaken for home. Table 15.2 gives an overview of different perceptual deficiency-related syndromes.

Subcortical VaD

SVD, small-vessel disease, is an underdiagnosed type of VaD (Wallin and Blennow, 1996). The term subcortical refers to lesions that predominately involve the basal ganglia, cerebral white matter and the brainstem. SVD incorporates lacunar infarct(s), the clinical entities of 'Binswanger's disease' and 'the lacunar state' (O'Brien et al, 2003). Lacunar infarcts or lacunes are small cavitated ischemic infarcts of less than 15 mm in diameter. They are typically located in the basal ganglia, internal capsule, thalamus, pons, corona radiata and centrum semiovale. Lacunes and white matter lesions are often seen together (Roman et al, 2002).

TIAs or stroke episodes may appear in SVD but are not always present. Hypertension, as well as hypotension, is associated with SVD, and these are often associated with diabetes mellitus and ischemic heart disease. In most cases, these multiple vascular disorders are pronounced and have peripheral complications. The course is seldom stepwise but usually continuous with an insidious onset and is slowly progressive (Pantoni et al, 1996).

Symptoms are caused by the interruption of prefrontal–subcortical circuits by ischemic lesions. These circuits are known to be involved in the executive control of working memory, organization, language, mood, regulation of attention, abstraction, conceptual flexibility, constructional skills, motivation, self-control and socially responsible behavior (Mega and Cummings, 1994). The patients with lesions in these areas may have problems with planning and sequencing, such as cooking, dressing, shopping, and housework. Typical symptoms of SVD are impairment of attention and executive functions, mental and motor slowness, extrapyramidal deficits (rigidity, hypokinesia), bilateral pyramidal deficits (short-step gait; increased reflexes in legs) and personality changes and emotional symptoms (Roman and Royall, 1999; Wallin and Blennow, 1996; Wallin et al, 1991, 2000). Positive masseter reflex may occur. There may be focal neurological symptoms in the form of inability to distinguish between the left and right sides but this finding is not as common as in MID. Emotional bluntness, which may be difficult to separate from mental slowness, is common. When emotional bluntness occurs with subcortical mental deficits, a frontosubcortical symptom pattern is present. Emotionalism or reduced control of emotions is a heightened tendency to cry (or rarely laugh), so that crying occurs more frequently, more easily, more vigorously or in circumstances that previously would have been out of character (Allman, 1991).

Personality change is the cardinal symptom of the frontal brain syndrome. This is also characterized by reduced initiative, impaired judgment, lack of awareness of one's illness, lack of insight, poor language skills, disorientation, perseveration, general disinhibition, loss of volition, disturbance of incentive, gross defects of integrative processes and changed oral and sexual behavior. This may of course lead to antisocial conduct and conflicts with the law. Disinhibition, which is often marked, is seen in social interactions and in some cases in sexual behavior. In some patients, the basic personality may be well preserved until late in the disease. The capacity for judgment may also persist, and a remarkable degree of insight is sometimes retained. In one study, patients with SVD showed relatively greater severe dysfunction of the frontal lobes, as expressed in specific psychiatric and neuropsychological changes, than AD patients matched for age, sex and severity of dementia. They had more severe anosognosia, emotional lability and more severe deficits in tests of planning, sequencing and verbal fluency (Starkstein et al, 1996). Verhey et al (1995) concluded, however, that depression, lack of insight and personality changes do not favor a diagnosis of VaD over that of AD. Reduced power of initiative, emotional lability and loss of insight are very common additional symptoms. The coexistence of apathy with subcortical pathology and cognitive impairment is seen in patients with multiple vascular insults to paramedian diencephalic structures (Marin, 1990). Unmotivated patients who fail to take part in their own rehabilitation may have lesions affecting the frontal lobes, the posterior limb of internal capsule and parts of the thalamus and caudate nucleus (Birkett, 1996). Subtle neurological defects, fatigue and depression may mimic apathy. Some patients may show akinesia and mutism, a state of aspontaneity. They may say 'My mind is empty' or 'I have nothing to say'. Robinson et al (1984) found apathy more strongly associated with lesions in the anterior part of the right hemisphere. Patients with VaD were often less energetic and more unreasonable. Typical early signs of dementia are loss of interest and initiative and inability to perform up to the usual standard. Despite full alertness and the preservation of normal levels of consciousness, the patient fatigues readily on mental effort.

Memory disturbances are present in all patients but do not predominate. Cortical symptoms, such as agnosia, aphasia and apraxia, are often absent. Lacunar dementia, which belongs to the SVD spectrum, may initially produce symptoms such as pure motor hemiparesis or pure sensory stroke or dysarthria (clumsy hand syndrome), homolateral ataxia or other clinical syndromes (Fisher, 1982). Recovery from each event is the rule but the neurological defects gradually accumulate to a state of dementia, combined with pyramidal, extrapyramidal, cerebellar or pseudobulbar symptoms. Bilateral thalamic lesions are characterized by attention deficits, slowing of thought processes, apathy, aphasia, agnosia and apraxia. Paramedian mesencephalic–diencephalic infarcts often cause impairments of ocular motility, co-ordination and gait, attention and mental control. There is a dramatic slowness of response, whether verbal or motor, and the patients are apathetic and lacking motivation. They often fall asleep when left alone but always awake easily (Katz et al, 1987). An association between white matter changes and cognitive function was found in studies that explicitly took into account syndromes reflecting disturbances of the anterior parts of the brain. De Groot et al (2000) found that tasks that involve speed of cognitive processes appear to be more affected by white matter changes than memory tasks.

Cognitive impairment in SVD with pronounced executive dysfunction may be clinically 'silent' to the physician but relatives or carers may report abnormal behavior resulting from lack of strategic planning and reduced speed of cognitive processing. As the disease progresses, patients limit their field of interest, show emotional instability, attention loss, decreased ability to make associations, and have difficulties in shifting from one idea to another, resulting in perseveration. Postural instability can later compromise gait initiation, turning and mobility.

Mixed-type dementia (AD + VaD)

The clinical differentiation of VaD from Alzheimer's disease (AD) with cerebrovascular disease can be difficult. Cerebrovascular disease may coexist with AD, and neurodegenerative AD changes may coexist with VaD (Snowdon et al, 1997). There is even evidence suggesting that mixed AD and VaD is more common than both 'pure' AD and 'pure' VaD (Wade et al, 1987). In studies using computerized tomography the frequency of white matter lesions (WMLs) has been reported to be about 70% in patients with VaD, about 30% in clinically diagnosed AD and about 15% in healthy elderly individuals (Tatemichi and Desmond, 1996). In studies using magnetic resonance imaging, the frequency of WMLs has been even higher. Although WMLs are a common phenomenon, their significance in dementia is unclear. More than 60% of older patients with AD present with incomplete white matter infarction and patients with anterior–choroidal–artery stroke may meet criteria for AD. Vascular risk factors predispose not only to VaD but also to the development of AD. Older patients with mild AD pathology and the presence of one or two basal ganglia lacunes have a much greater risk of clinical expression of dementia. In patients with lacunar stroke, the presence of extensive white matter lesions is a poor prognostic sign and increases the risk of recurrent stroke, dementia and death (Longstreth et al, 1998).

Summary

The variety of symptoms in patients with VaD may reflect the heterogeneity of the pathophysiological processes, as well as of the size, number and locations of the various tissue lesions in these patients. This appears to be true for the infarct-related dementia subtypes (MID and SID) but in SVD a more homogeneous symptom pattern, with emotional reduction, mental slowness and gait deficits seems to predominate. The difference may be explained by the variety of locations of brain lesions in the infarct-related dementias, whereas the subcortical region is the primary site of vascular damage in SVD.

The pronounced variety of symptoms in patients with VaD may also indicate that the phenomenological manifestations of VaD have not yet been clarified. In the view of the authors, an increased interest in the methodology of assessment and analysis of symptoms may contribute to a clearer description of the phenomenology of VaD and consequently to a better understanding of the disorder, including its subtypes and preliminary stages.

References

Allman P, Emotionalism following brain damage, *Behav Neurol* (1991) **4**:57–62.

Birkett P, *The Psychiatry of Stroke* (American Psychiatric Press: Washington DC, 1996) 154.

Bowler JV, Hachinski V, Vascular cognitive impairment: a new approach to vascular dementia, *Baillière's Clin Neurol* (1995) **4**:357–76.

Brodal A, Self-observations and neuro-anatomical considerations after a stroke, *Brain* (1973) **96**:675–94.

Brun A, Gustafson L, Zerebrovaskuläre Erkrankungen. Psychiatrie der Gegenwart, In: Kisker KP, Lauter H, Meyer J-E et al, eds, *Organische Psychosen*, Vol 6 (Springer-Verlag: Heidelberg, 1988) 253–95.

De Groot JC, De Leeuw F-E, Oudkerk M et al, Cerebral white matter lesions and cognitive function: the Rotterdam Scan Study, *Ann Neurol* (2000) **47**:145–51.

De Leeuw F-E, de Groot JC, Oudkerk M et al, Atrial fibrillation and the risk of cerebral white matter lesions, *Neurology* (2000) **54**:1795–800.

Erkinjuntti T, Types of multi-infarct dementia, *Acta Neurol Scand* (1987) **75**:391–9.

Erkinjuntti T, Vascular dementia: challenge of clinical diagnosis, *Int Psychogeriatr* (1997) **9**:51–8.

Fisher CM, Lacunar strokes and infarcts: a review, *Neurology* (1982) **32**:871–6.

Gustafson L, Hagberg B, Dementia with onset in the presenile period: a cross-sectional study, *Acta Psychiatr Scand* (1975) **257**:3–71.

Katz DI, Alexander MP, Mandell A, Dementia following strokes in the mesencephalon and diencephalon, *Arch Neurol* (1987) **44**:1127–33.

Kilander L, Andren B, Nyman H et al, Atrial fibrillation is an independent determinant of low cognitive function. A cross-sectional study in elderly men, *Stroke* (1998) **29**:1816–20.

Longstreth WT Jr, Bernick C, Manolio TA et al, Lacunar infarcts defined by magnetic resonance imaging of 3660 elderly people: the Cardiovascular Health Study, *Arch Neurol* (1998) **55**:1217–25.

Mahler ME, Cummings JL, The behavioural neurology of multi-infarct dementia, *Alzheimer Dis Assoc Disord* (1991) **5**:163–7.

Marin RS, Differential diagnosis and classification of apathy, *Am J Psychiatry* (1990) **147**:22–30.

Mayer-Gross W, Slater E, Roth M. In: *Clinical Psychiatry*, 3rd edn, (Ballière, Tindal & Cassell: London, 1969) 593–7.

Mega MS, Cummings JL, Frontal–subcortical circuits and neuropsychiatric disorders, *J Neuropsychiatry Clin Neurosci* (1994) **6**:358–70.

Newman MF, Kirchner JL, Phillips-Bute B et al, Longitudinal assessment of neurocognitive function after coronary-artery bypass surgery, *N Engl J Med* (2001) **344**:395–402.

O'Brien JT, Erkinjuntti T, Reisberg B et al, Vascular Cognitive Impairment. *Lancet Neurol* (2003) **2**:11–20.

Ott A, Breteler MMB, de Bruyne MC et al, Atrial fibrillation and dementia in a population-based study, *Stroke* (1997) **28**:316–21.

Pantoni L, Garcia JH, Brown GG, Vascular pathology in three cases of progressive cognitive deterioration, *J Neurol Sci* (1996) **135**:131–9.

Pullicino PM, Mifsud V, Wong EH et al, Hypoperfusion-related cerebral ischemia and cardiac left ventricular systolic dysfunction, *J Stroke Cerebrovasc Dis* (2001) **10**:178–82.

Robinson RG, Kubos KL, Starr LB et al, Mood disorders in stroke patients, *Brain* (1984) **107**:81–93.

Roman GC, Tatemichi TK, Erkinjuntti T et al, Vascular dementia: diagnostic criteria for research studies. Report of the NINDS-AIREN International Workshop, *Neurology* (1993) **43**:250–60.

Roman GC, Royall DR, Executive control function: a rational basis for the diagnosis of vascular dementia, *Alzheimer Dis Assoc Disord* (1999) **13**:S69–S80.

Roman GC, Erkinjuntti T, Wallin A et al, Subcortical ischaemic vascular dementia, *Lancet Neurology* (2002) **1**:426–36.

Roth M, The natural history of mental disorders arising in the senium, *J Ment Sci* (1955) **101**:281–301.

Snowdon DA, Greiner LH, Mortimer JA et al, Brain infarction and the clinical expression of Alzheimer disease. The Nun Study, *JAMA* (1997) **277**:813–17.

Starkstein SE, Sabe L, Vazquez S et al, Neuropsychological, psychiatric, and cerebral blood flow findings in vascular dementia and Alzheimer's disease, *Stroke* (1996) **27**:408–14.

Tagawa K, Nagata K, Shishido F, Occipital lobe infarction and positron emission tomography, *Tohoku J Exp Med* (1990) **161**:139–53.

Tatemichi TK, Desmond DW, Epidemiology of vascular dementia. In: Prohovnik I, Wade J, Knezevic S et al eds, *Vascular Dementia. Current Concepts* (Wiley: Chichester, 1996) 41–71.

Verhey FR, Ponds RW, Rozendaal N et al, Depression, insight, and personality changes in Alzheimer's disease and vascular dementia, *J Geriatr Psychiatry Neurol* (1995) **8**:23–7.

Wade JPH, Mirsen TR, Hachinski VC et al, The clinical diagnosis of Alzheimer's disease, *Arch Neurol* (1987) **44**:24–9.

Wallin A, Blennow K, Gottfries CG, Subcortical symptoms predominate in vascular dementia, *Int J Geriatr Psychiatry* (1991) **6**:137–45.

Wallin A, Edman Å, Blennow K et al, Stepwise comparative status analysis (STEP): a tool for identification of regional brain syndromes in dementia, *J Geriatr Psychiatry Neurol* (1996) **9**:185–99.

Wallin A, Blennow K, Clinical subgroups of the Alzheimer syndrome, *Acta Neurol Scand* (1996) **165**:51–7.

Wallin A, Sjögren M, Edman Å et al, Symptoms, vascular risk factors and blood–brain barrier function in relation to CT white-matter changes in dementia, *Eur Neurol* (2000) **44**:229–35.

Zuccala G, Onder G, Pedone C et al, Hypotension and cognitive impairment: Selective association in patients with heart failure, *Neurology* (2001) **57**:1986–92.

chapter 16

Vascular mild cognitive impairment and cognitive impairment after stroke

Sally Stephens, Stuart Sadler, Elise Rowan, Michael Bradbury and Clive Ballard

Introduction

The detection of preclinical dementia has become an important focus of clinical research to enable investigation and early treatment. Alzheimer's disease (AD) is the most common dementia accounting for at least 50% of cases. Operationalized criteria for dementia emphasize early and prominent memory loss. This assumption is not necessarily valid for those with mild cognitive deficits or dementia related to cerebrovascular disease.

Classification of vascular dementia

Vascular dementia (VaD) can be defined as a syndrome of acquired cognitive impairment due to cerebrovascular disorder (Tatemichi et al, 1994(a)). The NINDS AIREN criteria (Roman et al, 1993) describe a number of categories of VaD including multi-infarct dementia, strategic single infarct dementia, extensive white matter disease, hypoperfusion and hemorrhagic dementia, as in the following list.

1. Multi-infarct dementia involves multiple large complete infarcts usually from large vessel occlusions involving cortical and subcortical areas resulting in a clinical syndrome of dementia
2. Strategic single infarct dementia is due to small localized ischemic damage occurring in cortical and subcortical area of the brain that results in specific clinical syndromes. For example, infarcts to the angular gyrus

result in the onset of fluent aphasis, alexia with agraphia, memory disturbance, spatial disorientation and constructional disturbances.

3. Small vessel disease or microvascular disease results from lesions that
   occur in either cortical or subcortical areas of the brain and often involve
   white matter. The lesions result in an occlusion of a single arteriolar or
   arterial lumen that leads to complete lacuna infarct. Critical stenosis of
   multiple small vessels can also occur, resulting in hypoperfusion and
   complete infarcts.

4. White matter disease or leukoaraiosis is frequently noted on structural
   brain imaging. The frequency of white matter disease is found to rise
   steadily with age (Schmidt et al, 1991). It has been found to be associated
   with hypertension, cigarette smoking, low plasma vitamin E, lacunar
   infarcts, low education and hypoxic–ischemic disorders (Gorelick et al,
   1999).

5. Hypoperfusion results from a global brain ischemia secondary to cardiac
   arrest or profound hypertension, or from restricted ischemia that has
   occurred in the border zones between two main arterial territories. Hemorrhagic dementia occurs due to chronic subdural hematoma, sequelae of
   subarachnoid hemorrhage and a cerebral hematoma, and is often associated with amyloid angiopathy.

How cerebrovascular pathology leads to dementia or cognitive impairments
is not known. The volume of cerebral infarct is an important determinate of
cognitive impairment. In one series all patients experiencing dementia have
infarct volumes exceeding 50 ml (Tomlinson et al, 1970). However, Esiri et al
(1997) reported that microvascular disease rather than macroscopic
infarction was the main association of dementia in patients with cerebrovascular disease. In addition, the overlap of cerebrovascular and neurodegenerative pathologies (Snowdon et al, 1997) or concurrent cholinergic deficits
(Perry et al, 1978) are likely to be important. For example Del Ser et al (1990)
report that depending upon the definitions 60–90% of AD cases have cerebrovascular pathology. Vascular lesions worsen the level of cognitive deficits
in AD patients (Snowdon et al, 1997; Esiri et al, 1999). In addition, traditional vascular risk factors such as arteriosclerosis, hypertension, diabetes
mellitus and smoking are also risk factors for the development of AD (Skoog,
1998; Merchant et al, 1999; Kuusisto et al, 1997; Leibson et al, 1997).

Vascular cognitive impairment (VCI)

Hachinski and Bowler (1993) first described Vascular Cognitive Impairment (VCI) as an umbrella term encompassing all levels of cognitive decline related to cerebrovascular disease, from the earliest steps to severe dementia. Rockwood et al (1999) divided VCI into four groups: VCI which does not meet the criteria for dementia (i.e. aphasia following left middle cerebral artery infarction); vascular cognitive impairment, no dementia (CIND); VCI which meets the criteria for dementia (i.e. dementia in the setting of multiple cortical and subcortical strokes – VaD); and VCI presenting with other dementing illnesses (i.e. VCI plus AD or mixed AD/VaD). Since then the concept has been divided again into a collection of syndromes. These include vascular CIND, cortical VaD (equivalent to multi-infarct dementia), subcortical VaD, hyperfusion or cardiogenic dementia, hemorrhagic dementia, hereditary VaD and 'mixed' dementia (AD with evidence of CVD) (Rockwood, 2002). Much of the more recent literature, however, refers to VCI as a 'pre-dementia' syndrome in the context of cerebrovascular disease. This is useful in focusing upon a group of patients, probably at high risk of developing dementia (Rockwood, 2002), for whom there are no established diagnostic criteria.

Vascular CIND, utilizes a combination of clinical and global cognitive criteria to identify cognitive impairment in the absence of dementia and then assigns cases as vascular CIND on the basis of likely etiology. Graham et al (1997) diagnosed CIND in patients from the Canadian Study of Health and Aging (CSHA) study based on the exclusion of dementia and the presence of various categories of impairment identified in a clinical examination and in a battery of neuropsychological tests. CIND cases came from those who were below the modified Mini-Mental State Examination cut-off score but did not meet the criteria for dementia. Di Carlo et al (2000) utilized the concept CIND in a longitudinal study of an Italian population. Their criteria for CIND required the exclusion of dementia, a CAMCOG total score lower than 80 and a clinical judgment based on direct examination, evaluation of neuropsychological tests, informant interview, Hamilton Depression Scale and assessment of functional activities according to the Pfeffer Questionnaire.

Whilst these criteria have good face validity, their predictive value has not been fully established. In addition there are a number of other possible approaches which could have potential value. For example, concepts developed for the identification of 'pre-Alzheimer's disease might be usefully applied to the identification of VCI and to determine whether the specific profile of cognitive deficits related to cerebrovascular disease may improve the sensitivity of early identification.

Mild Cognitive Impairment and Alzheimer's disease

Mild Cognitive Impairment (MCI; Petersen et al, 1997) is the most widely used concept for the detection of people with early cognitive deficits who are at increased risk of Alzheimer's disease. The risk of subsequent AD has been estimated as between 4 and 12% p.a. (Petersen et al, 1999; Ritchie et al, 2001; Reisberg et al, 2000).

MCI patients perform memory tasks 1.5 standard deviations below an age-matched control population. MCI patients perform like unimpaired controls on measures of general cognition such as IQ tests. 25% of dementias developing in people with MCI are classified as VaD (Meyer et al, 2002), and in one study a substantial proportion of people with subcortical small vessel dementia exhibited prodromal MCI (Meyer et al, 2002).

As an attempt to address some of the limitations of the MCI concept, the International Pyschogeriatric Association (Levy, 1994) developed a set of criteria referred to as Age-Associated Cognitive Decline (AACD). The disorder is characterized by difficulties in *any* area of cognition, which could include memory and learning, attention and concentration, thinking/executive function (e.g. problem solving; abstraction), language (e.g. comprehension; word finding) or visuospatial functioning. AACD requires impairment of more than one standard deviation below the mean for age-matched controls. The prevalence can be influenced by the choice of cognitive domain and neuropsychological instrument (Hanninen et al, 1996). A large community study indicated that AACD had better predictive value for the development of dementia than MCI (Ritchie et al, 2001) although the predictive value within the context of VCI has not been determined.

Profile of cognitive impairment in vascular dementia and stroke

The cognitive deficits that are characteristic of AD include progressive loss of short-term and long-term memory, language and orientation. Constructional praxis, visual perception, attention and executive function are relatively unimpaired until the latter stages of AD (Huff et al, 1987; Becker et al,

1994). In comparison, VaD patients are likely to have a relative preservation of long-term memory and greater deficits in frontal executive functioning (planning; organization; abstraction; category fluency initiation; reasoning; mental flexibility; sequencing; fine motor performance; the allocation of attentional resources) than AD patients (e.g. Almkvist, 1993; Mendez and Ashla-Mendez, 1991; Villardita et al, 1992; Padovani et al, 1995; Lafosse et al, 1997).

A large proportion of studies have included a broad range of participants with cerebrovascular disease, with or without concurrent neurodegeneration. Around 25% of stroke survivors develop dementia within 12 months of having a stroke (Sacco et al, 1994; Barba et al, 2000; Desmond et al, 2000; Kokmen et al, 1996; Tatemichi et al, 1993), with even higher incidence rates in older stroke survivors (Pohjasvaara et al, 1997; Tatemichi et al, 1994(b)). Few studies have, however, examined the profile of cognitive impairment in these patients. Rao et al (1999) examined the profile of cognitive deficits in a small group of 25 stroke survivors, identifying greater impairment than controls across the majority of cognitive domains examined, including attention, planning and memory. In a much larger study where stroke patients with dementia were excluded, attention, memory, orientation and verbal fluency were all significantly more impaired in stroke patients than in the control group (Tatemichi et al, 1994(a)). More recently Leeds et al (2001) confirmed the presence of a dysexecutive syndrome after stroke. A preliminary report from a larger ongoing study conducted by our group in Newcastle (UK) described in detail the profile of cognitive impairments specifically in older stroke survivors (>75 years of age) without dementia (Ballard et al, 2003). The study sample consisted of 259 subjects (150 elderly stroke survivors, 57 AD, 22VaD and 30 elderly controls). Neuropsychological evaluations were undertaken using the Cambridge Examination for Mental Disorders in the Elderly (CAMCOG) and the Cognitive Drug Research computerized system. The CAMCOG is a 107-item standardized paper and pencil test, which has been shown to be well tolerated and sensitive for the identification of dementia in stroke patients. The schedule includes a detailed evaluation of memory on three subscales (new learning; remote memory; visual memory). The COGDRAS-D is a computerized assessment battery which has been widely used for the evaluation of attention/processing speed and executive function in dementia patients and elderly controls. Specific tasks include Simple Reaction Time (SRT), Choice Reaction Time (CRT), a numerical working memory task and a visuospatial working memory task.

In comparison with age-matched controls, global cognitive deficits are evident, although the most striking decrements are in cognitive processing speed, apparent on both attention and working memory tasks (the latter involving a strong component of executive functioning). In addition digit vigilance accuracy, an attentional task independent of processing speed, was also significantly more impaired in stroke patients. There were significant but less pronounced deficits of memory. The profile of cognitive impairment is summarized in Table 16.1.

To put this in context, the severity of deficits in cognitive processing speed and the magnitude of impairment in vigilance accuracy were similar in older stroke patients without dementia and patients with AD, although the stroke patients had much less pronounced impairment of memory.

Criteria for early cognitive impairment in stroke patients

There are several studies that have now attempted to examine the frequency of patients with VCI, prevalence rates varying from 15 to 20% in clinical settings (Rockwood et al, 2000; Szatmari et al, 1999). As part of an ongoing study in Newcastle, criteria for AACD, MCI and CIND were applied to the same sample of older stroke patients without dementia, to examine potential differences in the number of patients identified as having VCI. Age-related cut-offs on the appropriate cognitive tasks were obtained from an age matched control group. For each computerized task, performance one standard deviation below the performance level of the control group was taken to indicate the presence of AACD from that cognitive domain. Patients were defined as having MCI if they performed 1.5 standard deviations below the level of the control group on the total CAMCOG memory score. Patients were defined as having CIND if they scored less than 80 on the total CAMCOG score and met the clinical criteria (Di Carlo et al, 2000). The relative prevalence of mild but potentially significant VCI varied enormously depending upon the criteria and concept used, and which cognitive domain was assessed. Criteria based upon abnormalities of processing speed identify a much larger proportion of patients than criteria focusing upon memory. This is important in highlighting the different profile of early cognitive impairments in stroke patients compared to those typically reported in the context of Alzheimer's disease. The breakdown is shown in more detail in Table 16.2.

Table 16.1 Cognitive performance in older stroke survivors: a comparison with elderly controls and people with Alzheimer's disease

Cognitive task	Stroke survivors N = 150	Elderly controls N = 30	AD N = 57	Evaluation stroke vs controls	Evaluation stroke vs AD
CAMCOG total	83.2 ± 8.8	96.1 ± 7.4	64.8 ± 15.3	T = 7.5 p <0.0001	T = 8.5 p <0.0001
Memory	20.8 ± 3.1	23.4 ± 3.1	10.2 ± 5.7	T = 3.9 p <0.0001	T = 13.2 p <0.0001
SRT	619.1 ± 415.6	400.1 ± 103.1	634.4 ± 338.0	T = 5.6 p <0.0001	T = 0.25 p = 0.80
CRT	756.4 ± 279.9	569.9 ± 82.0	814.4 ± 415.6	T = 6.8 p <0.0001	T = 1.2 p = 0.26
Vigilance Accuracy	92.4 ± 15.5	98.9 ± 2.5	84.4 ± 5.6	T = 3.5 p = 0.001	T = 2.5 p = 0.01
Spatial working memory	2388.1 ± 1507.5	1480.1 ± 531.7	3194.0 ± 2379.4	T = 4.7 p <0.0001	T = 3.7 p <0.0001

SRT, simple reaction time; CRT, choice reaction time.

Table 16.2 Thresholds for early cognitive impairment in 150 older stroke survivors

Cognitive task	Threshold (1SD) from elderly control group (N = 30)	% Meeting specific sets of criteria for early cognitive deficits
Memory	CAMCOG memory < 20	MCI – 26 (17%)
Global cognition	CAMCOG total < 89	CIND – 48 (32%)
Choice reaction time	> 570 ms	AACD – 110 (73%)
Spatial working memory (accuracy)	< 61%	AACD – 31 (21%)
Spatial working memory (reaction time)	> 2781.1 ms	AACD – 21 (14%)
Digit vigilance accuracy	< 96.4	AACD – 67 (45%)

Patients with VaD or who have experienced strokes indicate that attention, processing speed and executive function are the most frequently and most severely impaired aspects of cognition. In addition, criteria utilizing these aspects of cognition identify higher frequencies of VCI, based upon a five-year follow-up of more than 100 patients with vascular CIND in the Canadian Study of Health and Aging (Ingles et al, 2002) – 44% of these patients developed dementia. Only baseline performance on memory and category fluency tasks was associated with incident dementia. There was no relationship with attentional or executive performance. Although this is a very important study, there are a number of important questions that remain unanswered. For example, as the comparative frequency of incident dementia was not examined in a group of patients with cerebrovascular disease but no evidence of cognitive dysfunction, it has not been clearly established that a diagnosis of vascular CIND identified a group at greater risk of subsequent cognitive decline than other individuals with cerebrovascular disease. In addition, memory dysfunction was significantly associated with the five-year incidence of dementia, the predictors of dementia over a shorter time course may have been different and the comparative value of vascular CIND and other criteria for VCI was not examined. These issues need further clarification in subsequent studies.

The substrates of mild cognitive deficits after stroke

Previous neuroimaging and neuropathological studies of cross-sectional design – comparing patients with and without dementia in the context of cerebrovascular disease – suggest that diffuse white matter changes and microvascular disease predict dementia in the context of cerebrovascular disease (Esiri et al, 1997), particularly in people with a small volume of cortical infarcts (Ballard et al, 2000). It is however evident from case series that strategic infarcts can result in dementia in some individuals (Tatemichi et al, 1992; Erkinjuntti et al, 1988). Several preliminary studies have been completed in patients with VCI. Bowler et al (2002) reported an association between VCI and atrophy but no correlation was seen with deep white matter hyperintensities. A trend towards an association was, however, seen between VCI and periventricular hyperintensities, which probably reflects ventricular enlargement as the two are strongly associated. Conversely, Garde et al (2000) reported an association between early VCI and deep white matter hyperintensities in the Rotterdam Study. In Newcastle we have reported preliminary findings from a study examining the relationship between atrophy and white matter hyperintensities on MRI and the profile of cognitive deficits amongst older stroke patients without dementia (Burton et al, 2003).

Significant associations were evident between cognitive impairments and both the severity of white matter lesions and atrophy in key frontostriatal areas. Processing speed, attentional measures and executive function were associated with hyperintensities in the internal capsule, caudate and thalamus. Lesions in these areas are likely to disrupt topographical fronto-striato–thalamofrontal circuits of which two, those involving the dorsolateral prefrontal cortex and anterior cingulate cortex, have been particularly implicated in executive function and attentional tasks (Alexander et al, 1986; Dubois and Pillon, 1997).

Summary

Perhaps a more fruitful way forward is to develop a better understanding of the relationship between specific lesions and specific aspects of cognition. For example, it could be hypothesized that medial temporal lobe atrophy may be associated with memory difficulties, whereas small vessel disease or atrophy in key frontosubcortical circuits may result in attentional and executive dysfunction. Refining these concepts on the basis of empirical data will perhaps enable us to create a meaningful group of subdivisions within the overall framework of VCI reflecting the predominant pattern of lesions and associated cognitive deficits in particular individuals. It is also possible that the best predictors of subsequent cognitive decline may differ between these subgroups.

References

Alexander GE, DeLong MR, Strick PL, Parallel organization of functional segregated circuits linking basal ganglia and cortex [Review] [128 refs], *Ann Rev Neurosci* (1986) 9:357–81.

Almkvist O, Backman L, Basun H, Wahlund LO, Patterns of neuropsychological performance in Alzheimer's disease and vascular dementia, *Cortex* (1993) 29:661–73.

Ballard C, McKeith I, O'Brien J et al, Neuropathological substrates of dementia and depression in vascular dementia, with a particular focus on cases with small infarct volumes, *Dementia* (2000) 11:59–65

Ballard C, Stephens S, Kenny R et al, Profile of neuropsychological deficits in older stroke survivors without dementia. *Dement Geriatr Cogn Disord* (2003) 16:52–6.

Barba R, Martinez-Espinosa S, Rodriguez-Garcia E et al, Post-stroke dementia. Clinical features and risk factors, *Stroke* (2000) 31:1494–501.

Becker JT, Boller F, Lopez OL et al, The natural history of Alzheimer's disease: Description of study cohort and accuracy of diagnosis, *Arch Neurol* (1994) 51:585–94.

Bowler JV, The concept of vascular cognitive impairment, *J Neurol Sci* (2002) 203–204: 11–15.

Burton EJ, Ballard C, Stephens S et al, Hyperintensities and fronto-subcortical atrophy on MRI are substrates of mild cognitive deficits after stroke, *Dement Geriatr Cogn Disord* (2003) 16:113–18.

Del Ser T, Bermejo F, Portera A et al, Vascular dementia: a clinicopathological study, *J Neurological Sci* (1990) 96:1–7.

Desmond DW, Moroney JT, Paik MC et al, Frequency and clinical determinants of dementia after ischemic stroke, *Neurology* (2000) 54:1124–31.

Di Carlo A, Baldersreschi M, Amaducci L et al, Cognitive impairment without dementia in older people: prevalence, vascular risk factors, impact on disability. The Italian Longitudinal Study on Aging, *J Am Geriatr Soc* (2000) 48:775–82.

Dubois B, Pillon B, Cognitive deficits in Parkinson's disease, *J Neurol* (1997) 244:2–8.

Esiri M, Wilcock GK, Morris JH, Neuropathological assessment of the lesions of significance in vascular dementia, *J Neurol Neurosurg Psychiatry* (1997) 63:749–53.

Esiri MM, Nagy Z, Smith MZ et al, Cerebrovascular disease and threshold for dementia in the early stages of Alzheimer's disease, *Lancet* (1999) 354:919–20.

Erkinjuntti T, Haltia M, Palo J, Ketonen L, Accuracy of the clinical diagnosis of vascular dementia: a prospective clinical and post-mortem neuropathological study, *J Neurol Neurosurg Psychiatry* (1988) 8:1037–44.

Garde E, Mortensen EL, Krabbe K et al, Relation between age-related decline in intelligence and cerebral white matter hyperintensities in healthy octogenarians: a longitudinal study, *Lancet* (2000) 356:628–34.

Gorelick PB, Erkinjuntti T, Hofman A et al, Prevention of vascular dementia, *Alzheimer Dis Assoc Disord* (1999) 13:S131–S139.

Graham JE, Rockwood K, Beattie L et al, Prevalence and severity of cognitive impairment with and without dementia in an elderly population, *Lancet* (1997) **349**:1793–6.

Hachinski VC, Bowler J, Vascular dementia, *Neurology* (1993) **43**:2159–60.

Hanninen T, Kolivisto K, Reinikainen KJ et al, Prevalence of ageing-associated cognitive decline in an elderly population, *Age Ageing* (1996) **3**:201–5.

Huff FJ, Belle SH, Nebes RD et al, Cognitive deficits and clinical diagnosis of Alzheimer's disease, *Neurology* (1987) **37**:1119–24.

Ingles JL, Wentzel C, Fisk JD, Rockwood K, Neuropsychological predictors of incident dementia in patients with vascular cognitive impairment, without dementia, *Stroke* (2002) **8**:1999–2002.

Kokmen E, Whisnant JP, O'Fallon WF et al, Dementia after ischemic stroke: a population-based study in Rochester, Minnesota (1960–1984), *Neurology* (1996) **46**:154–9.

Kuusisto J, Koivisto K, Mykkanen L et al, Association between features of the insulin resistance syndrome and Alzheimer's disease independently of apolipoprotein E4 phenotype: cross sectional population based study, *BMJ* (1997) **315**:1045–9.

Lafosse JM, Reed BR, Mungas D et al, Fluency and memory differences between ischemic vascular dementia and Alzheimer's disease, *Neuropsychology* (1997) **11**:514–22.

Leeds L, Meara RJ, Woods R, Hobson JP, A comparison of the new executive functioning domains of the CAMCOG-R with existing tests of executive function in elderly stroke survivors, *Age Ageing* (2001) **30**:251–4.

Leibson CL, Rocca WA, Hanson VA et al, Risk of dementia among persons with diabetes mellitus: A population-based cohort study, *Ann NY Acad Sci* (1997) **26**:422–7.

Levy R, Age-associated cognitive decline, *Int Psychogeriatr* (1994) **6**:63–8.

Mendez MF, Ashla-Mendez M, Differences between multi-infarct dementia and Alzheimer's disease on unstructured neuropsychological tasks, *J Clin Exper Neuropsychol* (1991) **13**:923–32.

Merchant C, Tang MX, Albert S et al, The influence of smoking on the risk of Alzheimer's Disease, *Neurology* (1999) **52**:1408–12.

Meyer JS, Xu G, Thornby J et al, Is mild cognitive impairment prodromal for vascular dementia like Alzheimer's disease? *Stroke* (2002) **33**:1981–5.

Ott A, Stolk RP, van Harskamp F et al, Diabetes mellitus and the risk of dementia: Rotterdam Study, *Neurology* (1999) **53**:1937–42.

Padovani A, Di Piero V, Bragoni M et al, Patterns of neuropsychological impairment in mild dementia: a comparison between Alzheimer's disease and multi-infarct dementia. *Acta Neurol Scand* (1995) **92**:433–42.

Perry EK, Perry RH, Blessed G, Tomlinson BE, Changes in brain cholinesterases in senile dementia of Alzheimer's type, *Neuropathol Appl Neurobiol* (1978) **4**:273–7.

Petersen RC, Smith GE, Waring SC et al, Mild cognitive impairment: Clinical charactersation and outcome, *Arch Neurol* (1999) **56**:303–8.

Petersen RC, Smith GE, Waring SC et al, Aging, memory, and mild cognitive impairment, *Int Psychogeriatr* (1997) **9**:65–9.

Pohjasvaara T, Erkinjuntti T, Vataja R, Kaste M, Dementia three months after stroke. Baseline frequency and effect of different definitions of dementia in the Helsinki Stroke Aging Memory Study (SAM) cohort, *Stroke* (1997) **28**:785–92.

Rao R, Jackson S, Howard R, Neuropsychological impairment in stroke, carotid stenosis, and peripheral vascular disease: A comparison with healthy community residents, *Stroke* (1999) **30**:2167–73.

Reisberg B, Franssen EH, Shah MA et al, Clinical diagnosis of dementia. In: Maj M and Sartorius N, eds, *Evidence and Experience in Psychiatry* (John Wiley: Chichester, 2000) 69–115.

Ritchie K, Artero S, and Touchon J, Classification criteria for mild cognitive impairment: a population-based validation study, *Neurology* (2001) **56**:37–42.

Rockwood K, Vascular cognitive impairment and vascular dementia, *J Neurol Sci* (2002) **203–4**:23–7.

Rockwood K, Bowler J, Erkinjuntti T et al, Subtypes of vascular dementia, *Alzheimer Dis Assoc Disord* (1999) **13**:S59–S65.

Rockwood K, Wentzel C, Hachinski V et al, Prevalence and outcomes of vascular cognitive impairment. Vascular Cognitive Impairment Investigators of the Canadian Study of Health and Aging, *Neurology* (2000) **54**:447–51.

Roman GC, Tatemichi T, Erkinjuntti T et al, Vascular Dementia: Diagnostic Criteria for Research Studies. Report of the NINCDS-AIREN International Workshop, *Neurology* (1993) **43**:250–60.

Sacco RL, Shi T, Zemenillo MC et al, Predictors of mortality and recurrence of dementia after hospitalized cerebral infarctions in an urban community: the Northern Manhattan Stroke Study, *Neurology* (1994) **44**:626–34.

Schmidt R, Fazekas F, Offenbacher H et al, Magnetic resonance imaging white matter lesions and cognitive impairment in hypertensive individuals, *Arch Neurol* (1991) **48**:417–20.

Skoog I, A review on blood pressure and ischaemic white matter lesions, *Dement Geriatr Cogn Disord* (1998) **9**:13–19.

Snowdon DA, Greiner LH, Mortimer JA et al, Brain infarction and the clinical expression of Alzheimer's disease: The Nun Study, *JAMA* (1997) **277**:813–17.

Szatmari S, Fekete I, Csiba L et al, Screening of vascular cognitive impairment on a Hungarian cohort, *Psychiatry Clin Neurosci* (1999) **53**:39–43.

Tatemichi TK, Desmond DW, Paik M et al, Clinical determinants of dementia related to stroke, *Ann Neurol* (1993) **33**:568–75.

Tatemichi TK, Desmond D, Prohovnik I et al, Confusion and memory loss from capsular genu infarction: a thalamocortical disconnection syndrome? *Neurology* (1992) **42**:1966–79.

Tatemichi TK, Desmond D, Stern Y et al, Cognitive impairment after stroke: frequency, pattern and relationship to functional abilities, *J Neurol Neurosurg Psychiatry* (1994a) **57**:202–7.

Tatemichi TK, Paik M, Bagiella E et al, Risk of dementia after stroke in a hospitalised cohort: results of a longitudinal study, *Neurology* (1994b) **44**:1885–91.

Tomlinson B, Blessed G, Roth M, Observations on the brains of demented old people, *J Neurol Sci* (1970) **11**:205–42.

Villardita C, Grioli S, Lomeo C et al, Clinical studies with oxiracetam in patients with dementia of Alzheimer type and multi-infarct dementia of mild to moderate degree, *Neuropsychobiology* (1992) **25**:24–8.

chapter 17

Cognition and neuropsychology

Tammy M Scott and Marshal Folstein

Introduction

Vascular dementia (VaD) is the second most common form of dementia in the USA and Europe, and is the most common form in Asia (Roman, 1991; Roman et al, 1993; Desmond, 1996). Until recently, research on VaD has been impeded by a lack of standards in diagnosis, classification, methodology and terminology, which created inconsistencies throughout the literature. During the 1990s, however, attempts were made to create diagnostic criteria allowing international comparison (Chui et al, 1992; Roman et al, 1993; Graham et al, 1996).

In 1991, a joint committee of the Neuroepidemiology Branch of the National Institute of Neurological Disorders and Stroke (NINDS) and the Association Internationale pour la Recherche et l'Enseignement en Neurosciences (AIREN) developed a definition of VaD and diagnostic criteria for neuroepidemiological studies. According to the criteria established by this NINDS-AIREN workshop, a neuropathological classification of VaD includes cases of dementia resulting from ischemic and hemorrhagic brain lesions, as well as from cerebral ischemic hypoxic lesions such as those due to cardiac arrest; it excludes cases due to pure asphyxia or respiratory failure (Roman et al, 1993). The definition of *dementia* adopted by the NINDS-AIREN committee is that of the ICD 10 (WHO, 1991), which specifies that cognitive decline should be demonstrated by loss of memory and deficits in *at least two other domains*. It also specifies that the decline in memory and intellectual abilities must cause impairment in functioning in daily living (Roman et al, 1993). It excludes cases of delirium, altered states of consciousness and other etiologic causes of dementia, as well as patients with conditions that interfere with assessment of intellectual functions. For better or worse, this last criterion requires the exclusion of patients with severe aphasia and significant sensorimotor deficits precluding testing. Undoubtedly this stringent criterion results in the false exclusion of many cases of VaD following stroke. Issues of sensitivity and specificity of these criteria are discussed later in this chapter.

The report of the NINDS-AIREN workshop prescribes a multidisciplinary approach to diagnosis and stresses the importance of a neuropsychological evaluation for the assessment of VaD. It suggests the following tests as being useful for screening for VaD: a four-word memory test with ten-minute delayed recall; a cube-drawing test for copy, a verbal fluency test (i.e. number of animals named in one minute), Luria's alternating hand sequence or finger rings; a letter cancelation test for neglect; a reaction time test; and the grooved pegboard test (Roman et al, 1993). While the report also suggests the use of the Mini-Mental States Examination (MMSE) (Folstein et al, 1975) as a screening tool for VaD, other studies suggest that a supplemental Mental Alternation Test be added to increase the sensitivity to subcortical dysfunction (Jones et al, 1993). Following the screening phase, the NINDS-AIREN committee recommends that suspected cases should be evaluated by a neuropsychologist, and that tests used should cover each major cognitive domain in order to fully evaluate the spectrum of neuropsychological abnormalities. In addition, they recommend that the neuropsychological testing battery used have sufficient sensitivity in detecting subcortical lesions and in evaluating language and motor functioning since subcortical structures are commonly affected in VaD (Roman et al, 1993).

Expanding on the neuropathological classifications outlined by the NINDS-AIREN report, Meyer et al (1996) proposed the following eight subtypes of VaD:

1. multi-infarct dementias
2. strategically placed infarctions causing dementia
3. multiple subcortical lacunar lesions
4. Binswanger's disease (arteriosclerotic subcortical leuko-encephalopathy)
5. mixtures of two or more of the above VaD subtypes
6. hemorrhagic lesions causing dementia
7. subcortical dementias due to cerebral autosomally dominant arteriolopathy with subcortical infarcts and leukoencephalopathy (CADASIL) or to familial amyloid angiopatheis and coagulopathies
8. mixtures of Alzheimer's disease (AD) and VaD.

The neuropsychiatric and cognitive patterns of impairments have been published for six of the eight subtypes, and are described below.

Multi-infarct dementia

The neuropathology of multi-infarct dementia (MID) includes multiple large cerebral infarcts caused by emboli or arising from occlusion by atherosclerotic plaques. The NINDS-AIREN criteria for MID specify that the cerebrovascular lesions associated with MID are multiple large *complete* infarcts that can involve cortical and subcortical areas. There have been a number of neuropsychological studies that have used clinical criteria consistent with the NINDS-AIREN criteria for MID.

The cognitive impairments associated with MID are necessarily dependent on the cortical or subcortical areas supplied by the affected blood vessels. For example, middle cerebral artery occlusions affecting the left hemisphere typically result in aphasia and apraxia (Benson and Geschwind, 1975; Geschwind, 1975; Benson, 1979); infarctions anterior to the Rolandic fissure result in nonfluent aphasias and lesions posterior to the central fissure are associated with fluent aphasia (Cummings and Benson, 1992). Right middle cerebral artery infarctions are usually associated with abnormalities in prosody, the ability to dress, and problems with visuospatial orientation and visuomotor performance (Hemphill and Klein, 1948; Ross, 1981). Since the definition of *dementia* specifies that multiple areas of cognition are impaired, pathology restricted to cortical areas usually require multiple bilateral infarcts in order to meet the diagnostic criteria (Cummings and Benson, 1992). In studies of the psychiatric sequelae of stroke, Starkstein et al (1987) found that those patients with left anterior lesions, either cortical or subcortical, had significantly greater frequency and severity of depression than patients with any other lesion location. In contrast, right hemisphere lesions were associated with a significantly higher incidence of excessive cheerfulness.

Strategically placed infarcts

Recent neuroimaging studies have shown that strategically located small infarctions are capable of creating deficits in multiple areas of cognitive functioning. While most of these regions are subcortical, infarcts to the angular gyrus have also been reported to result in multiple cognitive impairments.

The subcortical areas that result in a full dementia syndrome when infarcted include the basal ganglia, thalamus and genu of the internal capsule. These latter sites have pathways that project to the frontal or temporal lobes (Alexander et al, 1990; Tatemichi et al, 1992; Cummings, 1993), and it is thought that the cognitive and behavioral changes associated with infarcts to these areas result from interruptions of the circuits connecting subcortical and cortical regions (Tatemichi et al, 1995; McPherson and Cummings, 1996).

Angular gyrus

The clinical syndrome associated with infarct to the angular gyrus includes aphasia (with paraphasic errors), alexia with agraphia, Gerstmann's syndrome (acalculia, right–left disorientation, dysgraphia and finger agnosia) and constructional disturbance (Cummings and Benson, 1992). Patients with angular gyrus syndrome typically recognize their impairments and are frustrated by them. It is important to note that focal motor and/or sensory signs may be absent in these patients and that their lesions are not always detectable by computed tomography (CT). This often makes the syndrome difficult to distinguish from other types of dementia including AD (McPherson and Cummings, 1996).

Genu of the internal capsule

Small infarcts to the genu of the internal capsule have been shown to result in significant impairments in cognition. The main clinical features of this syndrome have been described as an acute confusional state soon after the stroke with fluctuating alertness, inattention, memory loss, apathy, abulia and psychomotor retardation (Tatemichi et al, 1995). Contralateral weakness appears to be mild or absent, with the severity of weakness correlated to the extent of the infarct in the posterior limb. The chronic phase of this syndrome in patients with dominant hemisphere lesions include significant verbal memory loss – along with other neuropsychological impairments such as naming and verbal fluency – despite an improved level of consciousness (Kooistra and Heilman, 1988; Markowitsch et al, 1990; Tatemichi et al, 1995). Persistence of symptoms as a result of nondominant hemisphere lesions appear to be more equivocal, with moderate impairment in visuospatial memory recovering within weeks in one patient (Tatemichi et al, 1995).

number of perseverations and intrusions (Schindler et al, 1984). Bennet et al (1994) compared patients with Binswanger's disease to those with AD and found that Binswanger's patients had relatively less profound impairments in episodic memory, more depressive symptomatology and a more variable rate of cognitive decline. One study, which compared performance on the Dementia Rating Scale (DRS; Mattis, 1988) in patients with AD, patients with single stroke and patients with MID, found that in general AD patients were more impaired on the memory subscale, while the stroke and MID patients were more impaired on DRS construction. Patients with MID were more impaired on the initiation/perseveration subscale than were AD patients, and AD patients scored lower on the conceptualization subscale compared to those patients with single stroke (Lukatela et al, 2000). In early-stage VaD and AD, VaD patients have been reported as having significantly better free recall, cued recall and recognition, but more perseverative errors during a card-sorting task than did the AD patients. The early-stage AD patients were shown to have more perseveration on a test of semantic fluency than did the patients with VaD (Traykov et al, 2002).

In a study comparing AD, VaD and senile dementia of Lewy body type (SDLT), Ballard et al (1996) found that patients with SDLT had significantly greater deterioration in verbal fluency than patients with AD or VaD, as well as a trend toward greater overall cognitive decline in the course of a year (as measured by the CAMCOG). Cherrier et al (1997) compared patients with frontotemporal dementia (FTD) with VaD, and found that FTD patients performed significantly better than the VaD patients on tests of digit span and constructions, while there was a trend that the VaD patients performed relatively less well on tests of verbal fluency and abstractions. There does not appear to be a neuropsychological literature on differentiating VaD from the dementias related to Parkinson's disease, Pick's disease, Creutzfeldt–Jakob disease, progressive supranuclear palsy and Huntington's disease. It is recommended that these etiologies be ruled out by detailed clinical history, neuroimaging and microscopic evaluation of adequately selected samples of brain parenchyma (Roman et al, 1993).

Summary

Neuropsychological testing is an invaluable tool for clinical assessment and research on the cognitive impairments associated with VaD. While there are a number of subcategories of VaD resulting from ischemic and hemorrhagic brain lesions, most variations are thought to create interruptions of subcorticofrontal pathways resulting in executive functioning impairments. Relative to AD, patients with VaD perform more poorly on tests influenced by frontal and subcortical mechanisms, particularly in self-regulation, planning, attention, verbal fluency and motor performance/fine motor co-ordination. In addition, patients with VaD have been shown to have more severe behavioral retardation, depression and anxiety than those with AD. The coincidence of AD and vascular disorders, however, is becoming increasingly recognized as a common occurrence, especially in older individuals.

References

Alexander GE, Crutcher MD, DeLong MR, Basal ganglia-thalamocortical circuits: parallel substrates for motor, oculomotor, 'prefrontal' and 'limbic' functions. In: Uylings HBM, Eden CGV, Bruin JPCD et al, eds, *Progress in Brain Research*, (Elsevier Science: New York, 1990) 119–46.

Almkvist O, Neuropsychological deficits in vascular dementia in relation to Alzheimer's disease: reviewing evidence for functional similarity or divergence, *Dementia* (1994) 5:203–9.

Babikian V, Ropper AH, Binswanger's disease: a review, *Stroke* (1987) 18:2–12.

Ballard C, Patel A, Oyebode F, Wilcock G, Cognitive decline in patients with Alzheimer's disease, vascular dementia and senile dementia of Lewy body type, *Age Ageing* (1996) 25:209–13.

Baudrimont M, Dubas F, Joutel A et al, Autosomal dominant leukoencephalopathy and subcortical ischemic stroke: a clinicopathological study, *Stroke* (1993) 24:122–5.

Bennett D, Gilley D, Lee S, Cochran E, White matter changes: neurobehavioral manifestations of Binswanger's disease and clinical correlates in Alzheimer's disease, *Dementia* (1994) 5:148–52.

Benson DF, *Aphasia, alexia, and agraphia* (Churchill Livingstone: New York, 1979).

Benson DF, Geschwind N, Psychiatric conditions associated with focal lesions of the central nervous system. In: Arieti S, Reiser M, eds *American Handbook of Psychiatry* (Basic Books: New York, 1975).

Bogousslavsky J, Ferrazzini M, Regli F et al, Manic delirium and frontal lobe syndrome with paramedian infarction of the right thalamus, *J Neurol Neurosurg Psychiatry* (1988) 51:116–19.

Boone K, Miller B, Lesser I et al, Neuropsychological correlates of white matter lesions in healthy elderly subjects, *Arch Neurol* (1992) 49:549–54.

Cherrier MM, Mendez MF, Perryman KM et al, Frontotemporal dementia versus vascular dementia: differential features on mental status examination, *J Am Geriatr Soc* (1997) 45:579–83.

Chui HC, Victoroff JI, Margolin D et al, Criteria for the diagnosis of ischemic vascular dementia proposed by the State of California Alzheimer's disease diagnostic and treatment centers, *Neurology* (1992) 42:473–80.

Corbet AJ, Bennett H, Kos S, Cognitive dysfunction following subcortical infarction, *Arch Neurol* (1994) 51:999–1007.

Cummings JL, Frontal–subcortical circuits and human behavior, *Arch Neurol* (1993) 50:873–80.

Cummings JL, Benson DF, *Dementia: A Clinical Approach*. (Butterworth-Heinemann: Boston, 1992).

DeCarli C, Murphy DGM, Tranh M et al, The effect of white matter hyperintensity volume on brain structure, cognitive performance, and cerebral metabolism of glucose in 51 healthy adults, *Neurology* (1995) **45**:2077–84.

De Groot JC, de Leeuw FE, Oudkerk M et al, Cerebral white matter lesions and cognitive function: the Rotterdam Scan Study, *Ann Neurol* (2000) **47**:145–51.

Desmond DW, Vascular dementia: a construct in evolution, *Cerebrovasc Brain Metab Rev* (1996) **8**:296–325.

Eslinger PJ, Warner GC, Grattan LM, Easton JD, 'Frontal Lobe' utilization behavior associated with paramedian thalamic infarction, *Neurology* (1991) **41**:450–2.

Exner C, Weniger G, Irle E, Implicit and explicit memory after focal thalamic lesions, *Neurology* (2001) **57**:2054–63.

Fischer P, Jellinger K, Gatterer G, Danielczyk W, Prospective neuropathological validation of Hachinski's Ischemic Score in dementias, *J Neurol Neurosurg Psychiatry* (1991) **54**:580–3.

Fisher CM, Binswanger's encephalopathy: a review, *J Neurol* (1989) **236**:65–79.

Folstein M, Folstein S, McHugh PR, Mini-Mental State: a practical method for grading the cognitive state of patients for the clinician, *J Psychiatr Res* (1975) **12**:189–98.

Frisoni GB, Bianchetti A, Govoni S et al, Association of apolipoprotein E E4 with vascular dementia, *JAMA* (1994) **271**:1317.

Gainotti G, Galtagirone C, Masullo C, Miceli G, Patterns of neuropsychologic impairment in various diagnostic groups of dementia. In: Amaducci L, Davidson AN, Antuono P, eds, *Aging of the Brain and Dementia: Aging*, Vol 13 (Raven Press: New York, 1980).

Gainotti G, Marra C, Villa G, A double dissociation between accuracy and time of execution on attentional tasks in Alzheimer's disease and multi-infarct dementia, *Brain* (2001) **124**:731–8.

Gentilini M, Renzi ED, Crisi G, Bilateral paramedian thalamic artery infarcts: report of eight cases, *J Neurol Neurosurg Psychiatry* (1987) **50**:900–9.

Geschwind N, The apraxias: neural mechanisms of disorders of learned movement, *Am Sci* 63:188–95.

Graham JE, Rockwood K, Beattie BL et al, Standardization of the diagnosis of dementia in the Canadian Study of Health and Aging, *Neuroepidemiology* (1996) **15**:246–56.

Hachinski V, Multi-infarct dementia, *Neurol Clin* (1983) **1**:27–36.

Hemphill RE, Klein R, Contribution to the dressing disability as a focal sign and to the imperception phenomena, *J Mental Sci* (1948) **94**:611–22.

Henon H, Pasquier F, Durieu I et al, Pre-existing dementia in stroke: baseline frequency, associated factors and outcome, *Stroke* (1997) **28**:2429–36.

Henon H, Durieu I, Guerouaou D et al, Post-stroke dementia: incidence and relationship to pre-stroke cognitive decline, *Neurology* (2001) **57**:1216–22.

Hier DB, Hagenlocker K, Schindler AG, Language disintegration in dementia: effects of etiology and severity, *Brain Lang* (1985) **25**:117–33.

Holmes C, Cairns N, Lantos P et al, Validity of current clinical criteria for Alzheimer's disease, vascular dementia and dementia with Lewy bodies, *Br J Psychiatry* (1999) **174**:45–50.

Jones BN, Teng EL, Folstein MF, Harrison KS, A new bedside test of cognition for patients with HIV infection, *Ann Intern Med* (1993) **119**:1001–4.

Kawamata J, Tanaka S, Shimohama S et al, Apolipoprotein E polymorphism in Japanese patients with Alzheimer's disease or vascular dementia, *J Neurol Neurosurg Psychiatry* (1994) **57**:1414–16.

Kertesz A, Clydesdale S, Neuropsychological deficits in vascular dementa vs Alzheimer's disease, *Arch Neurol* (1994) **51**:1226–31.

Kooistra CA, Heilman KM, Memory loss from a subcortical white matter infarct, *J Neurol Neurosurg Psychiatry* (1988) **51**:866–9.

Kumral E, Evyapan D, Balkir K, Acute caudate vascular lesions, *Stroke* (1999) **30**:100–8.

Kumral E, Evyapan D, Balkir K, Kutluhan S, Bilateral thalamic infarction; clinical etiological and MRI correlates, *Acta Neurol Scand* (2001) **103**:35–42.

Lafosse JM, Reed BR, Mungas D et al, Fluency and memory differences between ischemic vascular dementia and Alzheimer's disease, *Neuropsychology* (1997) **11**:514–22.

Loeb C, Meyer JS, Vascular dementia: still a debatable entity? *J Neurol Sci* (1996) **143**:31–40.

Longstreth W Jr, Manolio T, Arnold A et al, Clinical correlates of white matter findings on cranial magnetic resonance imaging of 3301 elderly people: the cardiovascular health study, *Stroke* (1996) **27**:1274–82.

Lotz PR, Ballinger WE Jr, Quisling RG, Subcortical arteriosclerotic encephalopathy: CT spectrum and pathologic correlation, *Am J Roentgenol* (1986) **147**:1209–14.

Lukatela K, Cohen RA, Kessler H et al, Dementia rating scale performance: a comparison of vascular and Alzheimer's dementia, *J Clin Experi Neuropsychol* (2000) **22**:445–54.

Markowitsch HJ, Cramon DY, Hormann E et al, Verbal memory deterioration after unilateral infarct of the internal capsule in an adulescent, *Cortex* (1990) **26**:597–609.

Mattis S, *Dementia Rating Scale* (Psychological Assessment Resources: Odessa, Florida, 1988).

McKhann G, Drachman D, Folstein M et al, Clinical diagnosis of Alzheimer's disease: report of the NINCDS-ADRDA Work Group under the auspices of department of health and human services task force on Alzheimer's disease, *Neurology* (1984) **34**:939–44.

McPherson S, Cummings J, Neuropsychological aspects of vascular dementia, *Brain Cogn* (1996) **31**:269–82.

Mendez MF, Adams NL, Lewandowski KS, Neurobehavioral changes associated with caudate lesions, *Neurology* (1989) **39**:349–54.

Meyer JS, Gelin X, Thornby J et al, Is mild cognitive impairment prodromal for vascular dementia like Alzheimer's disease? *Stroke* (2002) **33**:1981–5.

Meyer JS, Obara K, Muramatsu K et al, Cognitive performance after small strokes correlates with ischemia, not atrophy of the brain, *Dementia* (1995) **6**:312–22.

Meyer JS, Shirai T, Akiyama H, Neuroimaging for differentiating vascular from Alzheimer's dementias, *Cerebr Brain Metabol Rev* (1996) **8**:1–10.

Mirsen T, Hachinski V, Epidemiology and classification of vascular and multi-infarct dementia. In: Meyer JS, Lechner H, Marshall J, Toole JF, eds, *Vascular and Multi-Infarct Dementia* (Future Publishing: Mount Kisko, NY, 1988).

Moroney JT, Bagiella E, Desmond DW et al, Meta-analysis of the Hachinski Ischemic Score in pathologically verified dementias, *Neurology* (1997) **49**:1096–105.

Nichols FT, Mohr JP, Binswanger's subacute arteriosclerotic encephalopathy. In: Barnett HJM, Mohr JP, Stein VM, eds, *Stroke: Pathophysiology, Diagnosis, and Management* (Churchill Livingstone: New York, 1986).

Pedro-Botet J, Senti M, Nogues X, Lipoprotein and apolipoprotein profile in men with ischemic stroke. Role of lipoprotein(a), triglyceride-rich lipoproteins, and apolipoprotein E polymorphism, *Stroke* (1992) **23**:1556–62.

Powell AL, Cummings JL, Hill MA, Benson DF, Speech and language alterations in multi-infarct dementia, *Neurology* (1988) **38**:717–19.

Rockwood K, Parhad I, Hachinski VC et al, Diagnosis of vascular dementia: Consortium of Canadian Centres for Clinical Cognitive research concensus statement, *Can J Neurol Sci* (1994) **21**:358–64.

Roman GC, Senile dementia of the Binswanger type – a vascular form of dementia in the elderly, *JAMA* (1989) **258**:1782–8.

Roman GC, The epidemiology of vascular dementia. In: Hartmann A, Kuschinsky W, Hoyer S, eds, *Cerebral Ischemia and Dementia* (Springer-Verlag: Berlin, 1991) 9–15.

Roman GC, Tatemichi TK, Erkinjuntti T et al, Vascular dementia: diagnostic criteria for research studies – report of the NINDS-AIREN international Workshop, *Neurology* (1993) **43**:250–60.

Ross ED, The aphrosodias, *Arch Neurol* (1981) **38**:561–9.

Sabbadini G, Francia A, Calandriello L, Cerebral autosomal dominant arteriopathy with subcortical infarcts and leucoencephalopathy (CADASIL). Clinical, neuroimaging, pathological and genetic study of a large Italian family, *Brain* (1995) **118**:207–15.

Schindler AG, Caplan LR, Hier DB, Intrusions and perseverations, *Brain Language* (1984) **23**:148–58.

Shimano H, Ishibashi S, Murase T, Plasma apolipoproteins in patients with multi-infarct dementia, *Atherosclerosis* (1989) **79**:257–60.

Skoog I, Risk factors for vascular dementia: a review, *Dementia* (1994) **5**:137–44.

Snowdon DA, Greiner LH, Mortimer JA et al, Brain infarction and the clinical expression of Alzheimer's disease. The Nun Study, *JAMA* (1997) **277**:813–17.

Starkstein SE, Robinson RG, Price TR, Comparison of cortical and subcortical lesions in the production of poststroke mood disorders, *Brain* (1987) **110**:1045–59.

Starkstein SE, Sabe L, Vasquez S et al, Neuropsychological, psychiatric, and cerebral blood flow findings in vascular dementia and Alzheimer's disease, *Stroke* (1996) **27**:408–14.

Steinke W, Ley SC, Lacunar stroke is the major cause of progressive motor deficits, *Stroke* (2002) **33**:1510–16.

Strub RL, Frontal lobe syndrome in a patient with bilateral globus pallidus lesions, *Arch Neurol* (1989) **46**:1024–7.

Stuss DT, Guberman A, Nelson R, Larochelle S, The neuropsychology of paramedian thalamic infarction, *Brain Cogn* (1988) **8**:348–78.

Sultzer DL, Levin HS, Mahler ME et al, A comparison of psychiatric symptoms in vascular dementia and Alzheimer's disease, *Am J Psychiatry* (1993) **150**:1806–12.

Sultzer DL, Mahler ME, Cummings JL et al, Cortical abnormalities associated with subcortical lesions in vascular dementia, *Arch Neurol* (1995) **52**:773–80.

Tatemichi TK, Desmond DW, Mayeux R, Dementia after stroke: baseline frequency, risks, and clinical features in a hospitalized cohort, *Neurology* (1992) **42**:1185–93.

Tatemichi TK, Desmond DW, Prohovnik I, Strategic infarcts in vascular dementia. A clinical and brain imaging experience, *Arzneimittel-Forschung/Drug Res* (1995) **45**:371–85.

Tournier-Lasserve E, Joutel A, Melki J, Cerebral autosomal dominant arteriopathy with subcortical infarcts and leukoencephalopathy maps to chromosome 19q12, *Nat Genet* (1993) **3**:256–9.

Traykov L, Baudic S, Thibaudet MC et al, Neuropsychological deficit in early subcortical vascular dementia: comparison to Alzheimer's disease, *Demen Geriatr Cogn Disord* (2002) **14**:26–32.

Traykov L, Rigaud AS, Caputo L et al, Apolipoprotein E phenotypes in demented and cognitively impaired patients with and without cerebrovascular disease, *Euro J Neurol* (1999) **6**:415–21.

Villardita C, Alzheimer's disease compared with cerebrovascular dementia. Neuropsychological similarities and differences, *Acta Neurol Scand* (1993) **87**:299–308.

WHO, *The Neurological Adaptation of the International Classification of Diseases (ICD-10)* (draft). World Health Organization: Geneva, 1991).

Wolfe N, Linn R, Babikian VL, Albert ML, Frontal systems impairment following multiple lacunar infarcts, *Arch Neurol* (1990) **47**:129–32.

chapter 18

Noncognitive symptoms

Robert Barber

This chapter focuses on the emotional, psychological and behavioral changes associated with vascular brain disease. Specific attention will be given to these 'noncognitive' changes in patients with vascular dementia (VaD) and those with stroke disease without dementia.

Introduction: setting the scene

Noncognitive changes represent a diverse collection of symptoms for which there is no single etiology, mechanism or intervention. For a long time their significance has been overshadowed by the interest focused on cognitive changes but their clinical importance has now been underlined by studies demonstrating their impact on patients and their families, as summarized in Table 18.1. Importantly, these symptoms are often under recognized and under treated.

Vascular brain disease is associated with a multitude of noncognitive symptoms. Reported changes include affective and anxiety symptoms such as depression, generalized anxiety, agoraphobia, mania, emotional lability, catastrophic reactions, altered recognition of emotion, obsessive–compulsive symptoms, and post-traumatic stress disorder. Psychotic symptoms, delusions and hallucinations, can occur as well as behavioral changes such as agitation, aggression, restlessness, irritability, disinhibition, shouting, sexual dysfunction, apathy, fatigue, eating abnormalities and sleep disturbance. However, the vast majority of published work focuses on depression in stroke patients, and compared to Alzheimer's disease (AD), detailed study of noncognitive changes in VaD has been relatively neglected.

The reported prevalence of these symptoms varies, at times considerably,

Table 18.1 Summary of the clinical significance of noncognitive symptoms in cerebrovascular disease

	Associated with. . .
Patient	Distress
	Reduced quality of life and self-esteem
	Embarrassment
	Social avoidance and impaired quality of social contact
	Reduced daily functioning
	Premature institutionalization
	Possible impairment of cognitive function
	Risk factor for stroke and stroke-related mortality
	Interferes with the speed, extent and nature of stroke rehabilitation
Carers and family	Source of burden, stress and carer depression
	Reduced quality of life
	Reduced social networks
Institutional care	High prevalence of symptoms – impact on other residents and staff
Hospital care	Delayed discharge after stroke
	Increased length of hospital stay
General	Prime focus for intervention including drug treatments
	Increased financial costs

from study to study. This inconsistency often reflects differences in methodology including variations in diagnostic criteria, rating scales, recruitment and demography of subjects, the subtypes of VaD and stroke, and the imaging modality used to identify ischemic lesions. Studies also often lack a suitable reference or control group and vary in the duration and timing of assessments. Table 18.2 summarizes the published prevalence rates for the most widely documented noncognitive changes. As a general rule, noncognitive changes are more variable over time than cognitive changes.

An important factor that underpins the diversity of noncognitive symptoms in vascular disease, and to variation observed between studies, relates to the very nature of cerebrovascular disease. Cerebrovascular disease is pathologically and clinically heterogeneous (Roman, 2002). It incorporates a range of vascular mechanisms and changes that can impact in different brain areas. These changes interact with other non-vascular host factors including coexisting pathologies such as AD. This underlying pathological

Table 18.2 Summary of prevalence (%) of main types of noncognitive symptoms in vascular dementia and stroke disease

	Vascular dementia	*Stroke disease*
Depression	8–66%	14–60%
Generalised anxiety disorder	19–26%	1–27%
Agoraphobia	—	3%
Emotionalism	—	15–34%
Catastrophic reaction	—	20%
Hallucinations	Visual 13–25%	Rare
Delusions	Delusions 8–50%	Rare
Misidentifications	26–27%	Rare
Agitation	32%	—
Apathy	20–25%	20%
Mania	Rare	Rare
Irritability	18%	—
Disinhibition	11%	—

heterogeneity needs to be borne in mind when considering clinical phenotypes, including noncognitive symptoms.

There are, of course, many influences on the way people feel and behave. Current evidence falls short of a comprehensive biopsychosocial etiological model of noncognitive symptoms. Most noncognitive changes, such as depression and anxiety, are clearly not unique to patients with vascular disease, and are best construed as multifactorial in etiology. Other changes, such as catastrophic reactions and emotional lability, appear more selectively associated with brain damage, particularly vascular injury. The majority of published evidence emphasizes the potential role of neurobiological correlates of noncognitive changes. Not surprisingly, preliminary findings also point to the importance of other modifying factors. These factors, which may exert protective or negative influences, include patient variables such as personality, coping strategies, social functioning, concurrent medical and psychiatric factors and drug use, past personal and family psychiatric history, sensory deficits, age and cognitive status. Other social and environmental factors include life events, family and social supports, physical characteristics of the environment and, in care settings, the availability or otherwise of trained, skilled staff.

As more evidence emerges, the relationship between vascular disease and psychiatric disorders, in particular depression, is likely to prove to be more complex and far reaching than the primary focus of this chapter. Several lines of evidence support a bidirectional association between both cerebral and noncerebral vascular disease and depression. For example, psychological distress may be a predictor of fatal ischemic stroke (May et al, 2002) and more specifically depression can exert a negative influence on ischemic heart disease and stroke (Glassman and Shapiro, 1998; Simonsick et al, 1995). In turn, depression is associated with vascular risk factors, including ischemic white matter changes (Krishnan et al, 1997; Thomas et al, 2002), which can contribute to poor treatment outcomes (O'Brien et al, 1998). If a bidirectional relationship is confirmed, it could have major implications for the management of both psychiatric and vascular factors (Ballard and O'Brien, 2002; Carney and Freedland, 2002).

Finally, as a historical footnote, although there has been a recent surge of interest in noncognitive symptoms, especially in the context of dementia, in reality these changes are, of course, not new. For example, a particularly discerning account of these symptoms, as well as the relevance of vascular pathologies, was written by Thomas Coulston (1904). Informed by his experiences as Physician Superintendent of the Royal Edinburgh Asylum for the Insane in the late nineteenth century, his chapter 'Senile Insanity' states that patients experience 'loss of memory, irritability, excitement, night noise, restlessness, one third are melancholic, one third are maniacal' as well as psychotic symptoms. He considered the pathology of senile insanity to have 'a visible pathology in most cases; a gross lesion, 'softening' found in 42%; vascular disease is very common; atheroma and arteritis; atrophy in most cases. . . .'

Insightfully, on the treatment of senile insanity he wrote:

'. . . I can only lay down principles that I have found useful. The thing of first importance is undoubtedly to get a good nurse – a responsible, skilled, patient, experienced person. After a good nurse – and a daughter or relative sometimes make the best of all – comes the routine of management, diet, exercise and regime. Excitement, all new things or ways or places or persons should be avoided. Old people take best what they have been accustomed to. . . . Medications should only be used *occasionally* (his italics) so we can tide over a bad night comfortably. The use of this medication hath enabled relatives in many cases to keep an otherwise unmanageable case at home. . . . Few questions are so difficult to determine as the one of sending a person to an asylum or not. The feelings of everyone go against it if there is a good home, dutiful relatives and sufficient means. The best way is to try all other means first where there is money... Finally, I wish physicians in general practice who have to meet the smaller emergencies of senility would put their observations before the world more than they do. I find the management of most old cases is regarded without much interest.'

Captured in these observations are themes that are as relevant and challenging today as they were a hundred years ago. These include the importance of noncognitive symptoms, vascular pathologies, tailored drug interventions, psychological and supportive approaches to management, the role of family members and support networks, and the problems of carer burden, stigma, under detection and treatment, and the need to avoid institutionalization wherever possible.

Vascular dementia

In VaD, noncognitive symptoms are both common and clinically important. Overall an estimated 60% of subjects with VaD have one or more noncognitive symptoms (Lyketsos et al, 2000). Their importance is acknowledged in the main diagnostic criteria for VaD, which include personality and mood changes, abulia, depression, emotional incontinence and psychomotor retardation as supportive but not core features (Roman et al, 1993).

However, VaD has no single or unique signature of noncognitive symptoms. Indeed, given the heterogeneity inherent in VaD it has been argued that it is better thought of as several syndromes rather than as a disease (Rockwood et al, 1999). Subtypes of VaD include multi-infarct dementia, strategic single infarct dementia and small vessel disease with dementia, though other mechanisms exist as discussed in Chapter 9. Small vessel disease principally affects subcortical structures (and their links to the frontal lobes) with the primary lesions being lacunar infarct(s) and/or ischemic white matter lesions.

A more focused look at the subtypes of VaD has drawn attention to the particular prominence of noncognitive symptoms in subcortical vascular disease. This clinicopathological association is postulated to occur as a result of ischemic damage to key prefrontal–subcortical circuits. There are a number of loops linking subcortical structures and the frontal lobes but the main circuits thought to be involved in the genesis of noncognitive symptoms are the orbitofrontal circuit (leading to personality change, impaired social behavior, disinhibition, mania, impulsivity, irritability, and obsessive–compulsive symptoms), medial–frontal/anterior cingulate circuit (leading to impaired motivation, apathy and depression), and dorsolateral prefrontal circuit (leading to executive dysfunction, impersistence and low mood).

Depression

The weight of evidence indicates that depression is more common in VaD compared with AD (Ballard et al, 1996a). This finding is consistent across different clinical settings and confirmed in population samples (Newman, 1999; Lyketsos et al, 2000). Depression is also probably more severe and persistent in VaD than AD (Ballard et al, 1996a,b). Indeed, studies comparing a range of noncognitive variables in VaD and AD have found an increased prevalence of depressive symptoms to be one of the most important and consistent distinguishing features (Cooper and Mungas, 1993; Sultzer et al, 1993; Ballard et al, 2000; Groves et al, 2000).

One likely pathophysiological mechanism that helps to explain this difference relates to the differential distribution of pathology between VaD and AD. At the risk of oversimplification, AD results from a 'temporal–neocortical' pattern of pathology whilst VaD is associated with more damage to critical 'frontal-subcortical' areas. This is relevant because there is evidence that patients with dementia with established subcortical dysfunction are more susceptible to depressive symptoms (Lind et al, 2002). Indeed, overall depression is probably more common in patients with VaD affecting subcortical–frontal structures and in subjects with subcortical vascular disease compared to those with AD (Bennett et al, 1994; Cummings 1994; Aharon-Peretz et al, 2000).

The clinical correlates of depression in VaD are poorly understood. Depression may become more common in older patients and those with a past history of depression (Ballard et al, 2000). Reports differ as to whether depressive symptoms become more or less common with advancing illness.

Psychotic symptoms

Delusions and hallucinations also feature in VaD, though the evidence base is limited and once again prevalence rates vary between studies. Combining data from previous studies, Ballard and O'Brien (2002) found rates for delusions of 8–50%, visual hallucinations of 13–25% and delusional misidentification of 26–27%. With exceptions, studies generally indicate VaD and AD have a similar frequency, severity and content of psychotic symptoms (Binetti et al, 1993; Ballard et al, 2000). Delusions are usually paranoid in nature with elementary beliefs about theft or infidelity. More elaborate delusional misidentifications can also occur, including the belief that strangers are visiting or live in the house, that images such as those from a television are real or that one's reflection is another person, and the syndromes of Capgras and Fregoli.

The correlates of psychotic symptoms in VaD are also poorly understood. There is conflicting and inconclusive evidence of any specific link between psychotic symptoms and the severity and type of cognitive impairment, level of behavioral disturbance or stage of illness. In a small study by Cummings et al (1987) psychosis was more common in subjects with multiple and bilateral lesions.

Personality

There has been a degree of controversy and confusion regarding the nature of personality changes in VaD. Hachinski (1974) originally suggested a diagnosis of multi-infarct dementia be supported by the relative preservation of personality. Hachinski later refined this concept to 'the ability to experience and express emotion' (Mahler and Cummings, 1991), though this too is challenged by findings that subjects with VaD are less able to comprehend emotions than those with AD (Shimokawa et al, 2000). Further, 'personality change' is a now well-documented feature of VaD, as reflected in subsequent diagnostic criteria for VaD.

Problems also arise from the term 'personality'. It is inherently too broad and multifaceted to be used in a standardized way, and it can be difficult to define what really amounts to a true shift in personality. Nevertheless, the types of symptoms implied by 'personality change' are common and clinically important. They include changes in the way a person relates to other people, invariably leading to a decline in social functioning. These changes are often secondary to frontal lobe dysfunction and present as decreased drive, volition, apathy, emotional responsiveness and empathy, as well as disinhibition, irritability and loss of insight. These changes are similar but usually less severe than those observed in frontotemporal lobar degeneration (Bathgate et al, 2001).

Other noncognitive changes associated with vascular dementia

The evidence base for other symptoms is even less robust than that for depression and psychosis, so conclusions are limited. Agitation/aggression (32%), apathy (23%), irritability (18%) and disinhibition (11%) all feature in VaD (Lyketsos et al, 2000). In the same population-based study, 18% of subjects with VaD experienced anxiety symptoms, compared to 8% with AD. Two other studies also found higher rates in VaD than AD suggesting this is an important area for further study (Sultzer et al, 1993; Ballard et al, 2000).

Wandering, restlessness and aberrant motor behavior may be more common in AD than VaD (Cooper and Mungas, 1993; Lyketsos et al, 2002). However, these behaviors, along with agitation/aggression, become more evident with advancing dementia and are probably more influenced by the stage of dementia than a particular diagnosis (Lyketsos et al, 2000).

Noncognitive symptoms following stroke

Depression

The association between depressive symptoms and stroke disease has been extensively researched, indeed more than any other noncognitive symptom in cerebrovascular disease (Rao, 2000). Despite this, some key issues remain controversial and unresolved.

Depressive symptoms are common in stroke patients, and indeed their caregivers. Taken together, published prevalence studies consistently indicate depressive symptoms are more common in stroke patients than baseline population rates. However, due to different study designs, there is considerable divergence in the reported rates. Documented prevalence rates over time are 6–41% in the first two weeks, 47–53% at three to four months, 21–47% at one year, 19% at two years, 9–41% at three years, 35% at four years and 19% at seven years (Carota et al, 2002).

The headline rates usually describe the prevalence of all forms of depressive symptoms. Overall, rates for minor depression – commonly experienced as anxiety, worry, sleepiness and tearfulness – tend to be higher than rates for major depressive disorder, although again studies vary. On average, minor depressive illnesses also tend to be less enduring than major depression, e.g. mean duration of 12 vs 39 weeks respectively (Morris et al, 1990), though a proportion of patients with both minor and major depression will remain depressed for several years after stroke (Chemerinski and Robinson, 2000).

nitive decline. Such evidence clearly varies in its importance (hemiparesis or infarcts on imaging providing strong evidence while the presence of hypertension or coronary artery disease being weak). It may be found in the history (e.g. of stroke, transient ischemic attacks, falls or coronary artery disease), the physical examination (e.g. paresis or asymmetric reflexes) or special investigations (e.g. high cholesterol or infarcts on structural imaging). However, there are other features, possibly found in the assessment, which increase the likelihood that CVD may be an important factor. Generally speaking these features are related to damage to the frontal lobes and/or their connections with subcortical nuclei, since these areas are vulnerable to damage from CVD (Chui and Willis, 1999; Wolfe et al, 1990). Thus evidence in the history or mental state examination of emotional lability (House et al, 1989), depression (Alexopoulos et al, 1997; Ballard et al, 2000) or apathy (Wolfe et al, 1990) increases the probability that CVD is present, although such symptoms are also common in neurodegenerative diseases. On cognitive testing special effort should be made to seek evidence of executive dysfunction. This term is sometimes used interchangeably with frontal (or frontal-executive) lobe dysfunction, but it should be remembered that the frontal lobes subserve a much larger range of cognitive functions, e.g. language and memory, than executive functions, which map to the prefrontal areas and related frontal–subcortical circuits (Cummings, 1993). Executive function refers to planning, initiating, coordinating and monitoring goal-directed behavior and there are several commonly used neuropsychological tests for this, which are discussed in Chapter 16. Some suggestions for 'bedside' tests for use in the clinical assessment process are given below.

Differential diagnosis of vascular cognitive impairment

There are several reasons why someone might present with apparent cognitive impairment and which should be considered carefully during the assessment process. The dementing illnesses (vascular, neurodegenerative and other) are usually the main concern and assessment aims at determining whether dementia is present. The criteria for the dementia syndrome and the different dementias have been discussed in Chapter 2. Briefly, the clinician needs to establish that there are impairments in multiple cognitive domains (including amnesia) together with functional impairment. These must be chronic, occur in clear consciousness and represent a change.

If these criteria are met then the next question is whether this due to a neurodegenerative disease (AD; DLB; FTD), VaD or some combination of these? Details on distinguishing these are given elsewhere (Thomas and O'Brien, 2002) and in this chapter the focus is on the detection of CVD as a sole or contributory factor to the dementia. However, before proceeding down this road other confounders should be considered, especially in those with milder impairment. Delirium should be easily excluded in most cases in the clinical setting but the potential impact of depression and other 'functional' psychiatric disorders needs to be considered. Depression is a recognized cause of cognitive impairment in its own right (Abas et al, 1990) and also impairs everyday function (Alexopoulos et al, 1996). Schizophrenia impairs cognition globally and, like depression (Beats et al, 1996), this is especially true of executive function (Goldberg et al, 1987), whilst anxiety disorders can cause poor test performance. Mild cognitive impairment may result from brain insults, e.g. head injury (McAllister, 1992), and sensory deficits (deafness; blindness) also lead to poor scores on testing. Other organic factors (infections; alcohol or drug abuse; endocrine or metabolic disorders; vitamin deficiency) must be excluded by history, examination and investigations as contributory or primary factors. The potential influence of these conditions must be taken into account when determining whether and to what extent cognitive impairment is present and when interpreting results of standardized rating scales. This becomes all the more important when early forms of cognitive decline are being considered and the influence of such factors may be greater.

Finally, the 'diagnosis' of 'normality' needs to be considered. This can be very difficult when a patient appears to lie in the gray zone of mild objective cognitive impairment with minimal or no clear functional decline. The clinician has to try to determine whether the impairment is real and, if so, whether it genuinely reflects a change (deterioration) from the previous level. If so is this age-related rather than disease related? In practice it is frequently impossible to be sure about these issues following even the most thorough assessment process, in which case serial prospective (usually annual) assessments are often needed to answer the question.

The assessment process

Whilst service arrangements vary, especially the location of the assessment and the availability of special investigations, the assessment process outlined below follows the pattern of an initial clinical assessment, followed by further investigations before a final review and discussion.

Initial assessment

Clinical history

A good clinical history forms the foundation for any assessment as it not only supplies most of the information to be used but also shapes the rest of the assessment process and allows a good rapport to be formed with patients and informant. For those presenting with suspected cognitive impairment a history from an informant is essential as that from the patient may be unreliable and, without access to an informant account, the degree of unreliability is often difficult to determine. However, whilst it is prudent to ask for an informant to accompany the patient, judgment is needed about the extent to which they should be consulted. A patient with a complaint of memory loss may prove to have very little objective impairment and be able to give a reliable account of their difficulties and might regard consulting their spouse for information as insulting and a betrayal of the confidentiality they assumed they would enjoy. Such a situation is much more akin to that of the clinician assessing a patient with depression than that usually encountered in a dementia assessment. A careful and polite explanation of the reasons for seeking information from someone else will usually make the use of an informant acceptable.

The history should include a detailed list and description of the present problem(s) with their duration, development, pattern and severity. Did the memory just seem to gradually fade away or was it clearly temporally related to an event such as a fall or stroke? Whilst the classic insidious onset regarded as typical of AD does frequently occur in VaD, especially of the sub-cortical type, the opposite does not apply. That is, a history of cognitive impairment and deterioration related to probable vascular episodes makes pure AD very unlikely, unless the history is misleading. Having understood the present problems, careful questioning about any history of strokes, 'mini-strokes', falls and faints is essential, as are questions about wider vascular disease, e.g. hypertension, ischemic heart disease and peripheral vascular disease. Also of undoubted value is a careful review of medication. This frequently throws up medical problems, e.g. hypertension and diabetes mellitus, which might have been missed on the history and also allows the identification of treatments which may be exacerbating some of the problems, e.g. anticholinergic drugs (worsening confusion) and diuretics (causing hypotensive falls).

Once a history of cognitive decline has been established, it is necessary to determine its impact on social functioning. The questions asked about this should be guided by the level of cognitive decline. For someone who appears reasonably intact it is probably best to start by asking questions about instrumental activities of daily living (IADL), e.g. ability to handle money, self-administer medication and use a telephone. This is an opportune time to broach the subject of driving, as it may be necessary to advise that they stop doing so or be tested for safety if they wish to continue. For someone who is doing reasonably well in these areas of functioning then questions about self-care and toileting are probably inappropriate and vice versa. There are a variety of instruments used to measure activities of daily living (ADL) and it might be helpful to give one of these to the informant whilst other parts of the assessment are being completed with the patient. Examples include the Alzheimer's Disease Cooperative Study ADL scale, which is suitable for milder impairment, as it includes a high proportion of questions about IADL (Galasko et al, 1997), and the disability assessment in dementia scale, which is appropriate for moderate impairment (Gelinas et al, 1999).

Noncognitive features

Whilst psychiatric and behavioral disturbance is not a criterion for the diagnosis of dementia it is important to enquire about symptoms such as delusions and depression because they are extremely common in dementing illnesses (Lyketsos et al, 2000) and are therefore important problems in their own right. They can also help in distinguishing the likely cause of a dementia. For example, someone with early impairment and prominent visual hallucinations is much more likely to have DLB (Ballard et al, 1999); mood lability and depression both occur more commonly in VaD than AD (Ballard et al, 2000; Lyketsos et al, 2000). If time permits it can be helpful to use an instrument such as the NPI (Cummings et al, 1994) or BEHAVE–AD (Reisberg et al, 1987), which provide good coverage of the most common non-cognitive symptoms. In addition, since depression is both an important differential diagnosis and a common feature of dementia, the use of a depression scale can be useful, with the Cornell scale (Alexopoulos et al, 1988) being most appropriate as it is validated for use in dementia.

In summary, a thorough history should provide good evidence for the presence or absence of cognitive impairment in most cases and indicate whether CVD is a likely etiological factor. It is important to seek evidence of functional decline to establish the clinical significance of any cognitive impairment and to elucidate whether important and potentially treatable noncognitive symptoms are present. The later elements in the assessment process should be guided by the history.

Mental state examination

At interview the clinician should systematically examine the current mental state of the patient, including a thorough cognitive assessment. Evidence of overfamiliar or frankly disinhibited behavior or apathy indicates that frontal lobe damage may be present. Any evidence of a depressed or poorly reactive mood should lead to a probe for other symptoms consistent with a depression syndrome whilst delusional ideas or hallucinations should be sought as they can be treated. An important element to watch for throughout the interview is cognitive fluctuation. This phenomenon, which is a hallmark of DLB, may manifest itself with the patient drifting off during interview or showing frank drowsiness. However, alterations in concsiousness are often more subtle and if suspected the questions suggested by Walker et al (2000) can be used.

The depth and extent of the cognitive assessment depends on the service setting and the time and expertise available. The mini-mental state examination (MMSE) is commonly used as a screening instrument and in someone with moderate cognitive impairment this, together with an eclectic combination of other tests, may be sufficient. However, in people where the extent of the impairment is less clear, including those scoring over 23 on the MMSE this is inadequate. The MMSE suffers from ceiling effects and poorly assesses frontal–executive dysfunction, which is an important feature of vascular cognitive impairment. Thus in these patients a more thorough assessment is needed. However, in practice it is not usually feasible to complete a history, mental state examination and physical examination together with a thorough cognitive assessment in one sitting. One option is for the assessing clinician to extend the range of assessment by thoughtfully deploying several 'bedside' tests which tap into frontal lobe function and then follow this by arranging a fuller neuropsychological assessment at a separate visit. Verbal fluency can be tested briefly by using one letter from the FAS test, with less than 12 words in a minute being abnormal. Go-no-go tests with clapping (clap once, patient does nothing, clap twice patient claps once), drawing alternating sequences or multiple loops and alternating hands sequences (two-stage, with each hand alternating between fist and palm, or three-stage with one hand switching from fist to palm down to a side-down cut) can bring out repetitions indicating frontal lobe damage. Such tests can be extended as time permits and are simple but can indicate the likely presence of a dysexecutive syndrome and prompt more thorough testing later. Alternatively, the clinician might take the history and much of the behavioral and functional assessment from an informant whilst an assistant simultaneously conducts a battery of more detailed cognitive tests with the patient. Depending on the findings a separate visit may still be necessary to complete the cognitive assessment.

Physical examination

The rigor and focus of the physical examination will be guided by the findings in the history as it should aim to confirm or refute hypotheses generated from this. It should focus on seeking neurological and cardiovascular signs, remembering that in elderly people many findings which would be of concern in younger adults may be regarded as normal. There is debate about the boundaries of normality, how much is due to aging and how much to aging-related diseases, e.g. diabetes (Waite et al, 1996), but in the elderly normal findings include presbyacusis, presbyopia, mild loss of muscle bulk and strength, mildly flexed posture and gait changes (reduced stride length, reduced speed, wider base and reduced arm swing). Other signs reported as being acceptable as normal in older people include impaired vibration sense, loss of smooth ocular pursuit, reduction in vertical gaze and the presence of so-called 'primitive reflexes' (Jenkyn et al, 1985; Odenheimer et al, 1994). The latter are also known as frontal release signs and because frontal lobe features are common in CVD they are frequently regarded as useful in identifying frontal lobe damage due to CVD. However, 23% of young adults were found to have at least one reflex, with the frequency increasing with age and cognitive impairment and reaching 58% in people with dementia (Brown et al, 1998; Hogan and Ebly, 1995). The strongest predictor of dementia was the presence of multiple reflexes and the most useful individually were the glabellar and grasp reflexes, whilst the palmomental reflex was least helpful, being common at all ages.

Whilst being alert to more subtle abnormalities during the assessment it is probably wisest bearing the above in mind to seek evidence of focal neurological signs consistent with stroke disease and assess the cardiovascular system for abnormalities, which might be leading to CVD. Thus evidence of facial weakness with drooping of the corner of the mouth, a spastic increase in tone, hyperreflexia or paresis are important and any evidence of asymmetry should be regarded as abnormal. Gait abnormality, along with focal neurology, was found in a study of 1700 patients to best distinguish VaD from AD (Corey-Bloom et al, 1993), and was one of the NINDS-AIREN supporting criteria for probable VaD (Roman et al, 1993). Gait changes occur because of stroke disease (extended, abducting spastic limb with foot drop) and subcortical CVD (impaired initiation and locomotion with wide-based, ataxic, shuffling movements), although in milder forms the latter may be difficult to distinguish from normal aging. Extrapyramidal features were not found useful in separating VaD from AD (Corey-Bloom et al, 1993) but are important to seek as they suggest the presence of Lewy body disease.

A systematic cardiovascular assessment includes heart rate and rhythm, standing and lying blood pressure, auscultation for murmurs and bruits, presence of aortic aneurysm and absence of peripheral pulses with associated changes in skin temperature. Hypertension, including isolated systolic hypertension, and atrial fibrillation are especially important to identify as they are treatable risk factors for stroke. Evidence of hypotension or a history of unexplained falls should lead to further specialist assessment for one of the potentially treatable causes of neurocardiovascular instability (Kenny, 1996) whilst detection of a carotid bruit merits further specialist assessment to consider whether a carotid endarterectomy is indicated.

In conclusion, a thorough and systematic assessment involves careful history taking, a thorough mental state examination and a detailed physical assessment. Each element involves probing for evidence to support or refute the main diagnostic options so that at the end of the initial assessment a reasoned interpretation of the evidence allows probable diagnoses to be further investigated.

Further investigations

These are listed in Table 19.1. During the initial assessment a blood sample should be obtained to assess general physical health and potentially treatable factors which may be contributing to any impairment. The sample should be tested for full blood count, plasma viscosity, urea, creatinine and other electrolytes (including calcium), thyroid function, liver function, vitamin B_{12}, folate, glucose, cholesterol and syphilis serology. In addition a mid-stream urinalysis, chest radiograph, electrocardiogram and computed tomography or magnetic resonance imaging scan can be arranged before the review. Further investigations may be needed in some cases. Neuroimaging, including SPECT and PET, is fully dealt with in Chapter 20 and neuropsy-

Table 19.1 Recommendations for Investigations in assessing vascular cognitive impairment and dementia

All cases	*Selected cases*
Full blood count	EEG
Urea and creatinine	Neuropsychology
Calcium and other electrolytes	SPECT/PET scan
Plasma viscosity	MRI (if CT only available)
Thyroid function	
Liver function	
Vitamin B$_{12}$ and folate	
Random glucose	
Cholesterol	
Syphilis serology	
Urinalysis	
Chest X-ray	
ECG	
CT or MRI scan of head	

SPECT, single=photon emission computed tomography; PET, position emission tomography

chological assessment in Chapter 17. An electroencephalograph (EEG) can be helpful in some cases, and may be particularly useful in situations where there is not ready access to imaging. The EEG is a cheap, safe and noninvasive method for assessing the functional status of the brain, though its usefulness has declined in most centers with the advent of modern neuroimaging methods. It is important to remember that a normal EEG does not exclude dementia and that mildly abnormal EEGs do occur in healthy subjects. The EEG can be useful in assessing subjects with possible delirium, especially due to metabolic causes, as it usually shows widespread slowing with bursts of theta waves. It may also prove a useful investigation in patients with episodic symptoms which may have their basis in an underlying seizure disorder. In dementia the EEG usually shows an exaggeration of age-associated changes, with a diffuse slowing of the alpha rhythm and the emergence of theta and delta waves and these changes correlate with the severity of the dementia. Triphasic spikes are characteristic of the rare but important Creutzfeldt–Jakob disease while a normal EEG is particularly associated with frontotemporal dementia. VaD may be associated with focal slowing over areas of cortical infarction, though diffuse changes may be seen particularly with subcortical ischemic VaD.

Explanation of findings and management

Following all these investigations the assessment process is completed by reviewing all the evidence and arriving at a diagnosis and plan for future management and review. This should be discussed with the patient and, with their permission, with accompanying informants, although the detail and depth of this discussion will vary. Where a dementia diagnosis is clear then treatment with cholinesterase inhibitors or other antidementia medication will usually be indicated and any vascular disease identified should be treated. Similarly any noncognitive symptoms, e.g. depression, merit treatment with appropriate review. However, in many cases there may be no clear diagnosis of dementia or of milder cognitive impairment even after a thorough assessment. In some cases the clinician may be confident enough to reassure the patient that all is well but in others sufficient uncertainty will be present to make serial annual assessment the recommended outcome. In many cases only such prospective assessment will allow differentiation of a dementing illness, where there is evidence of deterioration over time, from a static impairment or no impairment. However, the assessing clinician always needs to humbly bear our continuing limitations in mind and accept that sometimes uncertainty may still remain. In spite of our technological advances and improved understanding of dementia and cognitive impairment we still frequently find ourselves unable after a single assessment or even serial prospective assessments to reach a diagnosis. In such cases careful follow-up, often at annual intervals, may be required.

References

Abas MA, Sahakian BJ, Levy R, Neuropsychological deficits and CT scan changes in elderly depressives, *Psychol Med* (1990) **20**:507–20.

Alexopoulos GS, Abrams RC, Young RC, Shamoian CA, Cornell Scale for Depression in Dementia, *Biol Psychiatry* (1988) **23**:271–84.

Alexopoulos GS, Meyers BS, Young RC et al, 'Vascular depression' hypothesis, *Arch Gen Psychiatry* (1997) **54**:915–22.

Alexopoulos GS, Vrontou C, Kakuma T et al, Disability in geriatric depression, *Am J Psychiatry* (1996) **153**:877–85.

Ballard C, Holmes C, McKeith I et al, Psychiatric morbidity in dementia with Lewy bodies: a prospective clinical and neuropathological comparative study with Alzheimer's disease, *Am J Psychiatry* (1999) **156**:1039–45.

Ballard C, Neill D, O'Brien J et al, Anxiety, depression and psychosis in vascular dementia: prevalence and associations, *J Affect Disord* (2000) **59**:97–106.

Beats BC, Sahakian BJ, Levy R, Cognitive performance in tests sensitive to frontal lobe dysfunction in the elderly depressed, *Psychol Med* (1996) **26**:591–603.

Brown DL, Smith TL, Knepper LE, Evaluation of five primitive reflexes in 240 young adults, *Neurology* (1998) **51**:322.

Chui H, Willis L, Vascular diseases of the frontal lobes. In: Miller BL, Cummings JL, eds, *The Human Frontal Lobes* (Guilford Publications: London, 1999), 370–401.

Corey-Bloom J, Galasko D, Hofstetter CR et al, Clinical features distinguishing large cohorts with possible AD, probable AD, and mixed dementia, *J Am Geriatr Soc* (1993) **41**:31–7.

Cummings JL, Frontal-subcortical circuits and human behavior, *Arch Neurol* (1993) **50**:873–80.

Cummings JL, Mega M, Gray K et al, The Neuropsychiatric Inventory: comprehensive assessment of psychopathology in dementia, *Neurology* (1994) **44**:2308–14.

Galasko D, Bennett D, Sano M et al, An inventory to assess activities of daily living for clinical trials in Alzheimer's disease. The Alzheimer's Disease Cooperative Study, *Alzheimer Dis Assoc Disord* (1997) **11**:S33–S39.

Gelinas I, Gauthier L, McIntyre M, Gauthier S, Development of a functional measure for persons with Alzheimer's disease: the disability assessment for dementia, *Am J Occup Ther* (1999) **53**:471–81.

Goldberg TE, Weinberger DR, Berman KF et al, Further evidence for dementia of the prefrontal type in schizophrenia? A controlled study of teaching the Wisconsin Card Sorting Test, *Arch Gen Psychiatry* (1987) **44**:1008–14.

Hogan DB, Ebly EM, Primitive reflexes and dementia: results from the Canadian Study of Health and Aging, *Age Ageing* (1995) **24**:375–81.

House A, Dennis M, Molyneux A et al, Emotionalism after stroke, *BMJ* (1989) **298**:991–4.

Jenkyn LR, Reeves AG, Warren T et al, Neurologic signs in senescence. *Arch Neurol* (1985) **42**:1154–7.

Kenny RA, *Syncope in the Older Patient: Causes, Investigations and Consequences of Syncope and Falls* (Chapman & Hall: London, 1996).

Lesser IM, Boone KB, Mehringer CM et al, Cognition and white matter hyperintensities in older depressed patients, *Am J Psychiatry* (1996) **153**:1280–7.

Levy R, Aging-associated cognitive decline, *Int Psychogeriatr* (1994) **6**:63–8.

Longstreth WT Jr, Bernick C, Manolio TA et al, Lacunar infarcts defined by magnetic resonance imaging of 3660 elderly people: the Cardiovascular Health Study, *Arch Neurol* (1998) **55**:1217–25.

Lyketsos CG, Steinberg M, Tschanz JT et al, Mental and behavioral disturbances in dementia: findings from the Cache County Study on Memory in Aging, *Am J Psychiatry* (2000) **157**:708–14.

McAllister TW, Neuropsychiatric sequelae of head injuries, *Psychiatric Clin N Am* (1992) **15**:395–413.

MRC/CFAS, Pathological correlates of late-onset dementia in a multicentre, community-based population in England and Wales, *Lancet* (2001) **357**:169–75.

Odenheimer G, Funkenstein HH, Beckett L et al, Comparison of neurologic changes in 'successfully aging' persons vs the total aging population, *Arch Neurol* (1994) **51**:573–80.

Petersen RC, Smith GE, Waring SC et al, Mild cognitive impairment: clinical characterization and outcome, *Arch Neurol* (1999) **56**:303–8.

Reisberg B, Borenstein J, Salob SP et al, Behavioral symptoms in Alzheimer's disease: phenomenology and treatment, *J Clin Psychiatry* (1987) **48**:9–15.

Roman GC, Tatemichi TK, Erkinjuntti T et al, Vascular dementia: diagnostic criteria for research studies. Report of the NINDS-AIREN International Workshop, *Neurology* (1993) **43**:250–60.

Thomas AJ, O'Brien JT, Alzheimer's disease. In: Jacoby R, Oppenheimer C, eds, *Psychiatry in the Elderly*, 3rd edn (Oxford University Press, Oxford, 2002) 508–32.

Waite LM, Broe GA, Creasey H et al, Neurological signs, aging, and the neurodegenerative syndromes, *Arch Neurol* (1996) **53**:498–502.

Walker MP, Ayre GA, Cummings JL et al, The Clinician Assessment of Fluctuation and the One Day Fluctuation Assessment Scale. Two methods to assess fluctuating confusion in dementia, *Br J Psychiatry* (2000) **177**:252–6.

Wolfe N, Linn R, Babikian VL et al, Frontal systems impairment following multiple lacunar infarcts, *Arch Neurol* (1990) **47**:129–32.

Ylikoski A, Erkinjuntti T, Raininko R et al, White matter hyperintensities on MRI in the neurologically nondiseased elderly. Analysis of cohorts of consecutive subjects aged 55 to 85 years living at home, *Stroke* (1995) **26**:1171–7.

chapter 20

Neuroimaging in vascular dementia

John O'Brien

Introduction

Neuroimaging is now an essential tool for the assessment and investigation of those with suspected vascular cognitive impairment (VCI) and vascular dementia (VaD). Traditionally used as a means of excluding any other intracranial lesion that may be responsible for dementia, it is increasingly necessary to add support and provide confirmation of the clinical diagnosis and to help determine the subtype of VaD (e.g. hemorrhagic vs ischemic; cortical vs subcortical; single strategic infarct vs multi-infarct) (Roman et al, 1993). Imaging can also be useful in individual cases to inform clinical understanding and management. As a number of different vascular pathologies can cause dementia, including hemorrhage, infarction (both single large and multiple small infarction) and diffuse white matter change (O'Brien et al, 2003), it is not surprising that there are no pathognomonic neuroimaging features of VaD. All these vascular changes can be visualized using the structural imaging techniques of computed tomography (CT) and magnetic resonance imaging (MRI), though it should be emphasized that the role of imaging is to provide confirmatory support for a diagnosis of VaD which has been formulated on clinical grounds. A diagnosis of VaD can and should never be made on the basis of scan appearances alone.

There are still many important areas which remain controversial, including the degree of vascular change on scanning needed to support a diagnosis of VaD, the relative significance of different types of vascular lesions and the contribution of functional as opposed to structural imaging. This chapter will review structural and functional brain imaging changes in VaD and summarize the neuroimaging evidence required to fulfill different sets of current diagnostic criteria for VaD.

Structural imaging in VaD

This consists of CT or MRI scanning. A detailed description of imaging modalities is outside the scope of this book but excellent summaries are contained elsewhere (Ames and Chiu, 1997). CT scanning involves the use of traditional radiography and a detector system which rotates around the head with reconstruction of the brain image, based on electron density, performed by back projection. Although recent hemorrhage (fresh blood) shows as areas of high attenuation (bright), after a few days both hemorrhage and infarction appear as areas of low attenuation (dark). CT scanning is cheap, widely available, quick (30 seconds per scan on modern spiral scanners), well tolerated and an effective way of showing cortical and subcortical infarcts as well as white matter changes.

In contrast to CT, MRI builds an image based on proton density and the physical properties of protons using a strong magnetic field (typically 1.5 Tesla) and a series of brief pulses of electromagnetic radiation. The image produced depends on three main properties: proton density and T1 and T2 relaxation times. Proton density, as the name implies, reflects the actual density of protons (largely water molecules) in the tissue. T1 is essentially the relaxation time (time taken for protons excited by a radiofrequency pulse to lose energy and return to normal) in three-dimensional space whilst T2 is the relaxation time reflecting loss of spin phase or coherence between adjacent protons (which initially spin in phase after a radiofrequency pulse). Both T1 and T2 depend on the physical and chemical environment of the protons, not just on their density. No image relies purely on just one of these properties, although scans weighted towards one parameter rather than another have different appearances and uses. Good anatomical resolution is provided by heavily T1-weighted images (for example, inversion recovery sequences) while proton density and T2-weighted images (for example, spin-echo sequences) are sensitive to changes in water content and provide good visualization of white matter lesions and smaller infarcts. Fluid attenuated inversion recovery (FLAIR) images provide excellent definition of white matter lesions and allow their separation from CSF, which is dark on FLAIR images but white on T2-weighted sequences.

MRI is less widely (though increasingly) available, more expensive (about three times the cost of CT), is unsuitable for patients with pacemakers or metallic implants in the head and can be claustrophobic, with about 10% patients unable to tolerate a scan. It does not visualize bone but provides superior resolution to CT, especially in the white matter. MRI, particularly using T2-weighted and FLAIR sequences, has been criticized as being too sensitive in detecting minor pathological changes, which may not always be of clinical significance (see below). Although MRI would be preferred to CT if both were equally available, in practice CT will usually be performed first in most clinical services, with MRI reserved for cases where CT is equivocal or uninformative or when better visualization of particular lesions (such as in the white matter or in subcortical areas) is required.

On structural imaging VaD, like Alzheimer's disease (AD), is associated with relatively nonspecific changes such as generalized cerebral atrophy and ventricular dilatation (Erkinjuntti et al, 1987; Aharon-Peretz et al, 1988; Loeb et al, 1988; Gorelick et al, 1992; Tatemichi et al, 1990). There may sometimes be focal atrophy, either cortical or ventricular, corresponding to focal infarction and subsequent local atrophy (Figure 20.1). A wide variety of other brain lesions can be seen including cortical infarcts, infarcts in strategic brain areas (basal ganglia and thalamus), multiple lacunes, extensive white matter change (or 'leukoaraiosis') or combinations thereof.

A major difficulty is the interpretation of the clinical significance of infarcts and, in particular, white matter changes seen on CT and MRI. Large

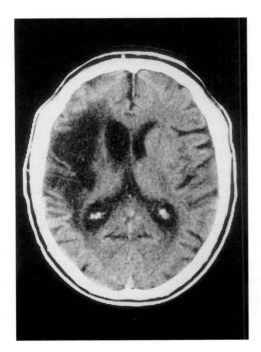

Figure 20.1 *Axial CT showing large areas of cortical and subcortical infarction in the right hemisphere. Note classic appearances of infarcts and the associated dilation of the right ventricle.*

infarcts, in keeping with the clinical symptoms and neuropsychological profile, may pose little problem. However, smaller infarcts, infarcts in 'silent' areas and more subtle white matter changes may be difficult to interpret (see 'Leukoaraiosis' below). The opposite difficulty is that many stroke patients have extensive scan evidence of cerebrovascular disease yet do not develop cognitive impairment. The essential question, therefore, in interpreting scan changes is in terms of the extent to which these are known to be robustly associated with VaD. This can be determined by considering (a) studies which have compared patients with VaD to other groups of patients and (b) studies which have compared stroke patients who subsequently develop dementia to those who remain cognitively intact

VaD compared to other disorders

Several studies have compared structural imaging changes between patients with VaD and AD. The degree of cortical atrophy or ventricular enlargement does not seem to separate groups, (Erkinjuntti et al, 1987; Aharon-Peretz et al, 1988) although VaD is invariably associated with an increased prevalence of infarcts and more extensive white matter change (Erkinjuntti et al, 1987; Aharon-Peretz et al, 1988; Pullicino et al, 1996). In contrast, focal atrophy of the frontal lobes occurs in approximately 50% of cases of frontal lobe dementia while focal atrophy of the medial temporal lobes on CT or MRI (especially of the hippocampus and entorhinal cortex), particularly with serial scanning, is associated with AD (Jobst et al, 1997; O'Brien et al, 1997; Fox et al, 1996) (Figure 20.2). In a comparison of CT and MRI in distinguishing between VaD and AD, Erkinjuntti et al (1987) found MRI more sensitive but CT more specific. Reed et al (1991) compared MRI changes in 25 patients with AD and 25 with multi-infarct dementia. Although there was overlap between groups, six MRI variables provided 84% correct diagnostic classification. These were ventricular to brain ratio, presence of subcortical infarcts, bifrontal ventricular ratio, bicaudate ventricular ratio, third ventricular ratio and the presence of diffuse periventricular high-intensity white matter lesions. Other studies also show overlap between diagnostic groups, for example, VaD can be associated with temporal lobe atrophy on CT or MRI (Jobst et al, 1997; Laakso et al, 1996; Barber et al, 1999a), while AD is associated with an increased prevalence of white matter changes (Scheltens et al, 1992; O'Brien et al, 1996). A study of progressive atrophy over a one-year period found rates of whole brain volume loss in VaD (1.9% per year) to

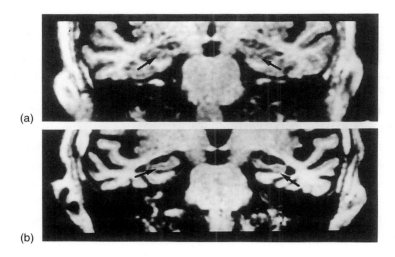

(a)

(b)

Figure 20.2 *Coronal T1-weighted MRI scan of subject with relatively normal temporal lobes and hippocampus (a) compared to subject with AD (b). Note the marked atrophy of the hippocampus (arrows), temporal horn and temporal lobe in the subject with AD.*

be remarkably similar to those in AD (2% per year) and dementia with Lewy bodies (DLB)(1.4% per year) (O'Brien et al, 2001). Whilst relative preservation of temporal lobe early in the disease process has been suggested as supportive of VaD rather than AD, caution is needed as temporal lobe preservation is also seen in DLB (Barber et al, 1999a, 2000), a disorder which can easily be mistaken for VaD because of the overlap in clinical features of neurological signs (parkinsonism), fluctuating cognitive impairments and visual hallucinations.

In summary, structural imaging studies which have compared VaD with AD find similar degrees of generalized cortical atrophy, ventricular enlargement and serial brain atrophy but generally confirm a higher prevalence of vascular lesions (particularly white matter change and infarction) in VaD compared to AD. In contrast, atrophy of the hippocampus and entorhinal cortex is associated with AD, especially when this is seen early in the disease process. The fact that studies to date have indicated that there are no pathognomonic imaging features specific to VaD again emphasizes the role of imaging in terms of providing confirmatory support to the diagnosis, rather than being an absolute diagnostic test.

The extent of vascular change necessary for dementia

There are two ways of approaching this subject. One is to consider the site of the lesion, the other the extent of the damage, although ultimately a combination of the two will undoubtedly be the variable of interest. The classic neuropathological study of Tomlinson et al (1970) found that a volume of infarction of at least 50 ml, and usually 100 ml, was necessary for VaD. However, patients with presumed VaD clinically but with smaller volumes of infarction are well recognized. Erkinjuntti et al (1988) studied 27 patients with VaD and found the mean volume of infarction was only 40 ml (range 1–229 ml) with an average of 3.4 infarctions (range 2–7) microscopically evident on neuropathological examination. Del Ser et al (1990) divided patients with evidence of cerebrovascular disease at autopsy into 28 who were demented during life and 12 who were not. Demented subjects had three times the infarct volume of nondemented subjects, although a volume of infarction of only 1% was sufficient to produce dementia in some cases. Such neuropathological studies have great relevance for understanding neuroimaging changes in VaD. If very small vascular changes can be associated with VaD in some cases, then very small and subtle vascular changes on imaging may sometimes be sufficient to support a clinical diagnosis of VaD.

Charletta et al (1995) compared 66 patients with VaD, 56 subjects who had had a stroke but who were not demented and 56 subjects with AD. Patients with VaD and stroke without dementia had a similar extent of white matter lesions but differed from each other by the size of the third ventricle. Gorelick et al (1992) compared CT findings in 58 patients with multi-infarct dementia and 74 patients who had had multiple infarcts without evidence of cognitive impairment. Dementia was associated with stroke severity, left cortical infarction, left ventricular enlargement and also level of education. In subjects with cerebrovascular disease, a number of studies have related both the extent of white matter change and cerebral atrophy to the presence of dementia (Gorelick et al, 1992; Tanaka et al, 1989; Figueroa et al, 1992). The total number of infarcts also appears to be important (Gorelick et al, 1992; Figueroa et al, 1992) as may left-sided or bilateral lesion location (Gorelick et al, 1992; Figueroa et al, 1992) or location in strategic areas such as the thalamus and anterior capsule (Figueroa et al, 1992). Just as there is now recognized to be an important interaction between degenerative and vascular pathology in the clinical expression of cognitive impairment (Snowdon et al, 1997) the same almost certainly exists with regard to imaging changes. For example, Fein et al (2000) found that it was the concurrent presence of hippocampal and cortical atrophy which explained the presence of dementia in those with ischemic subcortical vascular disease. Of importance, the absence of any evidence of cerebrovascular disease on structural imaging is strong evidence against the diagnosis of VaD (Roman et al, 1993; Erkinjuntti et al, 1999).

Imaging changes in poststroke dementia

Several studies have investigated lesion size and location in patients after stroke in relation to whether they subsequently develop dementia. In a series of 972 subjects who had undergone CT, dementia was associated with advancing age, number of infarcts, location of infarcts in temporoparietal areas and extent of white matter lesions (Tatemichi et al, 1990). No relationship was found between volume of infarct and dementia, which was consistent with some reports (Ladurner et al, 1982; Schmidt et al, 1992) but at variance with others (Figueroa et al, 1992; Censori et al, 1996; Liu et al, 1992). Most authors agree that location of lesions is important, with lesions in the thalamus (Ladurner et al, 1982), temporoparietal and temporo-occipital areas (Tatemichi et al, 1990), temporal lobes (Schmidt et al, 1992), frontal lobe and medial cerebral artery infarct location (Censori et al, 1996) and left cortical and parietal infarcts (Liu et al, 1992) all shown to be important. Several studies report an association between poststroke dementia and generalized measures such as cortical and central atrophy (Tatemichi et al, 1990; Figueroa et al, 1992; Schmidt et al, 1992; Censori et al, 1996; Liu et al, 1992; Hershey et al, 1987).

Pohjasvaara et al (1998) examined 337 patients aged 55–85 who, three months after ischemic stroke, had a comprehensive neuropsychological examination and MRI scan. Frequency of poststroke dementia at three months was 32% and was associated with advancing age, low level of education, past history of stroke and left hemisphere stroke location. The association between left-sided strokes and subsequent dementia has also been shown by others (Censori et al, 1996; Tatemichi et al, 1990). In a prospective study, Meyer et al (1995) compared repeat CT changes in 24 patients with VaD and 24 subjects with AD. Many VaD patients were treated with anti-platelet therapy and risk factor control. Cognitive decline amongst patients with VaD was associated with recurrent 'silent' strokes and perfusion changes (measured using xenon CT) in frontal white matter, and thalamic and internal capsule. Progressive cerebral atrophy and ventricular enlargement were much greater in the group with AD.

In summary, evidence from studies of patients with established VaD and poststroke dementia suggests that associations of VaD include cortical and central atrophy and indicate that both volume and location of lesion are important. In particular, bilaterality, left-sided lesions, diffuse white matter change and small infarcts in strategic areas may all be important. However, in addition to a 'lesion-based' view of VaD, clinical features such as age and level of education may play a significant role. Progressive cognitive decline in VaD may be associated with an increase in 'silent' cerebral infarction.

Leukoaraiosis

This term, meaning 'rarefaction of the white matter', was introduced by Hachinski and colleagues in 1987 (Hachinski et al, 1987) as a descriptive term for white matter changes seen on imaging which are not invariably associated with subcortical VaD or Binswanger's disease (BD). The nature and significance of such changes remains an area of uncertainty and controversy, and leukoaraiosis is one of the neuroimaging changes most widely misunderstood and misinterpreted. While BD – now usually subsumed by the term 'ischemic subcortical vascular dementia', which has clearly proposed diagnostic criteria (Erkinjuntti et al, 2000) – is likely to be associated with leukoaraiosis on scan, the converse does not apply. Leukoaraiosis, or white matter changes, can be associated with a number of different disorders including other types of VaD, AD, DLB, multiple sclerosis, hydrocephalus, various leukodystrophies, cerebral edema, neurosarcoid and conditions such as late-life depression. On CT, leukoaraiosis is seen as diffuse low-density areas in the white matter surrounding the cerebral ventricles (Figure 20.3). MRI, which builds an image based on proton rather than electron density, has greater sensitivity for demonstrating white matter lesions (Figures 20.4–20.6).

Although previously felt to be entirely nonspecific, it is now recognized that at least two types of white matter change can be demonstrated: periventricular and deep white matter lesions (see Figure 20.5). Periventricular lesions consist of, in milder forms, caps around the frontal and occipital horns of the lateral ventricles. More advanced periventricular change can be seen as a smooth halo surrounding the lateral ventricles, which extends a

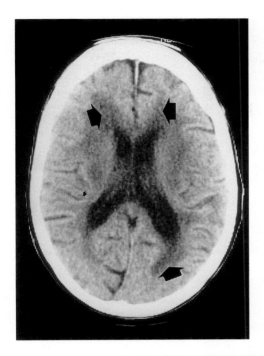

Figure 20.3 Axial CT scan showing severe leukoaraiosis extending into most of the white matter, particularly around the frontal and occipital horns and ventricles (arrows).

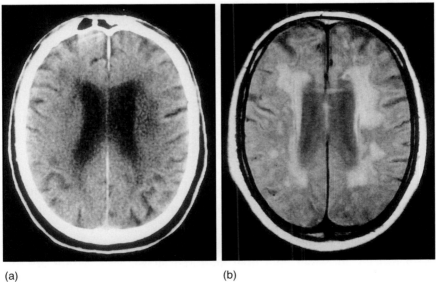

(a)   (b)

Figure 20.4 (a) Axial CT scan showing white matter change in a 73-year-old man with a clinical diagnosis of VaD. (b) Proton density MRI scan on same subject. Note the superior visualization of white matter change on the MRI scan compared to the CT scan.

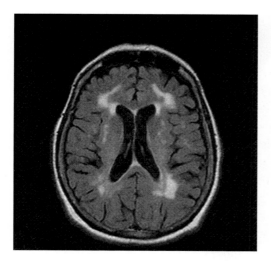

Figure 20.5 *Axial FLAIR (fluid attenuated inversion recovery) MRI scan showing periventricular (next to ventricles) and deep (separate from ventricles) white matter lesions. FLAIR sequences have advantages over traditional dual spin echo as fluid (CSF) appears dark rather than bright, easily allowing differentiation from white matter lesions.*

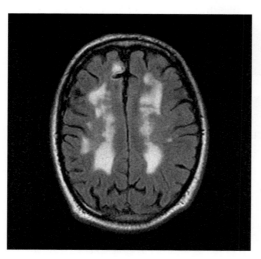

Figure 20.6 *Axial FLAIR (fluid attenuated inversion recovery) MRI scan showing extensive white matter change occupying more than 25% of the white matter and consistent with a clinical diagnosis of subcortical ischemic vascular dementia.*

variable distance into the white matter. Pathological studies have indicated that the pathogenesis of this periventricular type of lesion is essentially non-vascular (Awad et al, 1986; Fazekas et al, 1991, 1993; Scheltens et al, 1995). Periventricular changes are associated with loss of the ependymal lining of the ventricles, increased interstitial fluid and gliosis. Such lesions are not only common in the healthy elderly (where they are seen in up to 90% of subjects, depending on age) but are common in all types of dementia. For example, it has been shown that periventricular lesions occur with high but equal frequency in VaD, AD and DLB (Barber et al, 1999b).

In contrast, deep white matter lesions are separate from the ventricles (see Figure 20.5) and appear to have a different pathogenesis (Awad et al, 1986; Fazekas et al, 1991, 1993). A number of different pathologies have been related to deep white matter changes which is, perhaps, not surprising as these changes have been described in a number of different conditions including 'normal' aging and dementia. Very small punctate white matter lesions can be associated with small areas of demyelination or the pathological change of *état crible*, where dilatation of perivascular spaces and increased tortuosity of vessels is seen, not necessarily associated with atherosclerosis. Other possible causes of white matter change include focal cerebral edema, hypoxia and acidosis as well as chronic perfusion changes. More severe types of deep white matter change, however, can be associated with atherosclerotic disease. A useful guide to severity is to determine whether the white matter change occupies at least 25% of the white matter (see Figure 20.6). Change less than this is unlikely to be of clinical significance (Roman et al, 1993).

Given the variety of pathologies known to underlie white matter change, it is extremely important not to overinterpret imaging changes (particularly on FLAIR or proton density and T2-weighted MRI) with regard to vascular contribution to dementia. For example, prominent white matter changes are not invariably associated with demonstrable cognitive decline. However, in nondemented populations, including the healthy elderly (Schmidt et al, 1993; Boone et al, 1992; Breteler et al, 1994) and those with depression (Jenkins et al, 1998; Salloway et al, 1996; Simpson et al, 1997), minor degrees of white matter lesion may be associated with more subtle neuropsychological deficits, particularly with regard to impairments of attention, information processing and executive function.

Structural imaging requirements for the application of current diagnostic systems for VaD

These are summarized in Table 20.1. The Hachinski Ischemic Index (Hachinski et al, 1975) is composed of a number of clinical features and does not require any imaging information for its application. Requirements for ICD 10 (WHO, 1992) are open to interpretation. It is clear that structural neuroimaging is not mandatory for the diagnosis although the criteria do indicate that in some cases it will be needed. DSM-IV criteria (APA, 1994) require 'laboratory evidence of cerebrovascular disease', which may include

Table 20.1 Neuroimaging requirements for the application of widely used current diagnostic systems

Diagnostic criteria	Vascular brain changes required on structural imaging
Hachinski ischemic scale (Hachinski et al, 1975)	No requirement for brain imaging
ICD 10 (WHO, 1992)	In some cases, confirmation can be provided only by computerized axial tomography or, ultimately, neuropathological examination. In addition, the ICD 10 research diagnostic criteria require evidence from the history, examination or tests of significant cerebrovascular disease, which may reasonably be judged to be etiologically related to the dementia (e.g. history of stroke; evidence of cerebral infarction)
DSM-IV (APA, 1994)	There must be evidence of cerebrovascular disease (i.e. focal neurological signs and symptoms or laboratory evidence) that is judged to be etiologically related to the dementia. CT of the head and MRI usually demonstrate multiple vascular lesions of the cerebral cortex and subcortical structures. The extent of central nervous system lesions detected by CT and MRI in VaD typically exceeds the extent of changes detected in the brains of healthy elderly persons (e.g. periventricular and white matter hyperintensities noted on MRI scans). Lesions often appear in both white matter and gray matter structures, including subcortical regions and nuclei. Evidence of old infarctions (e.g. focal atrophy) may be detected, as well as findings of more recent disease
California criteria (Chui et al, 1992)	The criteria for the clinical diagnosis of probable ischemic VaD (IVD) include evidence of two or more ischemic strokes by history, neurological signs and/or neuroimaging studies (CT or T1-weighted MRI) and evidence of at least one infarct outside the cerebellum on CT or T1-weighted MRI. The diagnosis of probable IVD is supported by evidence of multiple infarcts in brain regions known to affect cognition. Features that are thought to be associated with IVD, but await further research, include

	periventricular and deep white matter changes on T2-weighted MRI that are excessive for age.
	A clinical diagnosis of possible IVD may be made when there is dementia and Binswanger's syndrome (without multiple strokes) that includes extensive white matter changes on neuroimaging
NINDS-AIREN criteria (Roman et al, 1993)	The criteria for the clinical diagnosis of probable VaD require the presence of cerebrovascular disease (CVD), defined by the presence of focal signs on neurological examination and evidence of relevant CVD by brain imaging (CT or MRI) including multiple large-vessel infarcts (angular gyrus, thalamus, basal forebrain or PCA or ACA territories), as well as multiple basal ganglia and white matter lesions, or combinations thereof. Features that make the diagnosis of VaD uncertain or unlikely include absence of cerebrovascular lesions on brain CT or MRI

imaging. They state that structural imaging 'usually' demonstrates multiple vascular lesions but this implies that diagnosis can still be made when scanning is normal or shows a single lesion. The California criteria for probable ischemic VaD (IVD) (Chui et al, 1992) require at least one infarct outside the cerebellum. A diagnosis of possible IVD does not require neuroimaging evidence of infarction. The NINDS-AIREN criteria (Roman et al, 1993) are the most rigorous with regard to the need for neuroimaging confirmation. The criteria for probable VaD include multiple infarcts or strategic single infarcts as well as multiple subcortical or white matter lesions. The criteria specifically state that the absence of cerebrovascular lesions on brain CT or MRI make the diagnosis of VaD uncertain. In the accompanying paper (Roman et al, 1993) it is stated that 'absence of cerebrovascular lesions CT or MRI is strong evidence against vascular aetiology and constitutes the most important brain imaging element to distinguish AD from VaD. There are no pathognomonic changes on brain CT or MRI of VaD.' The criteria adopt what seems to be, on the basis of previous work discussed above, a sensible approach which requires radiological findings to fulfill minimum standards for both severity and topography.

One difference between the NINDS-AIREN criteria and the California criteria is that the former recognize that a single lesion may cause VaD. They also accept that radiological lesions, regardless of location, may be taken as evidence of cerebrovascular disease. However, the criteria do exclude 'trivial' infarcts, for example, frontal horn capping or one or two lacunes. The brain imaging changes required for the NINDS-AIREN criteria are shown in Table 20.2. Perhaps one of the more difficult areas is the role of white matter change alone. The criteria deal with this by stating that white matter lesions on CT or MRI may be considered as evidence for cerebrovascular disease but for this to be the case they must be diffuse and extensive, extending to deep

Table 20.2 Brain imaging lesions associated with VaD (NINDS-AIREN criteria)

I. Topography

Radiological lesions associated with dementia include *any* of the following or combinations thereof:

1 Large-vessel strokes in the following territories:
    bilateral anterior cerebral artery
    posterior cerebral artery, including paramedian thalamic infarctions, inferior medial temporal lobe lesions
    association areas – parietotemporal, temporo-occipital territories (including angular gyrus)
    watershed carotid territories – superior frontal, parietal regions
2 Small-vessel disease:
    basal ganglia and frontal white matter lacunes
    extensive periventricular white matter lesions
    bilateral thalamic lesions

II. Severity

In addition to the above, relevant radiological lesions associated with dementia include:

    Large-vessel lesions of the dominant hemisphere
    Bilateral large-vessel hemispheric strokes
    Leukoencephalopathy involving at least one quarter of the total white matter

Although the volume of the lesion is weakly related to dementia, an additive effect may be present. White matter changes observed only on T2 MRI but not on T1 MRI or CT may not be significant. The absence of vascular lesions on brain CT/MRI rules out probable VaD.

white matter and fulfilling the '25% rule'. Changes observed only on T2 MRI are felt to be of doubtful significance.

However, the NINDS-AIREN criteria have also been criticized as being too dependent on the presence of changes on brain imaging for diagnosis. Frisoni et al (1995) examined 77 patients with AD and 17 with multi-infarct dementia (MID) according to DSM-III-R criteria. Seven (41%) of patients clinically diagnosed as having MID either had no lesion or insufficient lesions for diagnosis of probable VaD according to the NINDS-AIREN criteria. MID patients with CT evidence of cerebrovascular disease sufficient to meet probable VaD criteria were six times more likely to have a history of stroke than those without such lesions. Without large prospective studies to determine diagnostic accuracy it is difficult to assess whether the requirement for neuroimaging changes is sensible or not. It seems likely the NINDS-AIREN criteria will have high specificity but, if neuropathological work is correct in suggesting less than 1% infarction may be associated with dementia, sensitivity may be low.

Functional brain imaging in VaD

Functional brain imaging techniques include single photon emission tomography (SPET), which can use a number of tracers, most commonly a perfusion tracer like technetium 99-HMPAO. Positron emission tomography (PET) is primarily a research tool which can use a variety of ligands to look at cerebral metabolism and receptor changes in addition to blood flow. Other functional imaging techniques include magnetic resonance spectroscopy, diffusion weighted imaging, diffusion tensor imaging (DTI), functional MRI and EEG brain mapping.

The latter technique can demonstrate areas of power change, particularly slowing, which correspond to areas of ischemic damage. Changes with MRI spectroscopy are less clear. Several groups have demonstrated that neuronal loss occurring in AD is associated with reduced levels of N-acetyl aspartate (NAA), a putative neuronal marker (Shonk et al, 1995; Ernest et al, 1997; Schuff et al, 1997). More controversial is an increase in myoinositol (MI), although Shonk et al (1995) have suggested that the MI/NAA ratio can assist in differential diagnosis of AD from normal aging and frontal lobe dementia. The role spectroscopy could play in the recognition of VaD is unclear although preliminary evidence suggests that white matter lesions, irrespective of cause, may have similar spectroscopic appearances (MacKay et al,

1996). Diffusion weighted imaging and the closely related DTI offer exciting possibilities with regard to the assessment of patients with VaD (Fazekas et al, 2000). These techniques rely on demonstrating changes in the diffusivity of protons. Proton diffusion is not random and is limited by structural integrity, for example of axonal bundles. Diffusion is therefore more likely along a structurally intact fiber tract than along one whose integrity has been compromised by vascular damage. DTI, though still a research tool at present, has already been used to demonstrate fiber tract disruption associated with infarcts (Molko et al, 2001) and after stroke and to correlate changes with motor and cognitive symptoms (Gillard et al, 2001; Werring et al, 2000). Functional MRI (fMRI) is also largely a research tool at present. The most common type, blood oxygen level dependent (BOLD) fMRI, uses the change in paramagnetic properties between oxy- and deoxyhemoglobin to measure changes in blood flow in response to cortical activation caused by movement or the performance of cognitive tasks. BOLD fMRI has been able to document the degree of cortical reorganization after stroke (Feydy et al, 2002; Pineiro et al, 2001, 2002) and is likely to be a valuable tool in the investigation of cerebral substrates of cognitive impairment.

Studies using PET show that both blood flow and metabolic rate for oxygen decrease in parallel. Glucose metabolism in VaD generally shows asymmetric patterns reflecting regional abnormalities, particularly decreased metabolism in the transitional zone of temporal, parietal and occipital lobes (Duara et al, 1989; Meguro et al, 1991). In addition, diaschisis (a decrease in metabolism owing to distance effect) commonly occurs contralaterally in the cerebellum or cerebral hemisphere, thus complicating interpretation of changes.

For the foreseeable future SPET will remain the functional imaging technique most accessible to clinicians in their assessment of patients with VaD and VCI. Although structural imaging is undoubtedly the investigation of first choice to perform in the assessment of patients with vascular lesions, both to exclude some other intracranial cause for the cognitive impairment and to confirm the presence of vascular change, SPET can have a useful role in some cases. Numerous studies now demonstrate that SPET has high sensitivity and specificity (over 80%) in the distinction of patients with AD from age-matched controls (Jobst et al, 1997; O'Brien et al, 1992). Classically, bilateral temporoparietal patterns of hypoperfusion are seen (Figure 20.7), and with frontal perfusion in some cases, particularly with more severe disease. SPET is often considered the investigation of choice in supporting a diagnosis of dementia of frontal lobe type, where prominent hypoperfusion

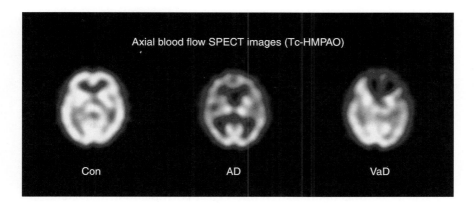

Figure 20.7 *Axial blood flow (Tc-HMPAO) SPET scans of control subject (left), AD subject (center) and vascular dementia (VaD) subject (right). Note the bilateral symmetric and posterior reduction in blood flow in the AD subjects compared with the asymmetric and focal frontal deficits (due to large cortical infarcts) in the vascular case.*

of frontal lobes is seen, with relative preservation (in most cases) of posterior perfusion. In VaD there is a variable pattern of perfusion. Classically, a 'patchy' multifocal pattern occurs, corresponding to perfusion deficits, but that will depend on the actual site of vascular lesions (see Figure 20.7). Large cortical infarcts are represented by areas of absent blood flow. More diffuse white matter change can be associated with more generalized cortical reduction in blood flow, with some regional variations which depend both on the site of lesion and the projection pathways. For example, infarcts in the basal ganglia can result in reduced cortical blood flow to frontal lobes, consistent with main projection pathways. As with PET, cerebellar and cerebral diaschisis can commonly be observed, especially after large infarcts.

Read et al (1995) compared results from SPET scanning against neuro-pathological diagnosis and found SPET could demonstrate abnormalities due to ischemic lesions not seen on structural imaging. Interestingly, two patients with a clinical diagnosis of multi-infarct dementia were found to have AD at autopsy; both had *in-vivo* SPET changes more consistent with AD. Other studies report similar findings (Jobst et al, 1997; Bonte et al, 1997) although the extent to which SPET is useful in routine clinical practice remains unclear (Pasquier et al, 1997) as most clinicopathological studies investigating the accuracy of SPET scanning in terms of diagnosis have been limited to a small number of subjects primarily with a diagnosis of AD. No large samples of patients with VaD have been reported. At present, it is probably sensible to reserve SPET as an investigation to use when information from structural imaging is not definitive enough to confirm or refute a diagnosis of VaD. Specific chemical ligands for PET and SPECT, increasingly becoming available, are still primarily research tools. Kuhl et al (1996) have shown profound loss of the choline transporter system (a putative presynaptic marker for cholinergic systems) in patients with AD and in patients with Parkinson's disease and dementia. The advent of such chemical imaging techniques offers the opportunity to investigate individual neurotransmitter systems by studying either receptor changes or presynaptic markers (or both) and, ultimately, offers great potential to investigate neuro-chemical correlates of ischemic lesions on scanning.

Mixed dementias

One difficulty with current classification systems is that they do not take account of mixed dementias, which are known to account for 10–20% of cases. The importance of mixed pathology was demonstrated by Snowdon et al (1997) who found that, among 61 subjects who met neuropathological criteria for AD, those with brain infarcts (particularly lacunar infarcts in the basal ganglia, thalamus or deep white matter) had poorer cognitive function and a higher prevalence of dementia than those without infarcts. Neuroimaging offers great potential to tease out mixed pathology as the vascular component to cognitive impairment can be demonstrated by structural imaging, with the necessary caveats regarding issues such as deep white matter change. The component of degenerative change to cognitive impairment is, perhaps, more difficult to quantify. However, it has been demonstrated that atrophy of the temporal lobe and hippocampus appears to be related to the presence of Alzheimer change, particularly tangle count in the medial temporal lobe (Huesgen et al, 1993; Harvey et al, 1999). Further prospective studies are needed to confirm this but it remains possible that selective volume change in medial temporal lobe areas may primarily reflect concurrent Alzheimer type pathology, whereas ischemic and other change would reflect vascular pathology. As such, imaging could prove a useful tool to help distinguish the contribution of different underlying pathologies to the clinical picture.

Imaging and the prediction of subsequent cognitive decline

With increasing emphasis on early detection and diagnosis, there is great interest in the possible role of imaging in the early detection of VaD and, in particular, in the assessment of VCI cases that may progress to VaD and even in detecting asymptomatic individuals at risk of subsequent VCI. There is reasonable evidence from a number of groups that atrophy of the hippocampus and entorhinal cortex on MRI and hypometabolism of the posterior cingulate and/or hippocampus on PET are predictive of subsequent progression to AD in those presenting with an amnestic type of mild cognitive impairment (MCI) (Convit et al, 2000; Jack et al, 1999; de Leon et al, 2001; Small et al, 2000). The literature on cognitive decline after stroke has already been reviewed. It has been speculated that for VCI it will be the presence of significant white matter changes that predict decline. However, a clear picture has not yet emerged. For example, while there is a relationship between white matter lesion load and lesion progression (the larger the lesions, the more likely they are to progress), a clear relationship between progression of white matter change and progression of cognitive impairment has not been demonstrated (Schmidt et al, 1999). Reasons for this may include the methodological difficulties still inherent in assessing the degree of white matter burden and its progression combined with the additional contribution of other changes such as cerebral atrophy. In summary, while some vascular imaging changes are more likely to be associated with cognitive progression than others (e.g. large white matter lesions or infarcts which are large, bilateral or in the dominant hemisphere), much more information on reliable predictors in individual cases is still required.

References

Aharon-Peretz J, Cummings JL, Hill MA, Vascular dementia and dementia of the Alzheimer type. Cognition, ventricular size, and leukoaraiosis, *Arch Neurol* (1988) **47**:719–21.

American Psychiatric Association, *Diagnostic and Statistical Manual of Mental Disorders*, 4th edn (American Psychiatric Association: Washington DC, 1994).

Ames D, Chiu E *Neuroimaging and the Psychiatry of Late Life* (Cambridge University Press: Cambridge, 1997).

Awad IA, Johnson PC, Spetzler RE et al, Incidental subcortical lesions identified on magnetic resonance imaging in the elderly. II. Postmortem pathological correlations, *Stroke* (1986) **17**:1090–7.

Barber R, Gholkar A, Scheltens et al, Medial temporal lobe atrophy on MRI in dementia with Lewy bodies, *Neurology* (1999a) **52**:1153–8.

Barber R, Gholkar A, Ballard C et al, White matter lesions on MRI in dementia with Lewy bodies, Alzheimer's disease, vascular dementia and normal ageing, *J Neurol Neurosurg Psychiatry* (1999b) **67**:66–93.

Barber R, Ballard C, McKeith IG et al, MRI volumetric study of dementia with Lewy bodies: a comparison with AD and vascular dementia, *Neurology* (2000) **54**:1304–9.

Bonte FJ, Weiner MF, Bigio EH et al, Brain blood flow in dementias: SPECT with histopathologic correlation in 54 patients, *Radiology* (1997) **202**:793–7.

Boone KB, Miller BL, Lesser JM et al, Neuropsychological correlates of white matter lesions in healthy elderly subjects. A threshold effect, *Arch Neurol* (1992) **49**:549–54.

Breteler MMB, van Amerongen NM, van Swieten JC et al, Cognitive correlates of ventricular enlargement and cerebral white matter lesions on magnetic resonance imaging, *Stroke* (1994) **25**:1109–15.

Censori B, Manara O, Agostinis C et al, Dementia after first stroke, *Stroke* (1996) **27**:1205–10.

Charletta D, Gorelick PB, Dollear TJ et al, CT and MRI findings among African-Americans with Alzheimer's disease, vascular dementia, and stroke without dementia, *Neurology* (1995) **45**:1456–61.

Chui HC, Victoroff JI, Margolin D et al, Criteria for the diagnosis of ischaemic vascular dementia proposed by the state of California Alzheimer's disease diagnostic and treatment centers, *Neurology* (1992) **42**:473–80.

Convit A, de Asis J, de Leon MJ et al, Atrophy of the medial occipitotemporal, inferior, and middle temporal gyri in non-demented elderly predict decline to Alzheimer's disease, *Neurobiol Aging* (2000) **21**:19–26.

De Leon MJ, Convit A, Wolf OT et al, Prediction of cognitive decline in normal elderly subjects with 2-[(18)F]fluoro-2-deoxy-D-glucose/positron-emission tomography (FDG/PET). *Proc Nat Acad Sci USA* (2001) **98**:10966–71.

Del Ser T, Bermejof B, Porteraa C et al, Vascular dementia: a clinical pathological study, *J Neurol Sci* (1990) **96**:1–17.

Duara R, Barker W, Loewenstein D et al, Sensitivity and specificity of positron emission tomography and magnetic resonance imaging studies in Alzheimer's disease and multi-infarct dementia, *Eur Neurol* (1989) **29** (Suppl 3):9–15.

Erkinjuntti T, Ketonen L, Sulkava R et al, CT in the differential diagnosis between Alzheimer's disease and vascular dementia, *Acta Neurol Scand* (1987) **75**:262–70.

Erkinjuntti T, Heltia M, Palo J et al, Accuracy of the clinical diagnosis of vascular dementia: a prospective clinical and post-mortem neuropathological study, *J Neurol Neurosurg Psychiatry* (1988) **51**:1037–44.

Erkinjuntti T, Bowler JV, DeCarli CS et al, Imaging of static brain lesions in vascular dementia: implications for clinical trials, *Alzheimer Dis Assoc Disord* (1999) **13** (Suppl 3):S81–S90.

Erkinjuntti T, Inzitari D, Pantoni L et al, Research criteria for subcortical vascular dementia in clinical trials. *J Neural Trans Suppl* (2000) **59**:23–30.

Ernest T, Chang C, Melchor R et al, Frontotemporal dementia and early Alzheimer's disease: differentiation with frontal lobe H-1 MR spectroscopy, *Radiology* (1997) **203**:829–36.

Fazekas F, Ropele S, Bammer R et al, Novel imaging technologies in the assessment of cerebral ageing and vascular dementia, *J Neural Trans Suppl* (2000) **59**:45–52.

Fazekas F, Kleinert R, Offenbacher H et al, The morphologic correlates of incidental punctate white matter hyperintensities on MR images, *Am J Neuroradiol* (1991) **12**:915–21.

Fazekas F, Kleinert R, Offenbacher H et al, Pathologic correlates of incidental MRI white matter signal hyperintensities, *Neurology* (1993) **43**:1683–9.

Fein G, Di Sclafani V, Tanabe J et al, Hippocampal and cortical atrophy predict dementia in subcortical ischemic vascular disease, *Neurology* (2000) **55**:1626–35.

Feydy A, Carlier R, Roby-Brami A et al, Longitudinal study of motor recovery after stroke: recruitment and focusing of brain activation. *Stroke* (2002) **33**:1610–17.

Figueroa M, Tatemichi TK, Cross DT et al, CT correlates of dementia after stroke, *Neurology* (1992) **42**:176.

Fox NC, Freeborough PA, Rossor MN, Visualisation and quantification of rates of atrophy in Alzheimer's disease, *Lancet* (1996) **348**:94–7.

Frisoni G, Beltramolloa, Binetti G et al, Computed tomography in the detection of the vascular component in dementia, *Gerontology* (1995) **41**:121–8.

Gillard JH, Papadakis NG, Martin K et al, MR diffusion tensor imaging of white matter tract disruption in stroke at 3 T, *Br J Radiol* (2001) **74**:642–7.

Gorelick P, Chatterjee A, Patel C et al, Cranial computed tomographic observations in multi-infarct dementia. A controlled study, *Stroke* (1992) **23**:801–11.

Hachinski VC, Potter P, Merskey H, Leukoaraiosis: an ancient term for a new problem, *Arch Neurol* (1987) **44**:21–3.

Hachinski VC, Iliff LD, Zilhka E et al, Cerebral blood flow in dementia, *Arch Neurol* (1975) **32**:632–7.

Harvey GT, O'Brien JT, Hughes J et al, Magnetic resonance imaging differences between dementia with Lewy bodies and Alzheimer's disease, *Psychol Med* (1999) **29**:181–7.

Hershey LA, Modic MT, Greenough PG et al, Magnetic resonance imaging in vascular dementia, *Neurology* (1987) **37**:29–36.

Huesgen CT, Burger PC, Crain BJ et al, In vitro MR microscopy of the hippocampus in Alzheimer's disease, *Neurology* (1993) **43**:145–52.

Jack CR, Petersen RC, Xu YC et al, Prediction of AD with MRI-based hippocampal volume in mild cognitive impairment, *Neurology* (1999) **52**:1397–403.

Jenkins M, Malloy P, Salloway S et al, Memory processes in depressed geriatric patients with and without subcortical hyperintensities on MRI, *J Neuroimaging* (1998) **8**:20–6.

Jobst KA, Barnetson LP, Shepstone BJ, Accurate prediction of histologically confirmed Alzheimer's disease and the differential diagnosis of dementia, *Int Psychogeriatr* (1997) **9** (Suppl 1):191–222.

Kuhl DE, Minoshima S, Fessler JA et al, In vivo mapping of cholinergic terminals in normal ageing, Alzheimer's disease, and Parkinson's disease, *Ann Neurol* (1996) **40**:399–410.

Laakso MP, Partanen K, Riekkinen P et al, Hippocampal volumes in Alzheimer's disease, Parkinson's disease with and without dementia, and in vascular dementia: an MRI study, *Neurology* (1996) **46**:678–81.

Ladurner G, Illiff LD, Lechner H, Clinical factors associated with dementia in ischaemic stroke, *J Neurol Neurosurg Psychiatry* (1982) **45**:97–101.

Liu CK, Miller BL, Cummings JL et al, A quantitative MRI study of vascular dementia, *Neurology* (1992) **42**:138–43.

Loeb C, Gandolfo C, Bino G, Intellectual impairment and cerebral lesions in multiple cerebral infarcts. A clinical computed tomography study, *Stroke* (1988) **19**:560–5.

MacKay S, Ezekiel F, Di Sclafani V et al, Alzheimer's disease and subcortical ischemic vascular dementia: evaluation by combining MR imaging segmentation and H-I MR spectroscopic imaging, *Radiology* (1996) **198**:537–45.

Meguro K, Doi C, Ueda M et al, Deceased cerebral glucose metabolism associated with mental deterioration in multi-infarct dementia, *Neuroradiology* (1991) **33**:305–9.

Meyer JS, Muramatsu K, Mortel KF et al, Prospective CT confirms differences between vascular and Alzheimer's dementia, *Stroke* (1995) **26**:735–42.

Molko N, Pappata S, Mangin JF et al, Diffusion tensor imaging study of subcortical gray matter in CADASIL, *Stroke* (2001) **32**:2049–54

O'Brien JT, Eagger S, Syed GMS et al, A study of regional cerebral blood flow and cognitive performance in Alzheimer's disease, *J Neurol Neurosurg Psychiatry* (1992) **55**:1182–7.

O'Brien JT, Desmond P, Ames D et al, A magnetic resonance imaging study of white matter lesions in depression and Alzheimer's disease, *Br J Psychiatry* (1996) **168**:477–85.

O'Brien JT, Desmond P, Ames D et al, Temporal lobe magnetic resonance imaging can differentiate Alzheimer's disease from normal ageing, depression, vascular dementia and other causes of cognitive impairment, *Psych Med* (1997) **27**:1267–75.

O'Brien JT, Paling S, Barber R et al, Progressive brain atrophy on serial MRI in dementia with Lewy bodies, AD, and vascular dementia, *Neurology* (2001) **56**:1386–8.

O'Brien JT, Erkinjuntti T, Reisberg B et al, Vascular cognitive impairment, *Lancet Neurol* (2003) **2**:11–20.

Pasquier F, Lavenue I, Lebert F et al, The use of SPECT in a multidisciplinary memory clinic, *Dement Geriatr Cog Disord* (1997) **8**:85–91.

Pineiro R, Pendlebury S, Johansen-Berg H, Matthews PM, Functional MRI detects posterior shifts in primary sensorimotor cortex activation after stroke: evidence of local adaptive reorganization? *Stroke* (2001) **32**:1134–9

Pineiro R, Pendlebury S, Johansen-Berg H, Matthews PM, Altered hemodynamic responses in patients after subcortical stroke measured by functional MRI, *Stroke* (2002) **33**:103–9.

Pohjasvaara T, Erkinjuntti T, Ylikoskir C et al, Clinical determinance of post-stroke dementia, *Stroke* (1998) **29**:75–81.

Pullicino P, Benedict RH, Capruso DX et al, Neuroimaging criteria for vascular dementia, *Arch Neurol* (1996) **53**:723–8.

Read SL, Miller BL, Mena I et al, SPECT in dementia: clinical and pathological correlation, *J Am Geriatr Soc* (1995) **43**:1243–7.

Reed K, Rogers R, Myer J, Cerebral magnetic resonance imaging compared in Alzheimer's and multi-infarct dementia, *J Neuropsychiatry Clin Neurosci* (1991) **3**:51–7.

Roman GC, Tatemichi T, Erkinjuntti T et al, Vascular dementia: diagnostic criteria for research studies. Report of the NINCDS-AIRENS International Workshop, *Neurology* (1993) **43**:250–60.

Salloway S, Malloy P, Kohn R et al, MRI and neuropsychological differences in early- and late-life-onset geriatric depression, *Neurology* (1996) **46**:1567–74.

Scheltens PH, Barkhof F, Valk J et al, White matter lesions of magnetic resonance imaging in Alzheimer's disease. Evidence for heterogeneity, *Brain* (1992) **115**:735–43.

Scheltens PH, Kamphorst W, Barkhof F et al, Histopathological correlates of white matter changes on MRI in Alzheimer's disease and normal ageing, *Neurology* (1995) **45**:883–8.

Schmidt R, Fazekas F, Offenbacher H et al, Neuropsychologic correlates of MRI white matter hyperintensities: a study of 150 normal volunteers, *Neurology* (1993) **43**:2490–4.

Schmidt R, Mechtler L, Kinkel PR et al, Cognitive impairment after hemispheric stroke: a clinical and computed tomographic study, *Neurology* (1992) **42** (Suppl 3):176.

Schmidt R, Fazekas F, Kapeller P et al, MRI white matter hyperintensities: three-year follow-up of the Austrian Stroke Prevention Study, *Neurology* (1999) **53**:132–9.

Schuff N, Amend D, Ezekiel F et al, Changes of hippocampal *N*-acetyl aspartate and volume in Alzheimer's disease: a proton MR spectroscopic imaging and MRI study, *Neurology* (1997) **49**:1513–21.

Shonk TK, Moats RA, Gifford P et al, Probable Alzheimer's disease: diagnosis with proton MR spectroscopy, *Radiology* (1995) **195**:65–72.

Simpson S, Jackson A, Baldwin RC et al, Subcortical hyperintensities in late-life depression; acute response to treatment and neuropsychological impairment, *Int Psychogeriatr* (1997) **3**:257–75.

Small G, Ercoli L, Silverman D et al, Influence of ApoE genotype and PET brain imaging on preclinical prediction of Alzheimer's disease, *Neurobiology of Aging* (2000) **21**(15):S74.

Snowdon DA, Greiner LH, Mortimer JA et al, Brain infarction and the clinical expression of Alzheimer disease, The Nun Study. *JAMA* (1997) **277**:813–17.

Tanaka Y, Tanaka O, Mizuno Y et al, A radiologic study of dynamic processes in lacunar dementia, *Stroke* (1989) **20**:1488–93.

Tatemichi TK, Foulkes MA, Mohr JP et al, Dementia in stroke survivors in the stroke data bank cohort, relevance, incidence, risk factors, and computed tomographic findings, *Stroke* (1990) **21**:858–66.

Tomlinson BE, Blessed G, Roth M, Observations on the brains of demented old people, *Neurol Sci* (1970) **11**:205–42.

Werring DJ, Toosy AT, Clark CA et al, Diffusion tensor imaging can detect and quantify corticospinal tract degeneration after stroke, *J Neurol Neurosurg Psychiatry* (2000) **69**:269–72.

World Health Organization, *International Classification of Diseases and Health Related Problems*, 10th rev (World Health Organization: Geneva, 1992).

Part VI

Management

chapter 21

Primary prevention

Stephen M Davis

Introduction

There is likely to be a huge increase in the prevalence of dementia, given the progressive aging of populations in both developed and developing countries. It is estimated that dementia affects 5% of individuals over the age of 65 years, increasing to 25% over 85 and 50% of those over 95 years of age (Tatemichi et al, 1990). In 1990, it was the eighth leading cause of disability and death in the world, and the disease burden from dementia is anticipated to increase 50% by 2020 (Skoog et al, 1996). Although Alzheimer's disease (AD) is the most common form of dementia in Western countries, vascular dementia (VaD) is more common than AD in Asia and other developing regions and may well be the commonest form of dementia worldwide (Gorelick and Roman, 1993). Despite the varied pathologies causing VaD, it is generally presumed to be the only preventable form of dementia (Hachinski, 1992; Butler et al, 1993).

The histological changes seen in VaD and AD show considerable overlap. Amyloid angiopathy is commonly associated with both conditions (Pasquier and Leys, 1997). The apolipoprotein-E genotype is associated with the pathogenesis of both atherosclerosis and Alzheimer's disease. (Hofman et al, 1997). Vascular risk factors such as systolic hypertension and hypercholesterolemia increase the risk of AD (Kivipelto et al, 2001). Vascular strategies appear useful for the prevention of AD as well as VaD.

Multiple cortical infarcts with cumulative brain volume loss have long been recognized as a major cause of VaD (Figure 21.1), but VaD can also be due to small, strategically located infarcts in the thalamus, caudate head or angular gyrus. Historically, lacunar infarcts and more diffuse white matter ischemic disease were first recognized by Binswanger as an important cause of VaD (Hachinski, 1991). Hachinski introduced the concept of leukoaraiosis in the 1980s to describe the clinical manifestations of subcortical white matter ischemia demonstrated on computed tomography (CT) and magnetic

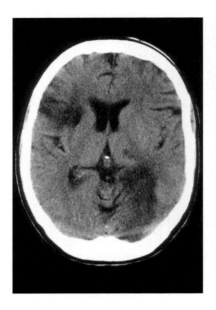

Figure 21.1 *An example of multiple cerebral infarcts shown on CT scan. Regions of cerebral infarction include infarction in the right middle cerebral and left posterior cerebral artery (PCA) territory. The left PCA infarct includes infarction in the thalamus, a common cause of memory abnormalities.*

resonance imaging (MRI) (Hachinski et al, 1987). It has been shown that the severity of these white matter changes correlates with cognitive impairment (Figure 21.2) (Breteler et al, 1994). The condition termed CADASIL (cerebral autosomal dominant arteriopathy with subcortical infarcts and leukoencephalopathy) represents a genetically determined cause of white matter pathology and dementia (Dichgans et al, 1998).

Poststroke dementia

Poststroke dementia is common. It has been estimated to affect over 20% of patients after stroke (Desmond et al, 2000), the relative risk of dementia being increased five- to nine-fold. In one study, over 50% of patients with poststroke dementia had the features of VaD, while a third had the clinical syndrome of AD (Desmond et al, 2000). Another study reported a lower incidence of poststroke dementia, affecting 5% of stroke patients over 60 at one year but increasing to 10% in those over 90 years old (Tatemichi et al, 1990). More advanced age at stroke onset and lower educational status were found to be significant covariates as was a low score on the Mini-Mental State Examination at baseline (Tatemichi et al, 1994). Another study showed a 50% increase in AD after the first year after a stroke, compared with community controls (Kokmen et al, 1996).

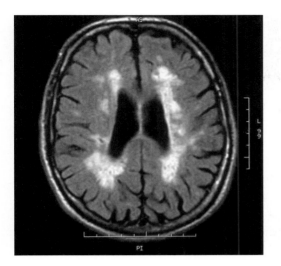

Figure 21.2 *MR scan showing multifocal white matter abnormalities as commonly seen in VaD.*

Prevention of VaD: an overall approach

In most Western countries, there has been an impressive fall in population-based stroke mortality over the past few decades (Bennett, 1995). However, with the ageing of the population and lack of decline in the incidence of stroke, a marked increase in stroke prevalence has been predicted (Jamrozik, 1997). Furthermore, age is the strongest independent risk factor for the development of VaD (Gorelick, 1997). The impressive advances in stroke prevention via a range of proven strategies should translate to a lowered risk of the development of VaD. There have been few studies to specifically test this hypothesis although there have been recent positive results from blood pressure-lowering trials. This chapter will review the major modifiable risk factors for stroke and the evidence concerning primary and secondary stroke prevention, based on the results of randomized, controlled clinical trials.

Stroke prevention involves primary and secondary strategies. Primary prevention includes treatment of risk factors and cerebrovascular lesions in individuals who have not experienced cerebrovascular symptoms. Secondary prevention involves strategies used after a stroke or transient ischemic attack (TIA), which should be tailored to the specific type of cerebrovascular pathology.

Primary prevention

Primary prevention strategies target the major risk factors for stroke (Table 21.1). In the consideration of risk factors and stroke, the population-attributable risk is a useful concept to evaluate the overall importance of a risk factor. This combines the relative risk of the individual factor and its prevalence (Whisnant, 1997).

Age and gender

In general, the frequency of stroke increases with advancing age, although there are important differences between stroke subtypes. For example, patients with subarachnoid hemorrhage are usually aged 30–60 years, often affecting young and middle-aged adults in their productive years. Conversely, cerebral infarcts due to extracranial vascular disease occurs in older individuals (Lefkovits et al, 1995). Overall, male gender is associated with increased stroke risk. Among older patients there is a slightly higher rate of stroke in females but this may simply reflect the greater longevity of women.

Table 21.1 Risk factors for ischemic stroke

Risk factor	Relative risk of stroke	Modifiable	Benefits proven
Age and gender	Increasing age; male gender	No	–
Smoking	1.0–4.0	Yes	Yes
Previous stroke; TIA	5.0–10.0	Yes	Yes
Hypertension	2.0–4.0	Yes	Yes
Diabetes	2.0–8.0	Yes	For vascular disease overall
Heart disease (particularly atrial fibrillation)	6.0–8.0	Yes	Yes
Hypercholesterolemia	1.0–2.0	Yes	Yes
Miscellaneous (obesity; lack of exercise; snoring; high hematocrit; elevated fibrinogen)	Variable	Yes	Some, e.g. exercise

Adapted with permission from Srikanth and Donnan, 1998.

Blood pressure and stroke

Hypertension is the most important risk factor for both cerebral infarction and hemorrhage (Rodgers et al, 1996; Whisnant, 1997), with a population attributable risk of 26% (Whisnant, 1997). Numerous population studies have demonstrated an increased frequency of stroke with both systolic and diastolic hypertension (MacMahon and Rodgers 1994). A meta-analysis of 14 randomized trials of antihypertensive therapy showed that modest blood pressure reduction of 5–6 mmHg reduces stroke risk by about 40% (Collins et al, 1990). This benefit also extends to those with mild hypertension. Recent studies indicate that blood pressure-lowering therapy also translates to a lower risk of VaD (see below).

Blood pressure, cognition and dementia

Cross-sectional and longitudinal studies have shown an association between hypertension and dementia, both VaD and AD types. A 15-year longitudinal study found associations between elevated systolic and diastolic blood pressure with both AD and VaD. Increased severity of white matter disease visualized on CT was thought to be a relevant mechanism linking blood pressure and dementia (Skoog et al, 1996). In follow-up of nearly 5000 individuals in the Honolulu Heart Program, midlife systolic blood pressure predicted reduced cognitive function in later life (Launer et al, 1995). In a Swedish population-based cohort study, higher diastolic blood pressure at baseline, insulin resistance and diabetes, all predicted later impairment of cognitive performance (Kilander et al, 1998). In a longitudinal study in Nantes, there was also an association between high blood pressure at baseline and cognitive decline over four years, which was highest in untreated hypertensive patients (Tzourio et al, 1999).

Lowering blood pressure and dementia

Few trials to date have specifically evaluated the effects of blood pressure reduction on dementia and cognitive impairment. These have been chiefly primary prevention studies, with the exception of the PROGRESS trial (PROGRESS Collaborative Group). The SHEP trial (Systolic Hypertension in the Elderly Program) was a large study evaluating antihypertensive treatment in elderly patients with systolic hypertension, who were randomized to active treatment with a diuretic and β-blocker, or placebo. Despite a substantial reduction in stroke and other secondary vascular endpoints with the antihypertensive therapy, the risks of cognitive impairment were similar in the two groups (SHEP Cooperative Research Group, 1991). However, further analysis indicated that there may have been a differential dropout from the study and that a benefit may have been missed (Di Bari et al, 2001). Another study, also using a combination of diuretic and β-blocker therapy over 4.5 years, similarly showed no overall benefit for cognitive outcomes (Prince et al, 1996).

In contrast, more recent studies have shown the benefits of blood pressure reduction in the attenuation of dementia and cognitive decline. In the Systolic Hypertension in Europe Trial (Syst-Eur), patients over 60 years of age with isolated systolic hypertension were randomised to receive active treatment with a calcium channel antagonist (some with additional enalapril and a thiazide), with a median follow-up of two years. There was a lower incidence of dementia in those on the antihypertensive therapy (Forette et al, 1998). The SCOPE trial (Study on Cognition and Prognosis in the Elderly) assessed the effects of the angiotensin II receptor antagonist, candesartin, on major cardiovascular events and cognitive function, in elderly patients with hypertension (Hansson et al, 1999). The candesartin group had a 28% reduction in the rate of nondisabling stroke and a small but significant attenuation of cognitive decline (Hansson and Lithell, 2002).

Cardiac disease

Valvular heart disease has long been recognized as a cause of cerebral embolism. The decline in rheumatic heart disease, associated with a 17-fold increase in stroke risk in those with atrial fibrillation, has probably contributed to the reduction in population-based stroke mortality. Attention has more recently been focused on other forms of cardiac disease, particularly nonvalvular atrial fibrillation (NVAF), the most common cause of cardiogenic embolic stroke in Western countries. It is associated with a 6–8 times increase in stroke risk (Risk factors for stroke and efficacy of antithrombotic therapy in atrial fibrillation. Analysis of pooled data from five randomized controlled trials, 1994). Atrial fibrillation represents an extraordinarily important opportunity for stroke prevention. An Australian study indicated a prevalence of atrial fibrillation of 11% of the population older than 75 years (Lake et al, 1989).

Clinical trials have demonstrated a relative risk reduction of about 70% in stroke using warfarin in patients with non-valvular atrial fibrillation, without prior cerebrovascular symptoms (Risk factors for stroke and efficacy of antithrombotic therapy in atrial fibrillation. Analysis of pooled data from five randomized controlled trials, 1994). There is also a modest therapeutic benefit with aspirin although it is only about half as effective as warfarin (Risk factors for stroke and efficacy of antithrombotic therapy in atrial fibrillation. Analysis of pooled data from five randomized controlled trials, 1994). In patients with valvular heart disease and atrial fibrillation, the risk of stroke is far higher than in those with NVAF (Risk factors for stroke and efficacy of antithrombotic therapy in atrial fibrillation. Analysis of pooled data from five randomized controlled trials, 1994). Warfarin is effective and is combined with aspirin to convey additional benefit in patients with prosthetic heart valves and atrial fibrillation or prior thrombo-embolism (Turpie et al, 1993).

Diabetes

Diabetes mellitus is associated with a two- to five-fold increase in the rate of stroke (Zimmet and Alberti, 1997). This is due to accelerated atherogenesis in the extracranial arteries (macrovascular disease) and the development of small vessel lacunar infarcts (microvascular disease). In addition, the prognosis of acute stroke in diabetic and other hyperglycemic patients is worse than in those with normal blood sugar levels, probably due to the production of excessive lactate and increased tissue damage (Kiers et al, 1992; Parsons et al, 2002). Optimal control of blood glucose is likely to reduce the vascular complications of diabetes.

Smoking

Smoking is an important specific risk factor for stroke, particularly ischemic stroke and subarachnoid hemorrhage (Shinton and Beevers, 1989; Donnan et al, 1993). It at least doubles stroke risk in both men and women (Robbins et al, 1994). There is a substantial reduction of stroke risk within two to four years of smoking cessation (Kawachi et al, 1993; Robbins et al, 1994). Chronic smoking also lowers cerebral blood flow. For these reasons, reduction in population-based smoking rates is an important public health strategy for stroke prevention and could potentially impact on the incidence of VaD (Jamrozik et al, 1994).

Hypercholesterolemia

Hypercholesterolemia is a somewhat weaker risk factor for stroke than for ischemic heart disease in epidemiological studies (Atkins et al, 1993). However, elevation of the low-density lipoprotein (LDL) cholesterol fraction is significantly related to increased cerebrovascular atherosclerosis. Recent trials of the HMG-CoA reductase inhibitors (the 'statins'), which lead to potent cholesterol reduction, have significantly reduced stroke risk in patients with ischemic heart disease and cholesterol ranging from normal to high levels (Blauw et al, 1997; Bucher et al, 1998). Some of the benefits of statins are thought to reflect pharmacological actions other than cholesterol lowering, such as antiplatelet actions and effects on atherosclerotic plaque. There is some evidence that use of statins is associated with a lower prevalence of dementia and attenuates progression of cognitive decline (Hajjar et al, 2002).

Heavy alcohol use

Heavy alcohol use is associated with an increased risk of both ischemic and hemorrhagic stroke, particularly subarachnoid hemorrhage. In contrast, some studies have suggested that low-to-moderate alcohol intake may actually be stroke protective (Jamrozik et al, 1994).

Miscellaneous factors

Polycythemia is an important and treatable risk factor for cerebral infarction. An elevated hematocrit, even in the upper 'physiological' range, is associated with increased stroke risk and stroke severity. Leisure-time physical activity has been linked with reduced risk of ischemic stroke (Sacco et al, 1998).

Asymptomatic carotid disease

There have been a number of trials to determine whether carotid endarterectomy (CEA) is beneficial in patients with severe asymptomatic carotid stenosis (Figure 21.3). The most definitive of these indicated that there was an 11% stroke rate over five years in the hemisphere ipsilateral to a 60% or greater carotid stenosis, reduced significantly to 5% by CEA in good surgical hands (Executive Committee for the Asymptomatic Carotid Atherosclerosis Study, 1995). However, this study also showed that the natural history of asymptomatic carotid stenosis was relatively benign. Therefore, a large number of operations would be required to prevent one stroke. The place of CEA for asymptomatic carotid stenosis therefore remains highly controversial (Prevention of Stroke, 1996).

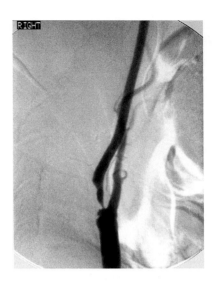

Figure 21.3 *Angiogram showing severe internal carotid stenosis.*

Secondary prevention

Secondary prevention strategies after stroke, unlike the primary prevention techniques, are tailored to the underlying stroke pathology. The range of secondary prevention strategies continues to expand (Table 21.2) (Davis and Donnan, 1998). The last decade has seen the proof of benefits derived from blood pressure lowering after stroke, the development of new antiplatelet strategies, proof of the efficacy of warfarin in patients with nonvalvular atrial fibrillation (both primary and secondary prevention), better delineation of the indications for carotid endarterectomy for symptomatic and asymptomatic disease, and the introduction of cerebrovascular stenting/angioplasty.

Blood pressure lowering after stroke

The PROGRESS Trial (Perindopril Protection Against Recurrent Stroke Study) was a landmark secondary prevention trial of blood pressure-lowering therapy in patients after stroke or TIA (PROGRESS Collaborative Group, 2001). Active treatments included the angiotensin-converting enzyme (ACE) inhibitor perindopril combined with indapamide, versus matching placebo(s). Over 50% of the PROGRESS cohort were normotensive at baseline, with the hypothesis that blood pressure lowering in patients at any baseline level of blood pressure would reduce stroke recurrence (Rodgers et al, 1996). Total stroke was reduced overall with active therapy by 28%.

Table 21.2 Therapeutic opportunities in secondary prevention

Strategy	Indication	Level of evidence
Antiplatelet and anticoagulant strategies		
Combination antiplatelet strategies	Ischemic stroke; TIA	II
		(combined aspirin/dipyramidole)
Aspirin	Ischemic stroke; TIA	I
Ticlopidine	Ischemic stroke; TIA	II
Clopidogrel	Ischemic stroke; TIA	II
Dipyramidole (combined with aspirin)	Ischemic stroke; TIA	II
Warfarin	Nonvalvular atrial fibrillation, valvular heart disease	I
Surgical and interventional strategies		
Carotid endarterectomy	Symptomatic carotid stenosis	I
Angioplasty stenting	Not yet proven; possibly patients with extracranial, intracranial symptomatic atherosclerotic stenosis	III (No randomized, controlled trials yet confirming benefits)

Quality of evidence ratings (Prevention of Stroke, 1996)
Level I.   Evidence is obtained from a systematic review of all relevant randomized controlled trials.
Level II.   Evidence is obtained from at least one properly designed randomized controlled trial.
Level III.   Evidence is obtained from well-designed controlled trials without randomization; from well-designed cohort or case-control analytic studies; preferably from more than one center or research group; from multiple time series with or without the intervention or from dramatic results in uncontrolled experiments.
Level IV.   Opinions of respected authorities, based on clinical experience, descriptive studies or reports of expert committees.

Dementia and cognitive function were both important secondary endpoints in PROGRESS. Over a mean follow-up of 3.9 years, active treatment reduced the risk of dementia by 12%, although this did not achieve statistical significance (95% CI: -8% to 28%; $P = 0.2$). There was a highly significant 34% reduction in the risk of dementia with recurrent stroke ($P = 0.03$). There was a significant overall reduction in cognitive decline of 19% ($P = 0.01$) in the patients receiving ACE-based therapy and the composite outcome of 'cognitive decline with recurrent stroke' was reduced by 45% ($P = 0.001$) (Tzourio et al, 2003).

Antiplatelet strategies

The benefits of aspirin were first established by pivotal studies nearly three decades ago, with a relative risk reduction of about 22% for the composite outcomes of stroke, death or MI (Antiplatelet Trialists Collaboration, 1994). Recent meta-analysis of the secondary prevention trials, where aspirin was tested against placebo, showed no discernible difference between high, medium and low doses of aspirin, effectively resolving a controversial issue for stroke clinicians (Algra and van Gijn, 1996).

The effectiveness of aspirin depends on the inhibition of platelet cyclo-oxygenase but other antiplatelet strategies with differing actions have also been proven to be effective in stroke prevention, with some benefits compared to aspirin. Ticlopidine, an ADP inhibitor, was shown to be superior to aspirin in a trial in high-risk patients (Hass et al, 1989). Ticlopidine has been largely replaced by clopidogrel because of its 1–2% risk of severe although reversible neutropenia. Clopidogrel, like ticlopidine, also inhibits platelet ADP but has not been associated with an increased risk of neutropenia. It was shown in the CAPRIE trial to be more effective than aspirin in stroke prevention (CAPRIE Steering Committee, 1996). The CAPRIE trial showed a relative risk reduction of 8.7% for clopidogrel over aspirin, although only a modest absolute risk reduction of 0.5%. Clopidogrel and aspirin have additive or synergistic effects because of their different actions. The combination was far more effective than aspirin alone in the CURE trial in patients with coronary artery syndromes (Yusuf et al, 2001). This combination approach is now being tested in stroke patients.

Dipyridamole reduces platelet aggregation by raising the antiaggregating effects of cyclic AMP and cyclic GMP. A synergistic effect between aspirin and dipyridamole was demonstrated in the ESPS 2 trial (Diener et al, 1996), In this factorial design, the relative risk of stroke was reduced by 18% with aspirin, 16% with dipyridamole, and an additive 37% with the combination of these two therapies. Aspirin and other antiplatelet therapies might have a role in the prevention and treatment of VaD (Freels et al, 2002), but convincing evidence is currently lacking and large controlled trials are needed (Williams et al, 2000).

Warfarin

The European Atrial Fibrillation trial (EAFT 1993), compared warfarin, aspirin and placebo in secondary stroke prevention. While both warfarin and aspirin were significantly effective in reducing stroke risk in patients with ischemic stroke and atrial fibrillation, warfarin was substantially more effective than aspirin and is the recommended strategy in appropriate anti-coagulation candidates.

Carotid endarterectomy

Two large trials (the North American Symptomatic Carotid Endarterectomy Trial – NASCET, and the European Carotid Surgery Trial – ECST) showed major benefits for carotid endarterectomy over optimal medical therapy in patients with greater than 70% carotid stenosis and either TIA or nondis-abling stroke (see Figure 21.3) (North American Symptomatic Carotid Endarterectomy Trial Collaborators, 1991; European Carotid Surgery Trialists Collaborative Group, 1991). In the NASCET study, an absolute risk reduction of 17% over 18 months was achieved, indicating that one stroke could be prevented for every six patients treated over this period (North American Symptomatic Carotid Endarterectomy Trial Collaborators, 1991). Hence, the indications for carotid endarterectomy are now based on a substantial evidence base.

Cerebrovascular angioplasty

Percutaneous transluminal angioplasty, of established value for coronary artery disease, has been more recently used for both symptomatic and asymptomatic carotid stenosis, usually combined with endovascular stenting (Bladin et al, 1998). The risks of the procedure are approximately equivalent to those of carotid endarterectomy. One trial showed no differences in the stroke rate, comparing CEA with angioplasty/stenting but this study was underpowered (Endovascular versus surgical treatment in patients with carotid stenosis in the Carotid and Vertebral Artery Transluminal Angio-plasty Study (CAVATAS): a randomised trial, 2001). Larger trials are now being conducted to compare the safety and efficacy of carotid angioplasty/stenting with carotid endarterectomy, in patients with sympto-matic carotid stenosis. The technique has also been used in small numbers of patients with surgically inaccessible, intracranial stenoses and may have a role in asymptomatic carotid stenosis.

Summary

Despite the heterogeneity of pathologies underlying VaD, most share common risk factors which can be modified by primary prevention strategies. To date, blood pressure lowering is the only interventional strategy that has been shown to reduce the risk of dementia and cognitive decline. Secondary prevention strategies should impact on relevant pathologies such as cardioembolic cerebral infarction, lacunar infarction and large vessel disease with thromboembolism. Most of these studies to date have recorded composite outcomes of death, stroke, MI and stroke-related disability, but have not evaluated the development of cognitive decline and dementia. Hence, more information is needed to gauge the efficacy of prevention strategies for VaD. In the next few years, more information should become available concerning the efficacy of strategies such as antiplatelet therapies and statins in the prevention of dementia. In the interim, promotion of primary and secondary vascular prevention strategies in public and professional education should emphasize the prevention of VaD as well as the conventional vascular endpoints of stroke, MI and vascular death.

References

Algra A, van Gijn J, Aspirin at any dose above 30 mg offers only modest protection after cerebral ischaemia. *J Neurol Neurosurg Psychiatry* (1996) **60**:197–9.

Antiplatelet Trialists Collaboration, Collaborative overview of randomised trials of antiplatelet treatment, Part 1. Prevention of death, myocardial infarction, and stroke by prolonged antiplatelet therapy in various categories of patients, *BMJ* (1994) **343**:139–42.

Atkins D, Psaty BM, Koepsell TD et al, Cholesterol reduction and the risk for stroke in men. A meta-analysis of randomized, controlled trials, *Ann Intern Med* (1993) **119**:136–45.

Bennett S, Cardiovascular risk factors in Australia: trends in socioeconomic inequalities, *J Epidemiol Community Health* (1995) **49**:363–72.

Bladin CF, Davis SM, Burton K et al, The use of percutaneous transluminal angioplasty (PTA) for the treatment of extracranial atherosclerotic vascular disease. The Australian Association of Neurologists (AAN), *Aus NZ J Med* (1998) **28**:654–6.

Blauw GJ, Lagaay AM, Smelt AH, Westendorp RG, Stroke, statins, and cholesterol. A meta-analysis of randomized, placebo-controlled, double-blind trials with HMG-CoA reductase inhibitors, *Stroke* (1997) **28**: 946–50.

Breteler MM, van Swieten JC, Bots ML et al, Cerebral white matter lesions, vascular risk factors, and cognitive function in a population-based study: the Rotterdam Study, *Neurology* (1994) **44**:1246–52.

Bucher HC, Griffith LE, Guyatt GH, Effect of HMGcoA reductase inhibitors on stroke. A meta-analysis of randomized, controlled trials, *Ann Intern Med* (1998) **128**:89–95.

Butler RN, Ahronheim J, Fillit H et al, Vascular dementia: stroke prevention takes on new urgency, *Geriatrics* (1993) **48**:40–2.

CAPRIE Steering Committee, A randomised, blinded trial of clopidogrel versus aspirin in patients at risk of ischaemic events (CAPRIE), *Lancet* (1996) **348**:1329–39.

Collins R, Peto R, MacMahon S et al, Blood pressure, stroke, and coronary heart disease. Part 2. Short-term reductions in blood pressure: overview of randomised drug trials in their epidemiological context, *Lancet* (1990) **335**:827–38.

Davis SM, Donnan GA, Secondary prevention for stroke after CAPRIE and ESPS-2. Opinion 1, *Cerebrovasc Dis* (1998) **8**:73–5, 77.

Desmond DW, Moroney JT, Paik MC et al, Frequency and clinical determinants of dementia after ischemic stroke, *Neurology* (2000) **54**:1124–31.

Di Bari M, Pahor M, Franse LV et al, Dementia and disability outcomes in large hypertension trial lessons learned from the systolic hypertension in the elderly program (SHEP) trial, *Am J Epidemiol* (2001) **153**:72–8.

Dichgans M, Mayer M, Uttner I et al, The phenotypic spectrum of CADASIL: clinical findings in 102 cases, *Ann Neurol* (1998) **44**:731–9.

Diener HC, Cunha L, Forbes C et al, European Stroke Prevention Study. 2. Dipyridamole and acetylsalicylic acid in the secondary prevention of stroke, *J Neurol Sci* (1996) **143**:1–13.

Donnan GA, You R, Thrift A, McNeil JJ, Smoking as a risk factor for stroke, *Cerebrovasc Dis* (1993) **3**:129–38.

EAFT (European Atrial Fibrillation Trial) Study Group, Secondary prevention in nonrheumatic atrial fibrillation after transient ischaemic attack or minor stroke, *Lancet* (1993) **342**:1255–62.

Endovascular versus surgical treatment in patients with carotid stenosis in the Carotid and Vertebral Artery Transluminal Angioplasty Study (CAVATAS): a randomised trial, *Lancet* (2001) **357**:1729–37.

European Carotid Surgery Trialists' Collaborative Group, MRC European Carotid Surgery Trial: interim results for symptomatic patients with severe (70–99%) or with mild (0–29%) carotid stenosis, *Lancet* (1991) **337**:1235–43.

Executive Committee for the Asymptomatic Carotid Atherosclerosis Study, Endarterectomy for asymptomatic carotid artery stenosis, *JAMA* (1995) **273**:1421–8.

Forette F, Seux ML, Staessen JA et al, Prevention of dementia in randomised double-blind placebo-controlled Systolic Hypertension in Europe (Syst-Eur) trial, *Lancet* (1998) **352**:1347–51.

Freels S, Nyenhuis DL, Gorelick PB, Predictors of survival in African American patients with AD, VaD, or stroke without dementia, *Neurology* (2002) **59**:1146–53.

Gorelick PB, Status of risk factors for dementia associated with stroke, *Stroke* (1997) **28**:459–63.

Gorelick PB, Roman GC, Vascular dementia: a time to 'seize the moment', *Neuroepidemiology* (1993) **12**:139–40.

Hachinski V, Binswanger's disease: neither Binswanger's nor a disease, *J Neurol Sci* (1991) **103**:1.

Hachinski V, Preventable senility: a call for action against the vascular dementias, *Lancet* (1992) **340**:645–8.

Hachinski VC, Potter P, Merskey H, Leuko-araiosis, *Arch Neurol* (1987) **44**:21–3.

Hajjar I, Schumpert J, Hirth V et al, The impact of the use of statins on the prevalence of dementia and the progression of cognitive impairment. *J Gerontol A Biol Sci Med Sci* (2002) **57**:M414–M418.

Hansson L, Lithell H, *SCOPE Results*, 19th Scientific Meeting of the International Society of Hypertension, Prague, Czech Republic, 2002.

Hansson L, Lithell H, Skoog I et al, Study on COgnition and Prognosis in the Elderly (SCOPE), *Blood Press* (1999) **8**:177–83.

Hass WK, Easton JD, Adams HP Jr et al, A randomized trial comparing ticlopidine hydrochloride with aspirin for the prevention of stroke in high-risk patients. Ticlopidine Aspirin Stroke Study Group, *N Engl J Med* (1989) **321**:501–7.

Hofman A, Ott A, Breteler MM et al, Atherosclerosis, apolipoprotein E, and prevalence of dementia and Alzheimer's disease in the Rotterdam Study, *Lancet* (1997) **349**:151–4.

Jamrozik K, Stroke. A looming epidemic? *Aus Fam Physician* (1997) **26**:1137–43.

Jamrozik K, Broadhurst RJ, Anderson CS, Stewart-Wynne EG, The role of lifestyle factors in the etiology of stroke. A population-based case-control study in Perth, Western Australia, *Stroke* (1994) **25**:51–9.

Kawachi I, Colditz GA, Stampfer MJ et al, Smoking cessation and decreased risk of stroke in women, *JAMA* (1993) **269**:232–6.

Kiers L, Davis SM, Larkins R et al, Stroke topography and outcome in relation to hyperglycaemia and diabetes, *J Neurol Neurosurg Psychiatry* (1992) **55**:263–70.

Kilander L, Nyman H, Boberg M et al, Hypertension is related to cognitive impairment: a 20-year follow-up of 999 men, *Hypertension* (1998) **31**:780–6.

Kivipelto M, Helkala EL, Laakso MP et al, Midlife vascular risk factors and Alzheimer's disease in later life: longitudinal, population-based study, *BMJ* (2001) **322**:1447–51.

Kokmen E, Whisnant JP, O'Fallon WM et al, Dementia after ischemic stroke: a population-based study in Rochester, Minnesota (1960–1984), *Neurology* (1996) **46**:154–9.

Lake FR, Cullen KJ, de Klerk NH et al, Atrial fibrillation and mortality in an elderly population, *Aus NZ J Med* (1989) **19**:321–6.

Launer LJ, Masaki K, Petrovitch H et al, The association between midlife blood pressure levels and late-life cognitive function. The Honolulu–Asia Aging Study, *JAMA* (1995) **274**:1846–51.

Lefkovits J, Plow EF, Topol EJ, Platelet glycoprotein IIb/IIIa receptors in cardiovascular medicine, *N Engl J Med* (1995) **332**:1553–9.

MacMahon S, Rodgers A, Antihypertensive agents and stroke prevention, *Cerebrovasc Dis* (1994) **4**:11–15.

North American Symptomatic Carotid Endarterectomy Trial Collaborators, Beneficial effect of carotid endarterectomy in symptomatic patients with high-grade carotid stenosis, *N Engl J Med* (1991) **325**:445–53.

National Health and Medical Research Council Working Party and Contractors (1996). *Prevention of stroke: clinical practice guidelines*. Canberra, Australian Government Publishing Service, Commonwealth of Australia.

Parsons MW, Barber PA, Desmond PM et al, Acute hyperglycemia adversely affects stroke outcome: a magnetic resonance imaging and spectroscopy study, *Ann Neurol* (2002) **52**:20–8.

Pasquier F, Leys D, Why are stroke patients prone to develop dementia? *J Neurol* (1997) **244**:135–42.

Prince MJ, Bird AS, Blizard RA, Mann AH, Is the cognitive function of older patients affected by antihypertensive treatment? Results from 54 months of the Medical Research Council's trial of hypertension in older adults, *BMJ* (1996) **312**:801–5.

PROGRESS Collaborative Group, Randomised trial of a perindopril-based blood pressure-lowering regimen among 6,105 individuals with previous stroke or transient ischaemic attack, *Lancet* (2001) **358**:1033–41.

Risk factors for stroke and efficacy of antithrombotic therapy in atrial fibrillation. Analysis of pooled data from five randomized controlled trials, *Arch Intern Med* (1994) **154**:1449–57.

Robbins AS, Manson JE, Lee IM et al, Cigarette smoking and stroke in a cohort of US male physicians, *Ann Intern Med* (1994) **120**:458–62.

Rodgers A, MacMahon S, Gamble G et al, Blood pressure and risk of stroke in patients with cerebrovascular disease. The United Kingdom Transient Ischaemic Attack Collaborative Group, *BMJ* (1996) **313**:147.

Sacco RL, Gan R, Boden-Albala et al, Leisure-time physical activity and ischemic stroke risk: the Northern Manhattan Stroke Study, *Stroke* (1998) **29**:380–7.

SHEP Cooperative Research Group, Prevention of stroke by antihypertensive drug treatment in older persons with isolated systolic hypertension. Final results of the Systolic Hypertension in the Elderly Program (SHEP), *JAMA* (1991) **265**:3255–64.

Shinton R, Beevers G, Meta-analysis of relation between cigarette smoking and stroke, *BMJ* (1989) **298**:789–94.

Skoog I, Lernfelt B, Landahl S et al, 15-year longitudinal study of blood pressure and dementia, *Lancet* (1996) **347**:1141–5.

Srikanth V, Donnan GA, Stroke: A current perspective, *Current Therapeutics* (1998) **39**:39–45.

Tatemichi TK, Foulkes MA, Mohr JP et al, Dementia in stroke survivors in the Stroke Data Bank cohort. Prevalence, incidence, risk factors, and computed tomographic findings, *Stroke* (1990) **21**:858–66.

Tatemichi TK, Paik M, Bagiella E et al, Risk of dementia after stroke in a hospitalized cohort: results of a longitudinal study, *Neurology* (1994) **44**:1885–91.

Turpie AG, Gent M, Laupacis A et al, A comparison of aspirin with placebo in patients treated with warfarin after heart-valve replacement, *N Engl J Med* (1993) **329**:524–9.

Tzourio C, Dufouil C, Ducimetiere P, Alperovitch A, Cognitive decline in individuals with high blood pressure: a longitudinal study in the elderly. EVA Study Group. Epidemiology of Vascular Aging, *Neurology* (1999) **53**:1948–52.

Tzourio C, Anderson C, Chapman N et al, for the PROGRESS Collaborative Group, Effects of blood pressure lowering with perindopril and indapamide on dementia and cognitive decline in patients with cerebrovascular disease, *Arch Intern Med* (2003) **163**:1069–75.

Whisnant JP, Modeling of risk factors for ischemic stroke. The Willis Lecture, *Stroke* (1997) **28**:1840–4.

Williams PS, Rands G, Orrel M, Spector A, Aspirin for vascular dementia. In: *Cochrane Database Syst Rev* (2000) **4**.

Yusuf S, Zhao F, Mehta SR et al, Effects of clopidogrel in addition to aspirin in patients with acute coronary syndromes without ST-segment elevation, *N Engl J Med* (2001) **345**:494–502.

Zimmet PZ, Alberti KGMM, The changing face of macrovascular disease in non-insulin-dependent diabetes mellitus: an epidemic in progress, *Lancet* (1997) **350**:1–4.

chapter 22

Secondary prevention: medical management of established cerebrovascular disease

Leon Flicker and Nicola T Lautenschlager

Introduction

Specific medical management focuses on the prevention of further cerebral damage. Most of the interventions discussed here have other benefits than purely on the outcome of cerebral damage. These include various vascular outcomes, particularly cardiac disease. Cerebrovascular disease is a marker for poor vascular health and there is now increasing evidence that these patients benefit from aggressive treatment, more so than those asymptomatic individuals who share similar magnitude of risk factors. This may be particularly so for patients with cerebrovascular disease and dementia. A study by Tatemichi et al (1994) demonstrated that the mortality rate was 19 deaths per 100 person-years for people who had a stroke that was complicated by dementia, compared to 6.9 deaths per hundred person-years who had a stroke which was uncomplicated by dementia. The relative risk for death associated with dementia was 3.9 (95% CI 1.8, 5.4). As well as mortality, dementia after stroke increases the risk of long term stroke recurrence (Moroney et al, 1997) with a relative risk of 2.7 (95% CI 1.4, 5.4) for recurrent stroke in those individuals who had dementia following their initial stroke.

This chapter focuses largely on the treatment and prevention of modifiable risk factors for cerebrovascular disease. Recognized risk factors can be divided into the categories of nonmodifiable and modifiable. Modifiable risk factors include hypertension, hypercholesterolemia, diabetes mellitus, physical inactivity, obesity and smoking. Nonmodifiable risk factors include advanced age, male sex, non-white race, positive family history (based probably on a mixture of genetic factors and shared common environmental risk factors) and cardiac diseases (Straus et al, 2002).

Control of hypertension

There have been numerous studies looking at the use of antihypertensives in elderly people. Many of these studies have now been systematically reviewed. For example, Mulrow et al (2002) reviewed 15 trials which included 21 908 elderly subjects. They found that treatment of hypertension in older people, 60 to 80 years of age, reduced cardiovascular morbidity and mortality from 177 to 126 (95% CI of the difference 31 to 73) events per 1000 participants over five years. Cardiovascular mortality was reduced from 69 to 50 deaths, total mortality was reduced from 129 to 111 deaths. They reviewed, separately, three trials which addressed the question of isolated systolic hypertension and found that cardiovascular morbidity and mortality were reduced over a five-year period from 157 to 104 events per 1000 participants (95% CI of the difference, 12 to 89). A more recent systematic review (Staessen et al, 2000) found that in patients with isolated systolic hypertension active treatment reduced mortality by 13% (CI of the difference 2–22%), reduced the incidence of stroke by 30% (CI of difference 18–41%) and reduced the incidence of all cardiovascular complications by 26% (CI of difference 17–34%). The effect of antihypertensive drugs has also been evaluated in people older than 80 years who participated in many of these large studies. Confining the analyses to these 1670 subjects suggested a reduction of 34% (CI of difference 8–52%) in the risk of stroke and a significant reduction of 22% in major cardiovascular outcome. However, there was little evidence of any effect on total mortality with an increase of 6% (95% CI of difference −5 to 18%) (Gueyffier et al, 1999). At this stage there appears to be clear evidence for treating healthy older people with either diastolic hypertension or isolated systolic hypertension.

There is also substantial evidence for the treatment of hypertension in people who have already sustained cerebrovascular damage. A meta-analysis demonstrated a 28% (CI of difference 15–39%) reduction in risk of stroke in those people who had survived a previous stroke (Gueyffier et al, 1997). However, the evidence for the aggressive treatment of hypertension in individuals who have already had vascular dementia (VaD) is scant. Because of disturbance in autoregulation it has been argued that excessive lowering of blood pressure may precipitate vascular damage. However, there seems to be little randomized trial evidence to confirm this impression (Konno et al, 1997).

One of the more exciting recent developments has been the reporting of several large studies of the use of antihypertensives, predominantly angiotensin-converting enzyme (ACE) inhibitors, and the effect on cognition. Forette et al (1998, 2002) reported a trial of 2418 patients with isolated systolic hypertension, aged 60 years and over, randomized to treatment with a possible combination of nitrendipine, enalapril and hydrochlorothiazide or placebo. In 1998 the authors reported a 50% reduction (95% CI of difference 0–76%) in the incidence of dementia from 7.7 to 3.8 cases per 1000 patient-years, detected with a mean treatment period of 2.0 years. In 2002, they reported results from an open-label extension phase increasing the follow-up period to 3.9 years. Antihypertensive therapy reduced the risk of dementia by 55% (95% CI of difference 16–76%) from 7.4 to 3.3 cases per 1000 patient-years. The predominant form of dementia in this study was Alzheimer's disease (AD). The pathophysiological mechanisms for this effect remain to be determined but it is heartening that the treatment of hypertension may have broader benefits on the cause of cognitive impairment than the prevention of strokes. In another landmark study, the PROGRESS Collaboration Group (2001) found that the use of the ACE inhibitor, perindopril, in some cases augmented by indapamide, in patients with previous strokes or TIAs, produced a reduction of 28% (CI of difference 17–38%) in the risk of further stroke. A recent report suggests a reduction in the risk of cognitive impairment and dementia, mainly due to a reduction in the risk of recurrent stroke. (PROGRESS Collaborative Group, 2003). These results are supported by the HOPE Study, which found, in those patients who were at high risk for stroke, that the ACE inhibitor ramipril was associated with a reduction of 32% (CI of difference of 16–44%) in the incidence of strokes (Bosch, 2002). Significantly fewer patients treated with ramipiril developed cognitive impairment after two years than those treated with placebo, a risk reduction of 41% (CI of difference 6–63%). In the HOPE Study, the patients were at high cardiovascular risk but had controlled blood pressure and the effect of treatment appeared to be independent of the antihypertensive effect of ACE inhibitors (Schrader and Lüders, 2002). It is important to emphasize that the excellent results of treatment in these highly monitored controlled trials may not be able to be replicated in routine clinical practice in patients with multiple co-morbidities and functional impairments.

Anticoagulation

There is substantial evidence available to address the question of treatment of nonembolic ischemic stroke or transient ischemic attack with anticoagulation, and this evidence has been systematically reviewed (Liu et al, 2002). Nine trials were available to be analyzed for a meta-analysis. The reviewers concluded that there was no evidence that anticoagulation significantly reduced the odds of death or dependency, with an odds ratio of 0.83 (95% CI 0.52–1.34) and it did not reduce the risk of ischemic or recurrent stroke, odds ratio 0.79 (95% CI 0.56–1.13). However, anti-coagulation did increase the odds of major bleeding with the risk for fatal intracranial hemorrhage increasing, odds ratio 2.54 (95% CI 1.19–5.45), and major extracranial hemorrhage, 4.87 (95%CI 2.50, 9.49). They concluded there was no clear evidence of benefit from long-term anticoagulation in patients with nonembolic stroke who were not in atrial fibrillation.

However, this is clearly not the case with those patients who have atrial fibrillation. A meta-analysis by Benavente et al (2002) showed that the risk for stroke for patients with atrial fibrillation from nonvalvular causes was reduced by the use of anticoagulation by 61% (95% CI 41–74%). In another meta-analysis the reduction in risk achieved by anticoagulation for patients with atrial fibrillation and previous cerebral ischemia appeared to be even greater, with a risk reduction of 64% (95% CI of difference 42–78%) (Koudstaal, 2002a). The clear recommendation following these analyses is that anticoagulants should be given to patients with nonrheumatic atrial fibrillation and that in those patients with recent cerebral ischemia this should be considered even more appropriate. However, many older patients have absolute contraindications to anticoagulation therapy and issues of compliance and relative contraindications such as risk of falls are even more common.

Antithrombotic treatment

Aspirin has been demonstrated in a meta-analysis of over 40 000 patients with acute ischemic stroke to reduce the risk of death or dependency following stroke by 6% (95% CI 2–7%) (Gubitz et al, 2002). However, in those patients with atrial fibrillation, aspirin is not as efficacious as anticoagulation, with anticoagulation resulting in a reduction in risk of recurrent stroke by 65% (95% CI of difference 41–78%) compared to aspirin (Koudstaal, 2002b). Caution must be exercised here as it is based on one trial of 455 subjects. Clearly antithrombotic therapy should be given to all patients with established cerebrovascular disease in sinus rhythm unless there are major contraindications. However, several questions remain.

Firstly, does dipyridamole add to the effect of aspirin? A recent meta-analysis (Antithrombotic Trialists' Collaboration, 2002) did not conclude that there were significant benefits of the combination of these two antithrombotic agents over aspirin alone. They found a nonsignificant 6% reduction in all serious vascular events for the combination therapy. It was noted that one study may have influenced the apparent benefit for the outcome of nonfatal stroke for the combination of the two agents. This study, the European Stroke Prevention Study, found benefits of a combination of dipyridamole and aspirin compared to aspirin (Diener et al, 1996). The stroke risk was reduced by 18% in patients with aspirin alone, 16% with dipyridamole alone and 37% with the combination. It should be noted that in this study, aspirin was used in a dose of 50 mg daily and the dipyridamole was used in a modified release form at a dose of 200 mg twice daily. This dose of aspirin may have been too small to produce comparable results to other studies.

Another question is whether thienopyridine derivatives such as ticlopidine and clopidogrel are more efficacious than aspirin in high-risk vascular patients. In a meta-analysis of 22 656 high-risk vascular patients (Hankey et al, 2002) there was a reduction in risk of stroke of 12% (95% CI of difference 2–21%) compared to aspirin. Ticlopidine was associated with a significant risk of neutropenia, and both ticlopidine and clopidrogel were associated with an increased risk of skin rash and diarrhea (more so with ticlopidine). Both clopidogrel and ticopidine were associated with less gastrointestinal bleeding. In general, the greater cost has limited the use of these agents for the prevention of further strokes in patients with established cerebrovascular disease. The question of using aspirin and clopidogrel together has been addressed in patients with acute coronary syndromes (Yusuf et al, 2001) but the effect may not be able to be translated to cerebrovascular disease (Albers and Amarenco, 2001). The cost-effectiveness for the treatment of established cerebrovascular disease with either clopidogrel alone, or in combination with aspirin, is difficult to evaluate at the time of writing.

Control of diabetes mellitus

Diabetes mellitus is a known risk factor for vascular diseases. Recent evidence would suggest that it is a potent risk factor for dementia. Ott et al (1996) analyzing data from the Rotterdam Study reported a positive association between diabetes and dementia with an odds ratio of 1.3 (95% CI 1.0, 1.9), even after adjusting for age and sex. More impressively, the risk of VaD was increased 5.4-fold, (95% CI 1.2, 23.8) for those people with diabetes treated with insulin and 3.2-fold (95% CI 1.4, 7.4) for those patients treated with oral medications. The overall risk for VaD associated with the presence of diabetes mellitus was 2.1 (95% CI 1.1, 4.0) but the risk of VaD was not increased for patients who had no drug treatment for diabetes. These results may reflect evidence for increased severity of diabetes associated with VaD, i.e. if patients have severe and longstanding diabetes they are more likely to develop VaD. However, it does raise the issue of whether high endogenous or exogenous insulin levels may be complicated by VaD. This has implications in the treatment of people with diabetes mellitus and VaD although evidence from the UK Prospective Diabetes Study Group (1998a) found benefits from intensive treatment of type 2 diabetes mellitus. The risk of any diabetes-related endpoint which included death, myocardial infarction, stroke or amputation, blindness or cataract was reduced by 12% with more intensive treatment. Using stroke as a single endpoint, there was no significant reduction in risk in the more intensively treated group for either fatal, (a 17% increase in relative risk: 95% CI 0.54–2.54) or nonfatal stroke (a 7% increase in risk: 95% CI 0.68–1.69). In this study, just as important as the control of type 2 diabetes was the control of hypertension with tight blood pressure control associated with a 44% reduction in strokes (95% CI of difference 11–65%) (UK PDSG, 1998b). Blood pressure treatments were found to be cost-effective (UK PDSG 1998c). At the time of writing there is good evidence for lowering blood pressure in those subjects with diabetes and established cerebrovascular disease, even for normotensive patients, (HOPE Study: Bosch et al, 2002) but not for more intensive treatments of diabetes mellitus.

Treatment of hyperlipidemia

The association between hypercholesterolemia and stroke has been relatively controversial. However, intervention studies seem to be less contentious.

Initially systematic reviews, for example Atkins et al (1993), failed to reveal a reduction in risk for fatal and nonfatal stroke. This may have been related to the earlier types of treatment, such as clofibrate or cholestyramine. A more recent meta-analysis by Herbert et al (1997) examined whether the use of HMG-CoA reductase inhibitors (statin drugs) reduce the risk of total mortality. A total of 16 individual trials with 29 000 subjects were analyzed, the average reduction in total cholesterol was 22%. The authors found a reduction in the risk of stroke of 29% (95%CI 14–41%) and an overall reduction in total mortality of 22% (95%CI 12–31%), which was attributable to a significant reduction in cardiovascular disease. An update of previous meta-analyses was performed and found a 25% reduction (95%CI 14–35%) in the risk of first onset fatal and nonfatal stroke (Straus et al, 2002). Although there is substantial evidence that statins may be more cost-effective for secondary prevention after coronary heart disease (Ebrahim et al, 1999), at the time of writing there is no evidence to support treatment for the secondary prevention of stroke. However, it would seem prudent to assume that for all patients in poor vascular health, treatment with statins may help to prevent strokes. Similarly, it is probably worthwhile to advise all patients with cerebrovascular disease to minimize the amount of saturated fat in the diet (Hooper et al, 2002).

Other measures

Large public health promotion programs have demonstrated the health benefits associated with smoking cessation (Ockene and Miller, 1997). It is now clear that smoking is not protective for the development of AD, but may in fact be positively associated with its development; previous studies were influenced by survival bias (Almeida et al, 2002). Unfortunately there are no randomized trials demonstrating that smoking cessation decreases the risk of recurrent stroke. However, observational data, e.g. Wannamethee et al (1995), suggest that the risk of stroke may decrease by 50% within five years of smoking cessation.

Elevated homocysteine levels may be a risk factor for cerebrovascular disease but at this stage there is no evidence that homocysteine lowering strategies, such as folate supplements, decrease the risk of stroke or other cardiovascular endpoints (Hankey, 2002). There are several trials underway addressing this question. Another potentially modifiable dietary factor relates to fatty acid intake. Unfortunately the data are largely observational and there may be complex relationships with outcomes such as dementia. For example, Barberger-Gateau et al, (2002) reported data from the PAQUID study that followed up a French cohort of 1416 older adults for a maximum period of seven years. Participants who ate seafood at least once a week had a reduced risk of developing dementia in the follow-up period (OR = 0.7, 95% CI 0.5–0.9). This 'protective' effect was only partly explained by higher education levels of seafood consumers. The omega-3 fatty acids contained in fish oil may either reduce vascular risk, and thus strokes, or alternatively reduce inflammatory processes in the brain.

Increased physical activity following stroke may have many benefits including physical fitness, functioning of the lower extremities and neurological performance (Batty and Lee, 2002). Unfortunately, there are no large randomized trials examining the potential effect at reducing the risk of recurrent stroke. The use of hormone replacement therapy (HRT) for the secondary prevention of stroke has been discouraged by the findings from the Women's Health Initiative (Writing group for Women's Health Initiative Investigators, 2002), suggesting an elevated risk of coronary heart disease, stroke and pulmonary embolism in women randomized to HRT.

Conclusions

At this stage the best evidence of the benefits of medical management for the prevention of further cerebrovascular damage is for the control of hypertension. In those patients with diabetes mellitus, antihypertensive treatment may even be more important than aggressive control of hyperglycemia, although modest benefits may be obtained from this intervention as well. It is not clear what the therapeutic target for antihypertensive treatment should be, and treatment with an ACE inhibitor, even for those people who are not overtly hypertensive, may be beneficial. The use of antiplatelet agents, and in particular aspirin, is efficacious and is preferred in patients without contraindications and who are not in atrial fibrillation. The potential use of dipyridamole and clopidogrel, with or without aspirin, as first-line therapy is uncertain. In those patients with atrial fibrillation, anti-coagulation should be utilized unless there are definite contraindications. In patients with hyperlipidemia, or perhaps even for other high-risk patients, 'statin' medications have a definite role. But as always, sensible lifestyle interventions should be attempted and in particular smoking cessation, maximizing physical activity and decreasing dietary saturated fats.

References

Albers GW, Amarenco P, Combination therapy with clopidogrel and aspirin: can the CURE results be extrapolated to cerebrovascular patients? *Stroke* (2001) **32**:2948–9

Almeida OP, Hulse GK, Lawrence D, Flicker L, Smoking as a risk factor for Alzheimer's disease: contrasting evidence from a systematic review of case-control and cohort studies, *Addiction* (2002) **97**:15–28.

Antithrombotic Trialists' Collaboration, Collaborative meta–analysis of randomised trials of antiplatelet therapy for prevention of death, myocardial infarction, and stroke in high risk patients, *BMJ* (2002) **324**:71–86.

Atkins D, Psaty BM, Koepsell TD et al, Cholesterol reduction and the risk of stroke in men: a meta-analysis of randomised,controlled trials, *Ann Int Med* (1993) **119**:136–45.

Barberger-Gateau P, Letenneur L, Deschamps V et al, Fish, meat, and risk of dementia: cohort study, *BMJ* (2002) **325**:932–3.

Batty GD, Lee IM, Physical activity for preventing strokes, *BMJ* (2002) **325**:350–1.

Benavente O, Hart R, Koudstaal P et al, Oral anticoagulants for preventing stroke in patients with non-valvular atrial fibrillation and no previous history of stroke or transient ischemic attacks (Cochrane Review). In: *The Cochrane Library*, Issue 4 (Oxford: Update Software, 2002).

Bosch J, Yusuf S, Pogue, J et al, Use of ramipiril in preventing stroke: double-blind randomised trial, *BMJ* (2002) **324**:1–5.

Diener HC, Cunha L, Forbes C et al, European stroke prevention study. 2. Dipyridamole and acetylsalicylic acid in the secondary prevention of stroke, *J Neurol Sci* (1996) **143**:1–13.

Ebrahim S, Davey Smith G, McCabe C et al, What role for statins: a review and economic model, *Health Technol Assess* (1999) **3**:1–91.

Forette F, Seux M-L, Staessen JA et al, Prevention of dementia in randomised double-blind placebo-controlled Systolic Hypertension in Europe (Syst-Eur) trial, *Lancet* (1998) **352**:1347–51.

Forette F, Seux M-L, Staessen JA et al, The prevention of dementia with antihypertensive treatment, *Arch Intern Med* (2002) **162**:2046–52.

Gubitz G, Sandercock P, Counsell C, Antiplatelet therapy for acute ischaemic stroke (Cochrane Review). In: *The Cochrane Library*, Issue 4 (Oxford: Update Software, 2002).

Gueyffier F, Boissel J, Boutitie F et al, Effect of antihypertensive treament in patients having already suffered from stroke: gathering the evidence, *Stroke* (1997) **28**:2557–62.

Gueyffier F, Bulpitt C, Boissel J et al, Antihypertensive drugs in very old people: a subgroup meta-analysis of randomised controlled trials, *Lancet* (1999) **353**:793–6.

Hankey GJ, Is homocysteine a causal and treatable risk factor for vascular disease of the brain (cognitive impairment and stroke, *Ann Neurol* (2002) **51**:279–80.

Hankey GJ, Sudlow CLM, Dunbabin DW, Thienopyridine derivatives (ticlopidine, clopidogrel) versus aspirin for preventing stroke and other serious vascular events in high vascular risk patients (Cochrane Review). In: *The Cochrane Library*, Issue 4 (Oxford: Update Software, 2002).

Herbert PR, Gaziano JM, Chan KS et al, Cholesterol lowering with statin drugs, risk of stroke and total mortality. An overview of randomized trials, *JAMA* (1997) **278**:313–21.

Hooper L, Summerbell CD, Higgins JPT et al, Reduced or modified dietary fat for preventing cardiovascular disease (Cochrane Review). In: *The Cochrane Library*, Issue 4 (Oxford: Update Software, 2002).

Konno S, Meyer JS, Terayama Y et al, Classification, diagnosis and treatment of vascular dementia, *Drugs Aging* (1997) **11**:361–73.

Koudstaal PJ, Anticoagulants for preventing stroke in patients with nonrheumatic atrial fibrillation and a history of stroke or transient ischemic attacks (Cochrane Review). In: *The Cochrane Library*, Issue 4 (Oxford: Update Software, 2002a).

Koudstaal PJ, Anticoagulants versus antiplatelet therapy for preventing stroke in patients with nonrheumatic atrial fibrillation and a history of stroke or transient ischemic attacks (Cochrane Review). In: *The Cochrane Library*, Issue 4 (Oxford: Update Software, 2002b).

Liu M, Counsell C, Sandercock P, Anticoagulants for preventing recurrence following ischaemic stroke or transient ischaemic attack (Cochrane Review). In: *The Cochrane Library*, (Oxford: Update Software, 2002).

Moroney JT, Bagiella E, Tatemichi TK et al, Dementia after stroke increases the risk of long-term stroke recurrence, *Neurology* (1997) 5:1317–25.

Mulrow C, Lau J, Cornell J, Brand M, Pharmacotherapy for hypertension in the elderly (Cochrane Review). In: *The Cochrane Library*, Issue 4 (Oxford: Update Software, 2002).

Ockene IS, Miller NH, Cigarette smoking, cardiovascular disease, and stroke, *Circulation* (1997) **96**:3243–7.

Ott A, Stolk RP, Hofman A et al, Association of diabetes mellitus and dementia: the Rotterdam Study, *Diabetologia* (1996) **39**:1392–7.

PROGRESS Collaborative Group, Randomised trial of a perindopril-based blood-pressure-lowering regimen among 6105 individuals with previous stroke or transient ischaemic attack, *Lancet* (2001) **358**:1033–41.

PROGRESS Collaborative Group, Effects of blood pressure lowering with perindopril and indapamide therapy on dementia and cognitive decline in patients with cerebrovascular disease, *Arch Int Med* (2003) **163**:1069–75.

Schrader J, Lüders S, Preventing stroke: high risk patients should receive ramipiril irrespective of their blood pressure, *BMJ* (2002) **324**:687–8.

Staessen JA, Gasowski J, Wang JG et al, Risks of untreated and treated isolated systolic hypertension in the elderly: meta-analysis of outcome trials, *Lancet* (2000) **355**:865–72.

Straus SE, Majumdar SR, McAlister FA, New evidence for stroke prevention – scientific review, *JAMA* (2002) **288**:1388–95.

Tatemichi TK, Paik M, Bagiella E et al, Risk of dementia after stroke in a hospitalised cohort: results of a longitudinal study, *Neurology* (1994) **44**:1885–91.

UK Prospective Diabetes Study (UKPDS) Group, Intensive blood-glucose control with sulphonylureas or insulin compared with conventional treatment and risk of complications in patients with type 2 diabetes: UKPDS 33, *Lancet* (1998a) **352**:837–53.

UK Prospective Diabetes Study Group, Tight blood pressure control and risk of macrovascular and microvascular complications in type 2 diabetes: UKPDS 38, *BMJ* (1998b) **317**:703–13.

UK Prospective Diabetes Study Group, Cost-effectiveness analysis of improved blood pressure control in hypertensive patients with type 2 diabetes: UKPDS 40, *BMJ* (1998c) **317**:720–6.

Wannamethee SG, Shaper AG, Whincup PH et al, Smoking cessation and the risk of stroke in middle-aged men, *JAMA* (1995) **274**:155–60.

Writing Group for the Women's Health Initiative Investigators, Risks and benefits of estrogen plus progestin in healthy postmenopausal women: principal results from the Women's Health Initiative Randomized Controlled Trial, *JAMA* (2002) **288**:321–33.

Yusuf S, Zhao F, Mehta SR et al, and the Clopidogrel in Unstable Angina to Prevent Recurrent Events Trial Investigators, Effects of clopidogrel in addition to aspirin in patients with acute coronary syndromes without ST-segment elevation, *N Engl J Med* (2001) **345**:494–502.

chapter 23

The treatment of cognitive impairment in vascular dementia

David Wilkinson

Introduction

Alzheimer's disease (AD) remains the dominant cause of dementia in the elderly. However, owing to the high prevalence of ischemic heart, and cerebrovascular, disease in this age group, the second most common cause of dementia or cognitive decline in the elderly is vascular dementia (VaD) (Rocca et al, 1991). Other chapters of this book give detailed descriptions of VaD, its etiology, whether resulting from ischemia, hypoperfusion or hemorrhagic cerebrovascular disease with or without additional cardiac or circulatory disorders. In any discussion on the treatment of cognitive decline in VaD the clinical relevance of its distinction from AD arises and is challenged by the evidence that it is not as great as was once supposed. In fact both pathologies occur together more commonly than VaD alone (Holmes et al, 1999). It follows then that current treatments for AD may have an important part to play in mixed dementia and consequently the attention of those preoccupied with the development of cholinesterase inhibitors (ChEIs) has included VaD in the last five years.

Differentiation is also difficult at the early stages of cognitive decline when the diagnosis of minimal cognitive impairment is made at a time when prophylactic treatments would be more effective if they treated both AD and VaD. The realization that cholinesterase inhibitors, the backbone of the current symptomatic treatment for Alzheimer's disease, do not treat the underlying disease process but rather treat the cholinergic deficit which causes some of the symptoms of dementia, has also led to the belief that ChEIs may be symptomatically effective in a number of other dementing disorders including VaD.

Treatment of mixed dementia

It is well known that stroke and vascular pathology often coexist in elderly patients with histological changes of AD (Galasko et al, 1994; Snowdon et al, 1997). Dementia, including VaD, is now one of the major public health goals in the Western world owing to the high estimated prevalence, which rises exponentially to the age of 90 (Jorm et al, 2001) to 50%, which is maintained even in centenarians (Obadia et al, 1997). The fact that the elderly is the fastest growing segment of the population has resulted in huge projected care costs and led to a search for strategies that would delay the onset of dementia or decrease the burden of institutionalization. An intervention that could delay the onset of AD by five years would reduce the number of cases by 50% by the year 2050 (Brookmeyer et al, 1998). Treatment of AD with cholinesterase inhibitors is now well established and has been shown repeatedly in numerous studies to improve cognition and global function and to help delay nursing home placement. Data now suggest that there are also likely to be effective pharmacological treatments for the large segment of patients with AD and VaD.

Rationale for cholinesterase inhibitor treatment in VaD

The use of cholinesterase inhibitors for the treatment of AD is based on the large body of preclinical and clinical evidence that cholinergic hypofunction is associated with AD (Bartus et al, 1982; Perry et al, 1978; Sato et al, 2002). Numerous studies now show that cholinergic deficits are also associated with VaD. The apparent reciprocal relationship between the cholinergic system and cerebral blood flow may be of particular relevance to VaD since cholinergic mechanisms play a role in modulation of regional cerebral blood flow (Biesold et al, 1989; Tanaka et al, 1994; Lacombe et al, 1997; Sato et al, 2002).

Observations from both post-mortem examinations and studies in living VaD patients suggest that cholinergic changes are associated with this condition, with the most profound deficits in hippocampus and the temporal cortex. One study found that the deficits showed a significant positive correlation with the severity of cognitive impairment (Waller et al, 1986). Cholinergic agents have been shown to be effective in increasing regional cerebral blood flow in humans (Blin et al, 1997). The decline in blood flow observed in AD patients can be restored or prevented by cholinesterase inhibitors (Nakano et al, 2001; Nordberg, 1999). Moreover the enhancement of cerebral blood flow observed in AD patients administered a cholinesterase inhibitor has also been correlated with cognitive performance (Vennerica et al, 2002). Cholinesterase inhibitors may improve cerebral blood flow by a direct effect on the vessels or by effects on neuronal activity, which secondarily increases blood flow.

Studies of several animal models of cerebral ischemia have demonstrated memory and/or behavior impairment, suggesting some usefulness as models of VaD (Naritomi, 1991). Observed effects in these models include increased expression of amyloid precursor protein found in focal stroke models (Shi et al, 2000), increased choline acetyl transferase (ChAT) activity observed in another VaD model (Yamada et al, 1984), and deposition of amyloid beta around cerebral blood vessels following cerebral hypoperfusion after lesions of the nucleus basalis of Meynert (NBM) (Roher et al, 2000). In general, older animals were more susceptible to these effects than young animals.

Studies in the spontaneously hypertensive stroke-prone (SHSP) rat, which exhibits behavioral and neuropathological changes similar to those observed in humans with VaD (Kimura et al, 2000), and in other animal models lend further support for the use of cholinesterase inhibitors in the treatment of VaD. SHSP rats showed a decrease in ACh in the CSF which increased with age (Togashi et al, 1994, 1996), a positive correlation between decreased hippocampal ACh release and impaired learning–memory function, and similar region-specific reductions in ACh levels as animals aged. ChEIs can restore cerebral blood flow that has been reduced subsequent to ablation of the NBM in young and old animals (Peruzzi et al, 2000). Inhibition of cholinesterase can result in enhanced cortical blood flow following hemorrhagic hypotension or during cerebral ischemia (Scremin et al, 1997). Acetyl cholinesterase inhibition has been reported to improve brain metabolism during ischemia, perhaps by facilitating appropriate cerebral blood flow regulation. Furthermore acetyl cholinesterase inhibition also protects against ischemia-induced changes in cholinergic markers (Tanaka et al, 1994).

The one common element emerging from ongoing research in VaD and AD is the role of cholinergic system deficits in the dementia of both disorders (Perry et al, 1978). Because the final common pathway of brain cortical pathology (loss of cerebral neuronal volume) in AD and VaD is similar, agents that increase cholinergic function in the central nervous system may be of therapeutic value in improving cognition in both disorders. There is therefore reason to believe that drugs that improve cognitive function in patients with AD will also benefit patients with VaD.

Clinical trial evidence for the effect of cholinesterase inhibitors on cognition in VaD

Galantamine

The first published study of a cholinesterase inhibitor in VaD patients was a study looking at galantamine in a mixed population of patients (Erkinjuntti et al, 2002). Patients were enrolled on the study if they had AD, according to the NINCDS-ADRDA criteria (McKhann et al, 1984), and some evidence, on brain imaging or physical examination, of cerebrovascular disease, or if they had VaD according to the NINDS-AIREN criteria (Roman et al, 1993). Approximately half the patients (n = 252) satisfied the criteria for probable VaD of whom two-thirds were assigned to active treatment. The study was a typical double-blind parallel group design with randomized allocation to either galantamine or placebo. After an initial titration phase up to 24 mg galantamine daily both groups were followed for six months and then were entered into an open-label extension for a further six months. The efficacy measures for cognition were the standard 11–point AD assessment scale (ADAS-cog) (Rosen et al, 1984) and the mini-mental state examination (MMSE) (Folstein et al, 1975).

The study showed that at the end of the study in a mixed group of AD and VaD patients there were statistically significant improvements on the ADAS and MMSE in favor of galantamine. However, this seemed to be largely due to the AD population, as the subgroup of VaD patients alone failed to reach significance at the 5% level. What was very interesting in this study, apart from the pragmatic help to practicing clinicians suggesting that patients with a doubtful diagnosis may well still respond to a ChEI, was the outcome in the placebo group. In the whole AD and VaD group the typical early improvement in the placebo group was followed by a decline in performance over the six months of one ADAS point compared with an improvement of 1.7 points in the galantamine group. The placebo arm of the VaD subgroup, however, was not significantly different from baseline at six months with an improvement of 0.4 rather than decline on the ADAS, giving a treatment difference of only 1.9 points rather than the 2.7 in the whole study population. This improvement in the treated arm of the VaD patients did not reach significance and whilst it was a trend it suggested that the effects of ChEIs might be somewhat attenuated in this type of dementia. The lack of deterioration over six months in the untreated VaD patients in a clinical trial implied that they did not have the progressive disease typical of AD (i.e. that a different population had indeed been identified by the NINDS-AIREN criteria) and suggested larger numbers or longer term studies may be needed to demonstrate whether the differences suggested by the trends in this study were indeed significant.

Donepezil

Two larger studies in pure VaD patients have recently completed and been reported using the ChEI donepezil (Black et al, 2003; Wilkinson et al, 2003). These studies each included over 600 patients randomly allocated to receive placebo, 5 mg donepezil or 10 mg donepezil daily for six months followed by a six-month open-label extension. The cognitive outcomes were again measured using the ADAS-cog and MMSE and again the placebo group failed to show any of the deterioration we have been so accustomed to see in studies in AD.

However, crucially in these two identical studies using different study sites, there were clear statistically significant improvements in cognition in favor of donepezil in this group of probable (75%) and possible (25%) VaD patients.

The effect of size was made up of a genuine improvement above baseline for both treatment doses as the placebo groups showed no change over the six months. In the pooled data for both studies the 10 mg group improved by 2.03 points, the 5 mg group by 1.57 and the placebo group by 0.18. The large sample size for the pooled data gave an effect size for the 10 mg group of 2.21 and for the 5 mg group of 1.75, and whilst there is a persistent numerical advantage for the higher dose it was not possible to demonstrate differences between groups in these studies, although there is a suggestion that as with the AD trials some patients may gain from treatment with the higher dose (Salloway et al, 2002).

Again what has been shown (Black et al, 2003; Wilkinson et al, 2003) in these studies is that using the NINDS-AIREN criteria a different population of dementia patients from the AD trials is identified: there are more men, they are somewhat older, less severe at baseline and with many more concomitant illnesses and drugs, mostly for cardiovascular indications, than the AD patients in clinical trials.

Another interesting finding from all three trials was the lack of cardiovascular adverse events with rates no greater than placebo.

No ChEI has at the time of writing gained a license for VaD but the fact that one study has shown efficacy in mixed AD/VaD and two studies have shown statistically significant improvements in cognition in VaD alone provide a clear evidence base for an effect. It seems likely that very soon, as further studies are completed, the regulators will be persuaded that VaD patients are an identifiable group and that they are likely to show improvements, rather than simply lack of decline, on ChEI treatment. Whether they then choose to turn the clock back and offer a license for dementia rather than for specific diseases remains to be seen but that was seen as a major problem with other compounds in the past in Europe.

Drugs targeting noncholinergic pathways

VaD has been assumed, though not universally, to be related to chronic cerebral hypoperfusion and so a number of drugs, which were seen as vasodilating, e.g. cyclandelate and nafronyl, were advocated as potential treatments. These and others have been reviewed by Cochrane (1979) and Yesavage et al (1979) and were found to produce no significant effects on cognition. Between then and the development and licensing of ChEIs many compounds were available for the treatment of neurodegenerative disorders, or in the case of hydergine in the USA for 'decline in mental capacity', and were given to patients who had cognitive impairment after stroke and with probable VaD (Olin et al, 1998). Several of these drugs have been recently studied in clinical trials to test efficacy but data have often not been robust enough and the regulators have started to resist licensing treatments for mixed diagnoses. However, some compounds are of interest and have some trial data.

Calcium channel inhibitors

Nimodipine is a calcium channel blocker that is used as an antihypertensive and for a time was the most frequently prescribed drug for the treatment of dementia in the world. It readily crosses the blood–brain barrier, produces vasodilatation of the small cerebral blood vessels and is postulated to prevent calcium influx into ischemic neurons (Greenberg et al, 1990).

Although the Cochrane review in 1998 concluded that, partly because the data was of limited quality, there was no convincing evidence of efficacy for nimodipine, some later studies have suggested that there may be some effect in small vessel disease. Overall the Scandinavian multi-infarct dementia trial of 259 patients over six months failed to demonstrate any significant effect of nimodipine on cognitive or any other outcomes. However, a *post-hoc* analysis of the 92 patients who, on the basis of their CT scans, were judged to have subcortical VaD, showed that they performed better than placebo on a majority of tests. The results were still not statistically significant, which was blamed on the sample size, but do evoke the noise of barrels being scraped (Pantoni et al, 2000a,b).

Nitrendipine, another calcium channel blocker, was used as the principal treatment in the Syst-Eur trial although enalapril, an ACE inhibitor, and a thiazide diuretic could be added if necessary (Forette et al, 1998). This VaD project investigated whether antihypertensive drug treatment could reduce the incidence of dementia. Cognitive function was assessed using the MMSE and the median follow-up was two years. Active treatment reduced the incidence of dementia by 50% from 21 in the placebo group to 11 in the nitrendipine group. Overall, however, there was no mean change in the MMSE scores in either group. In the active treatment group the MMSE seemed to increase slightly and correlated with the decrease in diastolic blood pressure. The conclusion of the investigators was that in elderly people with isolated systolic hypertension antihypertensive treatment was associated with a lower incidence of dementia.

Following this study a large prospective Study on Cognition and Prognosis in the Elderly (SCOPE) using the angiotensin II receptor antagonist candesartin cilexetil has started, which may help to evaluate the effectiveness of antihypertensive control on cognition in the elderly (Trenkwalder, 2002). Similar studies are also in progress with ACE inhibitors, e.g. PROGRESS (Tzourio and Anderson, 2000).

Statins

Statins which are (hydroxy-methylglutaryl-coenzyme A reductase inhibitors) have also been postulated to have an effect on reducing ischemic stroke through the stabilization of plaques, antithrombotic actions and effects on endothelial function, thus preserving regional blood flow. These may be unrelated to their effects on cholesterol so may have implications beyond VaD. Most of the evidence for an effect on reducing the risk of dementia is from retrospective observational studies, albeit using very large databases, but where the dementia diagnosis has not been specific and the reduction has mostly occurred in AD patients (Jick et al, 2000; Wolozin et al, 2000; Hajjar et al, 2002).

Propentofylline

Both VaD and AD involve pathological microglial activation with the production of cytokines, free radicals and excessive release of glutamate with loss of cholinergic neurons from consequent calcium influx. Propentofylline is a xanthine derivative, which inhibits adenosine uptake thus enhancing protective extracellular adenosine levels. It prevents the degradation of cAMP and cGMP through the inhibition of phosphodiesterase. It modulates the activation of microglia and is said to prevent neuronal damage. Doses of 300 mg three times a day have been shown to be well tolerated in placebo-controlled clinical trials of patients with AD, VaD and mixed diagnoses for up to one year (Noble and Wagstaff, 1997). The cognitive measures used in studies were the MMSE and the global Gottfries–Brane–Steen (GBS) scale (Gottfries et al, 1982), which has a weighting in favor of the cognitive portion. The studies were mostly in AD, or in mixed AD/VaD patients, but one study looked at VaD patients in a 12-week placebo-controlled trial using PET, which showed increased cerebral glucose metabolism after a verbal memory task in the propentofylline group, in contrast to a functional decline in the placebo group who had also deteriorated on the MMSE at the end of the study (Mielke et al, 1998). One study, again on a mixed population, included 90 patients with VaD (Marcusson et al, 1997). This was a 12-month double-blind placebo-controlled study and as with the ChEI vascular studies was surprising in that the placebo group patients maintained their cognitive function for the whole study. However, there were still statistically significant improvements in the MMSE, the Syndrom Kurztest (SKT) and the digit substitution test. The GBS was also significantly in favor of the treatment group and was heavily weighted by the intellectual subscore. The study did not have sufficient power to compare the AD/VaD groups but the VaD subgroup reached significance on all the primary efficacy variables whilst the AD group did only on the SKT. The fact that the whole group showed significant improvements on all measures was therefore influenced by the VaD subgroup and the proportion of VaD patients may explain the stability of the placebo group. It would seem likely then that propentofylline may have a particular role in the treatment of VaD patients but the results of further studies may answer this.

Memantine

Glutamate is an excitatory amino acid neurotransmitter found in cortical and hippocampal neurons. Evidence is accumulating to suggest that sustained elevations and/or increased sensitivity to glutamate may lead to influx of calcium, impairing neuronal homeostasis and causing eventual neurodegeneration resulting in cell death (Cacabelos et al, 1999; Lancelot et al, 1998; Greenamyre and Young, 1989). The NMDA receptor, which is known to be physiologically involved in memory and learning, is activated by glutamate and can be excessively stimulated as a result of ischemia resulting in excitotoxicity.

Memantine is an uncompetitive NMDA receptor antagonist that is said to act like magnesium in blocking the cation channel in the resting state, and continues to do so under ischemic stress but as it is voltage dependent it also allows normal synaptic transmission. It has been available in Germany for many years for use in neurodegenerative disorders and a number of clinical studies have shown memantine to improve cognition in various stages of dementia. These data have been sufficient to achieve a license in Europe for moderately severe and severe AD (Schmitt et al, 2002; Ditzler, 1991). However, in its early development its mode of action was seen as being relevant to the treatment of VaD. Two studies have recently been published on VaD, which had very similar designs.

The first (MMM 300) was a 28–week multicentre double-blind study conducted in France, which enrolled 321 patients with mild-to-moderate dementia (using DSM-III and MMSE 12–20) satisfying the criteria for probable VaD according to NINDS-AIREN (Orgogozo et al, 2002). Patients with AD were excluded according to the protocol.

Overall the results were rather equivocal with some numerical advantage for memantine in all parameters but with statistically significant improvements only on cognition using the ADAS-cog and MMSE. Once again this VaD group showed a lack of deterioration in the placebo group. Although there was some significance in the cognitive subscale of the GBS, overall the GBS, the CGI-C and NOSGER all failed to show a significant advantage for memantine.

The authors argue that the demonstration of a cognitive advantage in a VaD population was a proof of concept and that the lack of decline in the placebo group may have meant that the study was underpowered leading to the equivocal results.

The second study (MMM 500) was larger, perhaps giving the chance to test that assumption, randomizing 548 patients to either 20 mg memantine daily or placebo in a 28-week multicentre study in the UK (Wilcock et al, 2002). The same entry criteria were used for probable VaD but the mean

MMSE at entry was slightly higher (range 10–22). The results were in fact the same showing that whilst there was some slight advantage for memantine in a number of subanalyses, overall there were no significant improvements in any outcomes other than the ADAS-cog. In the placebo population the MMSE did not change over the 28 weeks in common with many VaD studies but neither did the memantine group.

Again subgroup analysis showed that there were greater benefits for the memantine by grouping the patients with more severe dementia as defined by entry MMSE and with small vessel disease on imaging. This latter finding was confirmed in a combined analysis of the two studies when the baseline CT/MRI findings were separated into those with larger cortical infarctions, or large vessel disease, and those with white matter lesions and lacunes, or small vessel disease (Mobius and Stoffler, 2002). Those with small vessel disease showed progressive decline in cognitive function compared with the large vessel group who showed no change after 28 weeks and as a result the symptomatic improvements were much greater in the small vessel group. This may suggest that whilst stroke and multiple infarctions are a risk factor for dementia they represent brain damage rather than dementia and the cognitive decline we see in VaD patient is caused by small vessel disease.

Summary

Many of the greatest medical advances have been the result of public health measures rather than direct medical interventions, and a significant reduction in the prevalence of VaD and even AD may be achieved through primary prevention. Vascular risk factors including arterial hypertension, unstable hypotension, coronary heart disease, atrial fibrillation, diabetes, obesity, hyperlipidemia and smoking have all been shown to increase the risk of cognitive impairment, primary prevention of these could significantly reduce the numbers of patients with VaD (Meyer et al, 1986; Passant et al, 1996). It seems from studies like Syst-Eur that treating hypertension in cognitively intact individuals in midlife could do a great deal to prevent the development of VaD and the use of calcium channel blockers, ACE inhibitors and statins may have more of an impact than any of the currently available treatments for cognitive decline. We have yet to see what effects these treatments will have on patients with established dementia. The clinical trials completed to date have nevertheless thrown up some interesting findings. It is clear now that ChEIs can and do have a significant impact on cognition in patients who have established VaD, with the NMDA antagonists and neuroprotectors having less clear effects. Clinical trials in well-defined VaD, as opposed to mixed dementia, have shown a lack of deterioration in the placebo-treated groups over six months. This lack of deterioration seems to be related to the multi-infarct or large vessel disease subgroups and the major drug effects seem to be in patients with small vessel disease, which is the group that also seems to show the more steady decline in cognitive function. This seems to suggest a more significant cholinergic deficit in those with more diffuse and widespread disease than the stroke patients who perhaps have more discrete brain injury. However, the lack of cognitive decline is, of course, a function of the tests we use to measure it. It may be that continued subcortical degeneration is not being detected by tests like the ADAS-cog and MMSE. Current VaD trials are using scales like Exit 25 (Royall et al, 1992), clock drawing (Royall et al, 1998) and the ADAS with the addition of a maze and digit substitution which do include a measure of executive function and may show that there is a more constant cognitive decline commensurate with the decline in function in the donepezil studies (Pratt et al, 2002a,b). Clinicians are still faced with a dilemma as VaD is a common diagnosis and whilst we have no licensed treatment, it seems that those patients with cerebrovascular disease showing a steady decline in cognition, who may be regarded as having a mixed dementia, will respond to treatment with ChEIs as well as those patients with VaD satisfying the NINDS-AIREN criteria. This does give some hope that there will soon be treatments available and current trials should soon give much greater clarity as how best to deal with those patients with vascular risk factors.

References

Bartus RT, Dean RL 3rd, Beer B, Lippa AS, The cholinergic hypothesis of geriatric memory dysfunction, *Science* (1982) 217:408–14.

Biesold D, Inanami O, Sato A, Sato Y, Stimulation of the nucleus basalis of Meynert increases cerebral cortical blood flow in rats, *Neurosci Lett* (1989) 98:39–44.

Black S, Roman GC, Geldmacher DS et al, Donepezil 307 Vascular Dementia Study Group. Efficacy and tolerability of donepezil in vascular dementia: positive results of a 24-week, multicenter, international, randomized, placebo-controlled clinical trial. *Stroke* 2003; 34:2323–30.

Blin J, Ivanoiu A, Coppens A et al, Cholinergic neurotransmission has different effects on cerebral glucose consumption and blood flow in young normals, aged normals, and Alzheimer's disease patients, *Neuroimage* (1997) 6:335–43.

Brookmeyer R, Gray S, Kawas C, Projections of Alzheimer's disease in the United States and the public health impact of delaying disease onset, *Am J Public Health* (1998) 88:1337–42.

Cacabelos R, Takeda M, Winblad B, The glutamatergic system and neurodegeneration in dementia: preventive strategies in Alzheimer's disease, *Int J Geriatr Psychiatry* (1999) **14**:3–47.

Cochrane AL, In: Tognoni G, Garattini S, eds, *Treatment and Prevention of Cerebrovascular Disorders* (Elsevier: Amsterdam, 1979): 453–5.

Erkinjuntti T, Kurz A, Gauthier S et al, Efficacy of galantamine in probable vascular dementia and Alzheimer's disease combined with cerebrovascular disease: a randomised trial, *Lancet* (2002) **359**:1283–90.

Folstein MF, Folstein FE, McHugh PR, Mini-mental state: a practical method for grading the cognitive state of patients for the clinician, *J Psychiatr Res* (1975) **12**:189–98.

Forette F, Seux M-L, Staessen JA et al, Prevention of dementia in randomized double-blind placebo-controlled Systolic Hypertension in Europe (Syst-Eur) Trial, *Lancet* (1998) **352**:1347–51.

Galasko D, Hansen LA, Katzman R et al, Clinical-neuropathological correlations in Alzheimer's disease and related dementias, *Arch Neurol* (1994) **51**:888–95.

Gottfries CG, Brane G, Steen B, GBS scale. In: Israel L, Kozarevic D, Sartorius N, eds, *Source Book of Geriatric Assessment* (Karger: Basel, 1982): 259–60.

Greenamyre J, Young A, Excitatory amino acids and Alzheimer's disease, *Neurobiol Aging* (1989) **10**:593–602.

Greenberg JH, Uematsu D, Araki N et al, Cytosolic free calcium during focal cerebral ischemia and the effects of nimodipine on calcium and histologic damage, *Stroke* (1990) **21**:72–7.

Hajjar I, Schumpert J, Hirth V et al, The impact of statins on the prevalence of dementia and the progression of cognitive impairment, *J Gerontol* (2002) **57**:414–18.

Holmes C, Cairns N, Lantos P, Mann A, Validity of current clinical criteria for Alzheimer's disease, vascular dementia and dementia with Lewy bodies, *Br J Psychiatry* (1999) **174**:45–50.

Jick H, Zornberg GL, Jick SS et al, Statins and the risk of dementia, *Lancet* (2000) **356**:1627–31.

Jorm AF, Jolley D, The incidence of dementia: a meta-analysis, *Neurology* (1998) **51**:728–33.

Kimura S, Saito H, Minami M et al, Pathogenesis of vascular dementia in stroke-prone spontaneously hypertensive rats, *Toxicology* (2000) **153**:167–78.

Kittner B, De Deyn PP, Erkinjuntti T, Investigating the natural course and treatment of vascular dementia and Alzheimers disease. Parallel study populations in two randomized, placebo-controlled trials, *Ann N Y Acad Sci* (2000) **903**:535–41.

Kumar V, Anand R, Messina J et al, An efficacy and safety analysis of Exelon in Alzheimer's patients with concurrent vascular risk factors, *Eur J Neurology* (2000) **7**: 159–69.

Lacombe P, Sercombe R, Vaucher E, Seylaz J, Reduced cortical vasodilatory response to stimulation of the nucleus basalis of Meynert in the aged rat and evidence for a control of the cerebral circulation, *Ann NY Acad Sci* (1997) **826**:410–15.

Marcusson J, Rother M, Kittner B et al, A 12-month randomized, placebo-controlled, trial of propentofylline (HWA285) in patients with dementia according to DSM-III-R, *Dementia* (1997) **8**:320–8.

McKhann G, Drachman D, Folstein M et al, Clinical diagnosis of Alzheimer's disease: report of the NINCDS-ADRDA Work Group under the auspices of Department of Health and Human Services Task Force on Alzheimer's Disease, *Neurology* (1984) **34**:939–44.

Meyer JS, Judd BW, Tawaklna T et al, Improved cognition after control of risk factors for multi-infarct dementia, *JAMA* (1986) **256**:2203–9.

Mielke R, Moller H-J, Erkinjuntti T et al, Propentofylline in the treatment of vascular dementia and Alzheimer type dementia: overview of phase 1 and phase 2 clinical trials, *Alzheimer Dis Assoc Disord* (1998); **12** (Suppl 2):S29–S35.

Mobius HJ, Stoffler A, New approaches to clinical trials in dementia: memantine in small vessel disease, *Cerebrovasc Dis* (2002); **13** (Suppl 2):61–6.

Nakano S, Asada T, Matsuda H et al, Donepezil hydrochloride preserves regional cerebral blood flow in patients with Alzheimer's disease, *J Nucl Med* (2001) **42**:1441–5.

Naritomi H, Experimental basis of multi-infarct dementia: memory impairments in rodent models of ischemia, *Alzheimer Dis Assoc Disord* (1991) **5**:103–11.

Noble S, Wagstaff AJ, Propentofylline, *CNS Drugs* (1997) **8**:257–66.

Nordberg A, PET studies and cholinergic therapy in Alzheimers disease, *Rev Neurol (Paris)* (1999); **155** (Suppl 4):S53–S63.

Obadia Y, Rotily M, Degrand-Guillaud A et al, The PREMAP Study: prevalence and risk factors of dementia and clinically diagnosed Alzheimers disease in Provence, France, *Eur J Epidemiol* (1997) **13**:247–53.

Olin J, Schneider L, Novit A, Luczac S, Efficacy of hydergine for dementia (Cochrane Review). In: *The Cochrane Library* (Oxford: Update Software, 1998) 3:1–31.

Orgogozo JM, Rigaud AS, Stoffler A et al, Efficacy and safety of memantine in patients with mild to moderate vascular dementia: a randomized, placebo-controlled trial (MMM 300), *Stroke* (2002) **33**:1834–9.

Pantoni L, Bianchi C, Beneke M et al, The Scandinavian Multi-Infarct Dementia Trial: a double-blind, placebo-controlled trial of nimodipine in multi-infarct dementia, *J Neurol Sci* (2000a) **175**:116–23.

Pantoni L, Rossi R, Inzitari D et al, Efficacy and safety of nimodipine in sub-cortical vascular dementia: a sub-group analysis of the Scandinavian Multi-Infarct Dementia Trial, *J Neurol Sci* (2000b) **175**:124–34.

Passant U, Warkentin S, Karlson S et al, Orthostatic hypotension in organic dementia: relationship between blood pressure, cortical blood flow and symptoms, *Clin Auton Res* (1996) **6**:29–36.

Perry EK, Tomlinson BE, Blessed G et al, Correlation of cholinergic abnormalities with senile plaques and mental test scores in senile dementia, *BMJ* (1978) **25**:1457–9.

Peruzzi P, von Euw D, Lacombe P, Differentiated cerebrovascular effects of physostigmine and tacrine in cortical areas deafferented from the nucleus basalis magnocellularis suggest involvement of basalocortical projections to microvessels, *Ann NY Acad Sci* (2000) **903**:394–406.

Rocca WA, Hofman A, Brayne C et al, The prevalence of vascular dementia in Europe: facts and fragments from 1980–1990 studies. EURODEM–Prevalence Research Group, *Ann Neurol* (1991) **30**:817–24.

Roher AE, Kuo YM, Potter PE et al, Cortical cholinergic denervation elicits vascular A beta deposition, *Ann NY Acad Sci* (2000) **903**:366–73.

Roman GC, Tatemichi TK, Erkinjuntti T et al, Vascular dementia: diagnostic criteria for research studies. Report of the NINDS-AIREN International Workshop, *Neurology* (1993) **43**:250–60.

Rosen WG, Mohs RC, Davis KL, A new rating scale for Alzheimer's disease, *Am J Psychiatry* (1984) **14**:1356–64.

Royall DR, Mahurin RK, Gray KF, Bedside assessment of executive cognitive impairment: the executive interview, *J Am Geriatr Soc* (1992) **40**:1221–6.

Royall DR, Cordes JA, Polk M, CLOX: an executive clock drawing task, *J Neurol Neurosurg Psychiatry* (1998) **64**:588–94.

Salloway SP, Pratt RD, Perdomo CA, *Donepezil is well tolerated in patients with vascular dementia: a comparison of tolerability in vascular dementia patients and Alzheimer's disease patients*, poster presentation, EFNS Vienna, 2002.

Sato A, Sato Y, Uchida S, Regulation of cerebral cortical blood flow by the basal forebrain cholinergic fibers and aging, *Auton Neurosci* (2002) **96**:13–19.

Schmitt FA, Cragar D, Ashford JW et al, Measuring cognition in advanced Alzheimer's disease for clinical trials, *J Neural Transm* (2002) **62**:135–48.

Scremin OU, Li MG, Scremin AM, Jenden DJ, Cholinesterase inhibition improves blood flow in the ischemic cerebral cortex, *Brain Res Bull* (1997) **42**:59–70.

Shi J, Yang SH, Stubley L et al, Hypoperfusion induces overexpression of beta-amyloid precursor protein mRNA in a focal ischemic rodent model, *Brain Res* (2000) **853**:1–4.

Snowdon DA, Greiner LH, Mortimer JA et al, Brain infarction and the clinical expression of Alzheimer disease. The Nun Study, *JAMA* (1997) **277**:813–17.

Tanaka K, Ogawa N, Mizukawa K et al, Acetyl-cholinesterase inhibitor ENA-713 protects against ischemia-induced decrease in pre- and postsynaptic cholinergic indices in the gerbil brain following transient ischemia, *Neurochem Res* (1994) **19**:117–22.

Togashi H, Matsumoto M, Yoshioka M et al, Neurochemical profiles in cerebrospinal fluid of stroke-prone spontaneously hypertensive rats, *Neurosci Lett* (1994) **166**:117–20.

Togashi H, Kimura S, Matsumoto M et al, Cholinergic changes in the hippocampus of stroke-prone spontaneously hypertensive rats, *Stroke* (1996) **27**:520–6.

Tohgi H, Abe T, Kimura M et al, Cerebrospinal fluid acetylcholine and choline in vascular dementia of Binswanger and multiple small infarct types as compared with Alzheimer-type dementia, *J Neural Transm* (1996) **103**:1211–20.

Trenkwalder P, Potential for antihypertensive treatment with an AT(1)–receptor blocker to reduce dementia in the elderly, *J Hum Hypertens* (2002); **16** (Suppl 3): S71–S75.

Tzourio C, Anderson C, Blood pressure reduction and risk of dementia in patients with stroke: Rationale of the dementia assessment in PROGRESS (Perindopril Protection Against Recurrent Stroke Study), *J Hypertens Suppl* (2000) **18**:S21–S24.

Vennerica A, Shanks MF, Staff RT et al, Cerebral blood flow and cognitive responses to rivastigmine treatment in Alzheimers disease, *Neuroreport* (2002) **13**:83–7.

Waller SB, Ball MJ, Reynolds MA, London ED, Muscarinic binding and choline acetyl-transferase in postmortem brains of demented patients, *Can J Neurol Sci* (1986): **13** (Suppl 4):528–32.

Wilcock G, Mobius HJ, Stoffler A on behalf of the MMM 500 group, A double-blind, placebo-controlled multicentre study of memantine in mild to moderate vascular dementia (MMM 500), *Int Clin Psychopharmacol* (2002) **17**:297–305.

Wilkinson D, Doody R, Helme R, Taubman K et al, and the donepezil 308 study group, Donepezil in vascular dementia: a randomized, placebo controlled study, *Neurology* (2003) **61**:479–86.

Wolozin B, Kellman W, Ruosseau P et al, Decreased prevalence of Alzheimer's disease associated with 3–hydroxy-3–methylglutaryl coenzyme A reductase inhibitors, *Arch Neurol* (2000) **57**:1439–43.

Yamada S, Ishima T, Hayashi M et al, Muscarinic cholinoceptors and choline acetyl-transferase activity in the hypothalamus of spontaneously hypertensive rats, *Life Sci* (1984) **34**:2151–8.

Yesavage JA, Tinklenberg JR, Hollister LE, Berger PA, Vasodilators in senile dementias. A review of the literature, *Arch Gen Psychiatry* (1979) **36**:220–3.

showed no benefit at all. Thus it seems sensible to consider the use of lithium for both initial and subsequent prophylactic treatment in poststroke mania. Antipsychotics may assist with the control of mania in this population, but because of the high likelihood of adverse effects from typical agents it would seem prudent to use novel agents with sedative properties in cautious initial doses (for example olanzapine 2.5–5 mg per day at first) and for a short duration.

Depression

Up to 22% of stroke patients may develop major and up to 17% non-major depression (Robinson, 1998). There is evidence of efficacy for antidepressant therapy from six double-blind placebo-controlled studies, all of which found active treatment to be superior to placebo. The studies are summarized in Table 24.1. However, the patient numbers and lengths of follow-up limit the weight of this evidence.

The most recent treatment study of this kind compared patients with poststroke major or minor depression receiving fluoxetine ($n = 23$), nortriptyline ($n = 16$) or placebo ($n = 17$) (Robinson et al, 2000). Patients in the nortriptyline group showed a significantly greater decline in Hamilton Depression Rating Scale (HDRS) scores than either the fluoxetine or placebo groups. The largest poststroke depression antidepressant study was undertaken by Andersen et al (1994). Sixty-six patients with poststroke depression were randomly allocated to treatment with citalopram ($n = 33$) or placebo ($n = 33$). Those on active treatment demonstrated significantly better outcomes than those on placebo. In patients whose strokes were relatively

Table 24.1 Double-blind placebo-controlled studies of antidepressant drugs given to poststroke patients

Study	No. of patients	Active treatment
Lipsey et al, 1984	39	Nortriptyline
Reding et al, 1985	27	Trazodone
Andersen et al, 1994	66	Citalopram
Kimura et al, 2000	47	Nortriptyline
Wiart et al, 2000	31	Fluoxetine
Robinson et al, 2000	56	Nortriptyline + fluoxetine

recent (<7 weeks), this effect was not significant, suggesting that depressive disorder could be very hard to distinguish from an acute reaction to the stress of having a stroke (Baldwin, 2002).

The prevention of poststroke depression has been studied by Narushima et al (2002). Forty-eight nondepressed poststroke patients were randomly allocated to receive nortriptyline, fluoxetine or placebo for three months following the stroke in a double-blind design. During the treatment period the treatment groups were significantly less depressed as measured by the HDRS when compared to the placebo group. However, six months following treatment cessation the two antidepressant groups showed significantly higher rates of depression than the placebo group! By 21 months after treatment cessation there were no intergroup differences. The authors rightly suggest that further studies lengthening the treatment period would shed greater light on this rather unexpected finding and the value (if any) of such prophylaxis.

The concept of 'vascular depression' has recently been proposed to account for a subgroup of patients with certain features distinguishing it from regular depression such as greater apathy, later onset and reduced insight together with demonstrable white matter and subcortical changes on imaging (Baldwin, 2002). As its etiology is felt to be due to cerebrovascular disease, Taragano et al (2001) undertook a double-blind, randomized trial examining augmentation with nimodipine (a calcium channel blocker) in cases of such vascular depression. Eighty-four patients already receiving antidepressant therapy were randomized to also receive either nimodipine or placebo. Those in the nimodipine group had significantly greater improvements in HDRS scores than members of the placebo group.

In two retrospective uncontroled case series of stroke patients receiving electroconvulsive therapy (ECT) covering a total of 34 patients, only three failed to show significant improvement and no patient in either study had a further stroke or worsening of their neurological impairment (Robinson, 1998).

There have been no formal trials of psychological treatment in those with poststroke depression, although individual case reports and accounts of therapies modified to accommodate the cognitive and linguistic deficits of stroke patients do exist (Birkett, 1996).

There is compelling evidence to indicate that the presence of cerebrovascular disease retards recovery and increases the risk of depressive relapse, death and dementia in elderly people with major depression (Baldwin, 2002; O'Brien et al, 1998).

When considering how and whether to treat a depressed patient who has had a stroke, practitioners must consider not only the possible adverse effects of the treatments they plan to use but also the fact that untreated poststroke depression is associated with worse rehabilitative outcome and reduced poststroke survival (Robinson, 1998). The poor outcome of older depressed people with cerebrovascular disease (O'Brien et al, 1998) is an argument for energetic early treatment not therapeutic nihilism. Where the syndrome meets criteria for major depression and is not improving over a two-week period and also where milder depressive syndromes are persisting and interfering with rehabilitation, it seems reasonable to commence therapy with a short-acting selective serotonin reuptake inhibitor (SSRI). Tricyclics should be reserved for resistant cases in view of the propensity of the older patient to experience anticholinergic effects and the risk of postural hypotension in an individual with established vascular disease. ECT will be indicated if depression is severe, especially when delusions are present, if life-threatening behaviors (such as suicide attempts or a failure to eat or drink) occur, or if the patient has a history of ECT-responsive depression. Despite reassuring research findings (Robinson, 1998), it seems prudent to delay ECT if possible for at least three months poststroke but clinical considerations will sometimes occasion earlier intervention. The fact that there is no specific evidence base in favor of psychological therapy should not deter practitioners from providing supportive therapy at least, and occasional cases may warrant an empirical trial of cognitive behavioral therapy or grief counseling.

From an examination of the research literature in this field it is clear that despite the relatively high prevalence of poststroke depression, there is a lack of quality treatment studies of large numbers of patients. Further studies of all modes of therapy are urgently needed. Indeed, services that see a high number of stroke patients have a duty to promote and execute treatment research in this field so that management strategies may be informed by quality evidence.

Emotional lability

Around one-fifth of all patients who have a stroke will experience pathological laughing and/or crying within the first year of the stroke event (Robinson, 1998). Although the condition may occur in association with an affective disorder, many patients are seen in whom emotional lability appears to occur independent of a depressive or manic disorder (Robinson, 1998); the condition seems to respond to antidepressants. There is some evidence that nortriptyline, sertraline, citalopram and fluoxetine produce improvement more often than placebo in such patients, although no study has randomized more that 28 patients (Burns et al, 1999; Robinson, 1998). One study found less emergence of pathological crying over one year among 47 stroke patients who were free of emotional lability at baseline or week of treatment, who were given sertraline for one year (0/47) than in a placebo treated group (6/43) (Rasmussen et al, 1999). Where emotional lability persists and causes distress a trial with a short half-life SSRI should be attempted.

Anxiety

Adopting a nonhierarchical approach to diagnosis, Burvill et al (1995b) found anxiety disorders in 12% of men and 28% of women followed up 12 months after a stroke (n = 294).

Sharpe et al (1990) reported that 12 out of 60 stroke patients suffered from anxiety disorders three to five years after their index stroke. However, far less research has been done on the management of poststroke anxiety and related disorders than on the management of poststroke depression.

The widespread use of benzodiazepines for poststroke anxiety should be discouraged in view of the potential of this class of agents to cause tolerance and dependence as well as the possible association of the longer-acting agents with hip fractures (Ray et al, 1989). Such drugs may accentuate disinhibition in those whose strokes have a frontal focus. Where a benzodiazepine is needed for control of anxiety or severe sleep disturbance in the poststroke period it is wise to employ shorter-acting agents such as oxazepam and to limit therapy to a maximum of four weeks or to use therapy intermittently (for example, temazepam 10 mg at night no more than three times a week).

There are no useful data on the use of buspirone in poststroke anxiety. This drug affects serotonergic transmission and its onset of action is over a two-week period. It does not cause drowsiness or addiction but is quite expensive.

Where phobic disorder or panic is prominent, one could take note of findings in patients with functional disorders of similar phenomenonology and undertake a trial of therapy with an SSRI (for example, sertraline 25 mg in the morning increasing to 50–100 mg according to tolerance or response). In occasional resistant cases a tricyclic antidepressant could be tried with caution.

Cognitive behavioral therapy (CBT) is now seen as the psychological treatment of choice for functional anxiety disorders but little systematic research has been conducted on those who experience such symptoms after stroke. In many health systems there is a gross shortage of available trained practitioners funded to provide such treatment. Nevertheless, where cognition is sufficiently preserved for the patient to engage in CBT and a therapist is available to undertake the treatment it should be the first intervention attempted. CBT may be used in combination with drugs as well as without them.

Summary

In reviewing the literature on psychiatric treatment of those with cerebrovascular disease for the second time in three years, we continue to be struck by the fact that despite the work of a few indefatigable researchers, what we do not know and need to find out far exceeds what we do know and can utilize in the care of our patients who have strokes and/or VaD. The interested reader will find more detailed expositions in very good books by Robinson (1998) and Birkett (1996). We hope that after reading them, some young researchers will dedicate themselves to this fascinating and important but still under-researched area.

References

Andersen G, Vestergaard K, Lauritzen L, Effective treatment of post stroke depression with the selective serotonin reuptake inhibitor citalopram, *Stroke* (1994) 25:1099–104.

Baldwin RC, Management of affective disorder in cerebrovascular disease. In: *Vascular Disease and Affective Disorders*, Chiu E, Ames D, Katona C, eds, (Martin Dunitz: London, 2002): 245–58.

Birkett DP, *The Psychiatry of Stroke* (American Psychiatric Press. Washington DC, 1996).

Brodaty H, Ames D, Snowdon J et al, A randomized placebo-controlled trial of risperidone for the treatment of aggression, agitation and psychosis of dementia, *J Clin Psychiatry* (2003) 64:134–43.

Brown TM, Boyle MF, Delirium, *BMJ* (2002) 325:644–7.

Burns A, Russell E, Stratton-Powell H et al, Sertraline in stroke-associated lability of mood, *Int J Geriatr Psychiatry* (1999) 14:681–5.

Burvill PW, Johnson GA, Jamorozik KD et al, Prevalence of depression after stroke: the Perth Community Stroke Study, *Br J Psychiatry* (1995a) 166:320–7.

Burvill PW, Johnson GA, Jamorozik KD et al, Anxiety disorders after stroke: results from the Perth Community Stroke Study, *Br J Psychiatry* (1995b) 166:328–32.

De Deyn PP, Rabheru K, Rasmussen A et al, A randomised trial of risperidone, placebo and haloperidol for behavioural symptoms of dementia, *Neurology* (1999) 53:946–55.

House A, Dennis M, Mogridge L et al, Mood disorders in the year after stroke, *Br J Psychiatry* (1991) **158**:183–92.

Katz IR, Jeste DV, Mintzer JE et al, Comparison of risperidone and placebo for psychosis and behavioural disturbances associated with dementia: a randomised, double-blind trial, *J Clin Psychiatry* (1999) **60**:107–15.

Kimura M, Robinson RG, Kosier JT, Treatment of cognitive impairment after poststroke depression: a double blind treatment trial, *Stroke* (2000) **31**:1482–6.

Kyomen HH, Satlin A, Hennen J, Wei JY, Estrogen therapy and aggressive behavior in elderly patients with moderate-to-severe dementia, *Am J Geriatr Psychiatry* (1999) **7**:339–48.

Kyomen HH, Hennen J, Gottlieb GL, Wei JY, Estrogen therapy and non-cognitive psychiatric signs and symptoms in elderly patients with dementia, *Am J Psychiatry* (2002) **159**:1225–7.

Levine DN, Finkelstein S, Delayed psychosis after right temporoparietal stroke or trauma: relation to epilepsy, *Neurology* (1982) **32**:267–73.

Levitsky AM, Owens NJ, Pharmacologic treatment of hypersexuality and paraphilias in nursing home residents, *J Am Geriatr Soc* (1999) **47**:231–4.

Lindesay J, Macdonald AJD, Starke I, *Delirium and the Elderly* (Oxford University Press: Oxford, 1990).

Lipsey JR, Robinson GD, Rao K, Price TR, Nortryptyline treatment of post-stroke depression: a double blind study, *Lancet* (1984) **333**:297–300.

Lothstein LM, Fogg-Waberski J, Reynolds P, Risk management and treatment of sexual disinhibition in geriatric patients, *Connecticut Med* (1997) **61**:609–18.

Narushima K, Kosier T, Robinson RG, Preventing poststroke depression: a 12-week double-blind randomised treatment trial and 21–month follow-up, *J Nerv Men Dis* (2002) **190**:296–303.

O'Brien J, Ames D, Chiu E et al, Severe deep white matter lesions and outcome in elderly patients with major depressive disorder: follow-up study, *BMJ* (1998) **317**:982–4.

Rasmussen A, Klysner R, Mellerup E, Post-stroke emotional lability: a double-blind psychopharmacological treatment with sertraline, *Ninth Congress of the International Psychogeriatric Association: Abstracts* (1999): 114–15.

Ray WA, Griffin MR, Downey W, Benzodiazepines of long and short elimination half-life and the risk of hip fracture, *JAMA* (1989) **62**:3303–7.

Reding M, Haycox J, Blass J, Depression in patients referred to a dementia clinic, *Archives of Neurology* (1985) **42**:894–6.

Robinson RG, *The Clinical Neuropsychiatry of Stroke* (Cambridge University Press: Cambridge, 1998).

Robinson RG, Schultz SK, Castillo C et al, Nortriptyline versus fluoxetine in the treatment of depression and in short-term recovery after stroke: a placebo controlled, double-blind study, *Am J Psychiatry* (2000) **157**:351–9.

Sharpe M, Hawton K, House A et al, Mood disorders in long-term survivors of stroke: associations with brain lesion location and volume, *Psychol Med* (1990) **20**:815–22.

Starkstein SE, Fredoroff JP, Berthier ML, Robinson RG, Manic depressive and pure manic states after brain lesions, *Biol Psychiatry* (1991) **29**:149–58.

Street JS, Clark WS, Gannon KS et al, Olanzapine treatment of psychotic and behavioural symptoms in patients with Alzheimer's disease in nursing care facilities, *Arch Gen Psychiatry* (2000) **57**:968–76.

Taragano FE, Allegri R, Vicario A et al, A double-blind, randomised clinical trial assessing the efficacy and safety of augmenting standard antidepressant therapy with nimodipine in the treatment of 'vascular depression', *Int J Geriatr Psychiatry* (2001) **16**:254–60.

Wiart L, Petit H, Joseph PA et al, Fluoxetine in early post-stroke depression: a double blind placebo controlled study, *Stroke* (2000) **31**:1829–32.

chapter 25

Vascular dementia: consequences for family carers and implications for management

Henry Brodaty, Alisa Green and Lee-Fay Low

There is an aphorism in geriatric medicine that when a person is diagnosed with dementia there is usually a second patient, the family carer. Such recognition has resulted in a vast literature on carers and dementia. However, much less has been written about carers and vascular dementia (VaD) or on carers and stroke. This chapter attempts to redress this.

The impact of dementia on the family carer

Living with a person with a mental disability is an unremitting burden (Anderson, 1987). The decline in cognitive abilities, the loss of functional capacity, the dwindling companionship and the increasing demands of physical care impose escalating stresses on family carers (Brodaty and Hadzi-Pavlovic, 1990).

Such stresses manifest psychologically, physically, socially, financially and by the increased use of health services (Brodaty and Hadzi-Pavlovic, 1990). Research indicates that carers have high levels and rates of psychological distress and depression (Brodaty and Hadzi-Pavlovic, 1990; Mittelman et al, 1995; Morris et al, 1988; Poulshock and Deimling, 1984) and a corresponding decline in physical health (Haley, 1997), exacerbation of pre-existing medical conditions, such as hypertension (Schulz et al, 1990; Vedhara et al, 1999), and compromised immune function (Kiecolt-Glaser et al, 1987).

The provision of care to a spouse or parent with dementia often requires the carer to leave or reduce paid employment (Stone et al, 1987), as what may initially be part-time assistance can often become an all-encompassing role (Aneshensel et al, 1995). This is reflected in the findings of one study that (primary) family carers spent an average of 60 hours per week on their caring responsibilities (Max et al, 1995). Carers must cope with restrictions on social and leisure activities, disruption of household and work routines, conflicting multiple role demands, disruption of family relationships, and lack of support and assistance from other family members and from health and agency professionals (Biegel et al, 1991).

Effects of stroke on the family carer

Stroke, which is often the harbinger of VaD, may have distinct effects on carers, who are likely to be particularly stressed at several points on the post-stroke trajectory (Holbrook, 1982):

- immediately after the stroke when the carer has to come to terms with an event that is usually dramatically sudden and potentially life threatening
- during the treatment phase and inpatient care
- at the time of discharge from hospital when the carer realizes that she or he is suddenly to be given responsibility for the patient
- in the weeks and months following hospital discharge when professional support dwindles and the carer may become exhausted.

Carers may already have feelings of guilt about the stroke, e.g. did they give the patient the wrong diet or could they have called for help earlier. Subsequently they may fear leaving the patient alone or become overprotective (Warlow et al, 1996).

Predictors of stress in carers of persons with stroke

Factors associated with carer stress up to six months after a stroke include the objective severity of the stroke (Wade et al, 1986; Brocklehurst et al, 1981; Shultz et al, 1988) behavioral or mood disturbances in the stroke patient, physical disability (Shultz et al,1988; Wade et al, 1986; Grant et al, 2000), lack of social support for the carer (Grant et al, 2000) and concerns by the carer over the future care of the stroke patient (Schulz et al, 1988). From six months after a stroke, additional factors associated with stress in carers include dissatisfaction with their social life (Schulz et al, 1988; Carnwath and Johnson, 1987; Draper et al, 1992), poor physical health (Schulz et al, 1988), less family support (Silliman et al, 1986) and demographic variables such as income and occupation. Increased levels of depression and psychological distress in carers have been found to persist for up to three years after the stroke (Silliman et al, 1986; Nolan et al, 1996; Vitaliano et al, 1991).

Comparison of the effects of VaD and Alzheimer's disease

Research into carers' needs has mainly focused on dementia in general, or Alzheimer's disease (AD) in particular (Brodaty and Hadzi-Pavlovic, 1990; Aneshensel et al, 1995; Nolan et al, 1996). However, there is a growing recognition that the demands of caring and the needs of the care recipient differ according to the type of dementia (Vitaliano et al, 1991; Hoffman and Platt, 1991).

AD and VaD together account for approximately 80% of dementia cases in the elderly (Evans et al, 1989). Though similar in many ways, there are clinical reasons why their impacts may differ. These disorders vary in their antecedent risk factors, onset, nature of disease progression, neuropsychological profile, neurological features and associated physical ill health (Nolan et al, 1986). In addition, risk factors for VaD such as hypertension, cardiovascular disease, cerebrovascular disease (CVD) and diabetes mellitus have their own morbidity and may have independent effects on family members prior to the onset of stroke or VaD (Leys et al, 2002). Finally, the common occurrence of mixed VaD and AD can be interpreted by caregivers as doubly distressing.

Differences in onset and progression

The sudden onset of VaD can have an immediate and marked impact on the family, leaving them devoid of time to prepare for the changes (Hoffman and Platt, 1991). By contrast, the usual progression of AD is gradual and allows more time for carers to adapt to their role (Nolan et al, 1996). By contrast, carers of persons with VaD, especially of those with multi-infarct dementia (MID), must repeatedly adapt to unexpected sudden deteriorations inherent in that dementia's 'stepwise' decline. Further, the patient's fluctuating mental state, more typical of VaD, may be confusing to carers.

Differences in patients' psychological and physical disabilities

VaD is more likely than AD to leave the individual's personality superficially intact, so that persons with VaD may not seem to other family members and friends to have changed much (Vitaliano et al, 1991). This may lessen carer burden or paradoxically make it more difficult for family carers coping with cognitive decline in a person perceived by others to be functioning normally. Similarly, physical disability, which is more likely to complicate the picture in VaD, may increase the burden on family carers but may also legitimize the carer role. Finally, depression is a more common feature of VaD than AD (Mega et al, 1996; Donaldson et al, 1998). Depression in such cases is directly associated with psychological morbidity in carers (Brodaty and Luscombe, 1996, 1998).

In a large retrospective cohort (n = 161 106) it was found that across different levels of cognitive function, AD is associated with less physical comorbidity (even including nonvascular conditions) than VaD (Landi et al, 1999). VaD patients are significantly more likely to be hospitalized than AD patients, and this risk is not influenced by level of cognitive impairment (Landi et al, 1999).

Given that behavioral and psychological symptoms of dementia (BPSD) are powerful mediators of caregiver psychological distress (Brodaty, 1996), differences in BPSD between dementia types may affect the level of stress experienced by caregivers. While some studies have found that AD patients are more likely to have agitation and delusions than VaD patients (Lyketsos et al, 2000; Bernard et al, 1998) and VaD patients are more likely to have depression (Lyketsos et al, 2000), others have found no difference in a range of troublesome and disruptive behaviors or on depression between AD, VaD and mixed AD and VaD subjects (Swearer et al, 1988; Draper et al, 1998).

Differences in effects on carers

Despite clinical differences, empirical evidence that there are differential effects on carers of VaD, stroke and AD is equivocal. In a comparison of stroke and dementia carers, Draper et al (1992) found that subjective burden and psychological morbidity in carers were independent of the patient's diagnosis. A subsequent study by the same group reported that the risk factors identified for carer stress in stroke and dementia care were similar (Draper et al, 1996). However, Reese et al. (1994) found that AD carers reported significantly greater feelings of burden than stroke carers or a control group of noncarers. Other studies have found that AD carers may be less satisfied with the assistance they receive from family and friends than carers of stroke patients (Draper et al, 1992), have less social support (Franks and Stephens, 1996) and have fewer social resources even after controling for age and socioeconomic status (Reese et al, 1994). This may result in part from the common perception that AD is a mental illness (Aronson, 1988) while stroke is clearly identified as a physical disorder.

A cross-sectional study comparing carers ($n = 72$) of AD and VaD patients showed that in patients with mild-to-moderate dementia, VaD carers had similar or slightly higher burden scores to AD carers, but carers of severely demented AD patients were significantly more burdened than carers of severely demented VaD patients (Vetter et al, 1999). VaD patients were also reported to be a greater financial burden than AD patients (Vetter et al, 1999). Another study of AD and VaD caregivers ($n = 79$) at 'breaking point' when patients were on the waiting list for group-living units, also found no difference in level of burden (Annerstedt et al, 2000).

A study of carers of frail elders has shown that reduction in hours of employment by carers of stroke and dementia subjects was similar (Covinski et al, 2001). Twenty six per cent of carers of subjects with a history of stroke reduced their work hours [Odds ratio (OR) = 1.42, 95% confidence interval (CI) = 1.16–1.73], as did 23% of carers of subjects with dementia without behavioral disturbance (OR = 1.31, 95% CI 1.06–1.63) and 27.4% of carers of subjects with behavioral disturbance (OR = 1.68, 95% CI = 1.31–2.17) (Covinski et al, 2001).

The disparate findings of these studies could reflect amalgamation of different subtypes of dementia and disability – physical, cognitive and behavioral. For instance Draper et al (1992) compared patients with dementia (including MID) to those with stroke without dementia, and Reese et al (1994) compared AD and stroke patients.

Ethnic and cultural influences on the management of VaD

Ethnic and cultural factors must be considered in the management of dementia. The prevalence of AD and VaD differ in different countries or ethnic groups, as do the ways in which these diseases present themselves, and the ways in which families respond. Whereas AD is more common in Western countries, VaD tends to be the more prevalent subtype of dementia in Asian countries (White et al, 1996; Ueda et al, 1992; Yoshitake et al, 1995). These findings may reflect methodological, genetic, social, cultural or environmental differences (White et al, 1996; Mayreux et al, 1993; Hendrie et al, 1995) and the difficulties with diagnosis resulting from language differences and cultural bias inherent in many diagnostic instruments.

Family attitudes vary with ethnicity and strongly influence care and management. For instance, minority family carers in the USA, particularly African-American carers, are more likely to maintain their elderly at home, rather than admit them to nursing homes (Wallsten, 1997). Even within ethnic groups, minor nuances of cultural variations in family custom can become important, e.g. in some groups, such as Italian-Americans, the family eats together at set times. This practice can cause tension if a patient is unable to eat in a socially acceptable way (Birkett, 1996).

Carers from different cultures appear to experience the stresses of caregiving independent of dementia subtype. In the USA African-American carers experience lower rates of depression and subjective burden than Caucasian carers (Lawton et al, 1992). They also appear to find caring tasks less stressful and consider themselves more effective, in contrast to Caucasian carers (Haley, 1997). Such differences may reflect cultural variation in factors such as expectations about caring and previous experiences with adversity (Haley, 1997) as well as socioeconomic status (Wallsten, 1997).

Cultural variance also appears to affect the way that family members approach and view their caring role and responsibilities. In some cultures, traditional gender role expectations may mean that the older son or his wife, rather than a daughter, may take on the major burden of caring, or that sons may be the ones responsible for making decisions, while daughters provide day-to-day care (Yeo, 1996; Johnson, 1995). Different cultures vary in the extent to which families will place relatives in nursing homes (Wallsten, 1997; Lawton et al, 1992). In some, placing an elderly relative in a nursing home is considered abandonment and therefore unthinkable, even in cases of extreme stress and burden to the carer (Yeo, 1996).

Thus, diverse minority and ethnic groups often require special services to meet their unique needs, which may easily be overlooked or poorly understood. Awareness of the needs of different cultural groups can assist in the establishment of more culturally appropriate services that are also more valued by the individuals in need of such services (Larson and Imai, 1996).

However, multiple barriers impede access to necessary services: language; dependence upon others for translation; lack of cultural relevance of services; and misconceptions that mean that behaviors related to dementia evoke little concern until symptoms are quite advanced (Valle, 1989). Many cultures view confusion, disorientation and memory loss as normal parts of aging, while others regard these as signs of 'craziness' (Yeo, 1996). For example, in India depression is construed as a normal part of aging and is attributed to abuse, neglect or lack of love from children (Patel and Prince, 2001). The most frequent obstacle to diagnosis and management of dementia is lack of a common language. For instance, ethnic carers may be unable to understand medical instructions, which can lead to incorrect medication administration or noncompliance (Espino and Lewis, 1998).

In English-speaking countries, non-English-speaking elders depend on their Anglophone relatives to learn about and make use of services (Valle, 1989). Access to services for ethnic populations can be facilitated by locating programs within the ethnic community, using personnel who are culturally compatible with the target group, and providing social and health services alongside existing services in the community. Close working relationships with community agencies already serving minority populations (e.g. within a neighborhood health facility where the residents are accustomed to receiving primary medical care) help strengthen and encourage referrals, and provide training and education for staff members (Hart et al, 1996).

Management of VaD together with the family

Until dementia can be reversed or 'cured', management aims to maximize the quality of life of the patient and, where there is a family, that of the carer. Management planning requires a longterm view and the establishment of partnerships between the principal protagonists – patients, families and clinicians. The family is critical to both diagnosis and management.

A knowledge of the likely trajectory of the dementia assists in planning. The greater variability and unpredictability of VaD forces variation from the 'staged management' model (Brodaty, 1999). For example, the shock of the sudden development of dementia following a stroke, the uncertainty of how much improvement will occur in the longterm and the fact that sometimes the patient has a more severe dementia right from the start without ever evolving through the stages of early dementia, may exacerbate the carer's distress and make care more difficult. Even so, it is useful to conceptualize the course of VaD as progressing through early, middle and late stages. New challenges arise for the family in each stage and management can be formulated accordingly (Brodaty, 1999).

Many of the interventions for dementia caregivers, especially during the early-to-middle stages are targeted at those looking after AD patients. Intervention studies that have specifically included VaD caregivers or caregivers for any type of dementia have demonstrated efficacy in reducing caregiver burden and delaying institutionalization (Brodaty et al, 1993; Hepburn et al, 2001). We have been unable to locate any published reports of education or caregiver support interventions specifically for the caregivers of VaD patients.

Early stage of dementia

The first concern after making a diagnosis is how to inform the patient and the family. This is a sensitive and delicate process which requires the clinician to determine the extent to which each wishes to be informed of the diagnosis and its implications, and thus to 'titrate' the amount of information provided against the patient's and carer's reactions. Patients have a right to know their diagnosis but, equally, not to have this forced on them if they do not wish to know. Family members may express strong views about withholding the diagnosis from the patient, though, paradoxically, wishing to be informed were they in the same situation (Maguire et al, 1996). This may run counter to the clinician's duty to the patient. Usually it is possible to resolve this impasse by alleviating the family's fears through discussion and/or by allowing the family time to consider the matter further. Well-judged disclosures rarely distress patients and may even afford relief, as they can then understand why they have been experiencing difficulties.

Assessment is more than mere diagnosis – it requires an evaluation of the patient's particular capabilities and deficits. This will guide management, which should build on strengths and compensate for deficits, for example, the use of memory aids such as a notebook by the phone for messages and the establishment of a daily routine.

In the early stage of dementia family members may undergo a reaction similar to grieving or bereavement – for the loss of the person they knew or in anticipation of such a loss. It is important to allow family members the opportunity to voice their concerns; referral to a local support group may be of assistance. The patient and family members may differ in the extent to which they wish to learn about dementia; questions are often best answered

Barclay LL, Zemcov A, Blass JP, Sansone J, Survival in Alzheimer's disease and vascular dementias, *Neurology* (1985) **35**:834–40.

Bernard BA, Wilson RS, Gilley DW et al, Affective and behavioral symptoms in African Americans with Alzheimer's disease or vascular dementia, *J Mental Health Aging* (1998) **4**:97–104.

Biegel DE, Sales E, Schulz R, *Family Caregiving in Chronic Illness: Alzheimer's Disease, Cancer, Heart Disease, Mental Illness, and Stroke* (Sage Publications: Thousand Oaks, California, 1991).

Birkett DP, The family. In: Birkett DP, ed, *The Psychiatry of Stroke* (American Psychiatric Press: Washington DC, 1996) 311–19.

Brocklehurst JC, Morris P, Andrews K et al, Social effects of stroke, *Soc Sci Med* (1981) **15A**:35–9.

Brodaty H, Caregivers and behavioral disturbances: effects and interventions, *Int Psychogeriatrics* (1996) **8**:455–8.

Brodaty H, *Managing Alzheimer's Disease in Primary Care* (Science Press: London, 1999).

Brodaty H, Hadzi-Pavlovic D, Psychosocial effects on carers living with persons with dementia, *Aust NZ J Psychiatry* (1990) **24**:351–61.

Brodaty H, Luscombe G, Depression in persons with dementia, *Int Psychogeriatrics* (1996) **8**:609–22.

Brodaty H, Luscombe G, Psychological morbidity in caregivers is associated with depression in patients with dementia, *Alzheim Dis Assoc Disord* (1998) **12**:62–70.

Brodaty H, Griffin D, Hadzi-Pavlovic D, A survey of dementia carers: doctor's communications, problem behaviours, and institutional care, *Aust NZ J Psychiatry* (1990) **24**:362–70.

Brodaty H, McGilchrist CA, Harris L, Peters KE, Time until institutionalisation and death in patients with dementia, *Arch Neurol* (1993) **50**:643–50.

Brodaty H, Gresham M, Luscombe G, The Prince Henry Hospital dementia caregivers training programme, *Int J Geriatr Psychiatry* (1997) **12**:183–92.

Carnwath TC, Johnson DA, Psychiatric morbidity among spouses of patients with stroke, *BMJ* (1987) **294**:409–11.

Carrier L, Brodaty H, Mood and behavior management. In: Gauthier S, ed, *Clinical Diagnosis and Management of Alzheimer's Disease*, 2nd edn (Martin Dunitz: London, 1999) 206–20.

Covinski KE, Eng C, Lui L-Y et al, Reduced employment in caregivers of frail elders: impact of ethnicity, patient clinical characteristics and caregiver characteristics, *J Gerontol A Biol* (2001) **56A**:M707–M713.

Donaldson C, Tarrier N, Burns A, Determinants of carer stress in Alzheimer's disease, *Int J Geriatr Psychiatry* (1998) **13**:48–56.

Drachman DA, O'Donnell BF, Lew RA, Swearer JM, The prognosis in Alzheimer's disease: 'how far' rather than 'how fast' best predicts the course, *Arch Neurol* (1990) **47**:851–6.

Draper B, Poulos CJ, Cole AMD et al, A comparison of caregivers for elderly stroke and dementia victims, *J Am Geriatr Soc* (1992) **40**:896–901.

Draper B, Poulos R, Poulos CJ, Ehrlich F, Risk factors for stress in elderly caregivers, *Int J Geriatr Psychiatry* (1996) **11**:227–31.

Draper B, MacCuspie-Moore C, Brodaty H, Suicidal ideation and the 'wish to die' in dementia patients: the role of depression, *Age Ageing* (1998) **27**:503–7.

Erkinjuntti T, Kurz A, Gauthier S et al, Efficacy of galantamine in probable vascular dementia and Alzheimer's disease combined with cerebrovascular disease: a randomised trial, *Lancet* (2002) **359**:1283–90.

Espino DV, Lewis R, Dementia in older minority populations, *Am J Geriatr Psychiatry* (1998) **6**:S19–S25.

Evans DA, Funkenstein HH, Albert MS et al, Prevalence of Alzheimer's disease in a community of older persons. Higher than previously reported, *JAMA* (1989) 262:2551–6.

Franks MM, Stephens MAP, Social support in the context of caregiving: husbands' provision of support to wives involved in parent care, *J Gerontol B Psychol* (1996) 51B:P43–P52.

Fratiglioni L, Forsell Y, Aguero-Torres H, Winblad B, Severity of dementia and institutionalisation in the elderly: prevalence data from an urban area in Sweden, *Neuroepidemiology* (1994) 13:79–88.

Geldmacher DS, Whitehouse PJ, Current concepts: evaluation of dementia, *N Engl J Med* (1996) 335:330–6.

Grant JS, Bartolucci AA, Elliot TR, Giger J, Sociodemographic, physical and psychosocial characteristics of depressed and non-depressed family caregivers of stroke survivors, *Brain Injury* (2000) 14:1289–300.

Grant JS, Elliott TR, Weaver M et al, Telephone intervention with family caregivers of stroke survivors after rehabilitation, *Stroke* (2002) 33:2060–5.

Haley WE, The family caregiver's role in Alzheimer's disease, *Neurology* (1997) 48(Suppl 6):S25–S29.

Hart VR, Gallagher-Thompson D, Davies HD et al, Strategies for increasing participation of ethnic minorities in Alzheimer's disease diagnostic centers: a multifaceted approach in California, *Gerontologist* (1996) 36:259–62.

Haupt M, Kurz A, Predictors of nursing home placement in patients with Alzheimer's disease, *Int J Geriat Psychiatry* (1993) 8:741–6.

Hendrie HC, Osuntokun BO, Hall KS et al, Prevalence of Alzheimer's disease and dementia in two communities: Nigerian Africans and African Americans, *Am J Psychiatry* (1995) 152:1485–92.

Hepburn KW, Tornatore J, Center B, Ostwald SW, Dementia family caregiver training: affecting beliefs about caregiving and caregiver outcomes, *J Am Geriatr Soc* (2001) 49:450–7.

Herbert R, Brayne C, Epidemiology of vascular dementia, *Neuroepidemiology* (1995) 14:240–57.

Hier DB, Warach JD, Gorelick PB, Thomas J, Predictors of survival in clinically diagnosed Alzheimer's disease and multi-infarct dementia, *Arch Neurol* (1989) 46:1213–16.

Hoffman SB, Platt CA, *Comforting the Confused: Strategies for Managing Dementia* (Springer: New York, 1991).

Holbrook M, Stroke: social and emotional outcome, *J Roy Coll Phys Lond* (1982) 116:100–4.

Hope T, Keene J, Gedling K et al, Predictors of institutionalization for people with dementia living at home with a carer, *Int J Geriat Psychiatry* (1998) 13:682–90.

Johnson TW, Utilising culture in work with aging families. In: Smith GC, Tobin SS, Robertson-Tchabo EA, Power PW, eds, *Strengthening Aging Families* (Sage Publications: Thousand Oaks, California, 1995) 175–95.

Katzman R, Hill LR, Yu ESH et al, The malignancy of dementia: predictors of mortality in clinically diagnosed dementia in a population survey of Shanghai, China, *Arch Neurol* (1994) 51:1220–5.

Kiecolt-Glaser JK, Glaser R, Shuttleworth EC et al, Chronic stress and immunity in family caregivers of Alzheimer's disease victims, *Psychosom Med* (1987) 49:523–5.

Landi F, Gambassi G, Lapane KL et al, on behalf of the SAGE Study Group, Impact of the type and severity of dementia on the hospitalization and survival of the elderly, *Dement Geriatr Cogn* (1999) 10:121–9.

Larson EB, Imai Y, An overview of dementia and ethnicity with special emphasis on the epidemiology of dementia. In: Yeo G, Gallagher-Thompson D, eds, *Ethnicity and the Dementias* (Taylor & Francis: Bristol, 1996) 9–20.

Lawton MP, Rajagopal D, Brody E, Kleban MH, The dynamics of caregiving for demented elder among black and white families, *J Gerontol Psychol* (1992) **47**:S156–S164.

Leys D, Englund E, Erkinjuntti T, Vascular dementia. In: Qizilbash N, Schneider LS, Chiu H et al, eds, *Evidence-Based Dementia Practise* (Blackwell Science: Oxford, 2002) 260–87.

Lyketsos CG, Steinberg M, Tschanz JT et al, Mental and behavioral disturbances in dementia: findings from the Cache County Study on Memory in Aging, *Am J Psychiatry* (2000) **157**:708–14.

Maguire CP, Kirby M, Cohen R et al, Family members' attitudes toward telling the patient with Alzheimer's disease their diagnosis. *BMJ* (1996) **313**:529–30.

Mant J, Carter J, Wade DT, Winner S, Family support for stroke: a randomised controlled trial, *Lancet* (2000) **356**:808–13.

Max W, Webber P, Fox P, Alzheimer's disease: the unpaid burden of caring, *J Aging Health* (1995) **7**:179–99.

Mayreux R, Stern Y, Ottman R et al, The apolipoprotein epsilon 4 allele in patients with Alzheimer's disease, *Ann Neurol* (1993) **34**:752–4.

Mega MS, Cummings JL, Fiorello T, Gornbein J, The spectrum of behavioral changes in Alzheimer's disease, *Neurology* (1996) **46**:130–5.

Mittelman MS, Ferris SH, Shulman E et al, A comprehensive support program: effect on depression in spouse-caregivers of AD patients, *Gerontologist* (1995) **35**:792–802.

Morris RG, Morris LW, Britton PG, Factors affecting the emotional well-being of the caregivers of dementia sufferers, *Br J Psychiatry* (1988) **53**:147–56.

Nolan BH, Swihart AA, Pirozzolo FJ, The neuropsychology of normal aging and dementia: an introduction. In: Wedding D, Horton AM, Webster J, eds, *The Neuropsychology Handbook: Behavioral and Clinical Perspectives* (Springer: New York, 1986) 410–40.

Nolan M, Grant G, Keady J, *Understanding Family Care* (Open University Press: Buckingham, 1996).

Patel V, Prince M, Ageing and mental health in a developing country: who cares? Qualitative studies from Goa, India, *Psychol Med* (2001) **31**:29–38.

Peisah C, Brodaty H, Practical guidelines for the treatment of behavioural complications of dementia, *Med J Aust* (1994) **161**:558–63.

Poulshock SW, Deimling GT, Families caring for elders in residence: issues in the measurement of burden, *J Gerontol* (1984) **39**:230–9.

Reese D, Gross AM, Smalley DL, Meeser SC, Caregivers of Alzheimer's disease and stroke patients: immunological and psychological considerations, *Gerontologist* (1994) **34**:534–40.

Schulz R, Tompkins CA, Rau MT, A longitudinal study of the psychosocial impact of stroke on primary support persons, *Psychol Aging* (1988) **3**:131–41.

Schulz R, Visintainer P, Williamson G, Psychiatric and physical morbidity effects of caregiving, *J Gerontol* (1990) **45**:181–91.

Silliman RA, Fletcher RH, Earp JL, Wagner EH, Families of elderly stroke patients. Effects of home care, *J Am Geriatr Soc* (1986) **34**:643–8.

Stone R, Cafferata GL, Sangel J, Caregivers of the frail elderly: a national profile, *Gerontologist* (1987) **27**:616–25.

Swearer JM, Drachman DA, O'Donnell BF, Mitchell AL, Troublesome and disruptive behaviors in dementia. Relationships to diagnosis and disease severity, *J Am Geriatr Soc* (1988) **36**:784–90.

Teri L, Logsdon R, Uomoto J, McCurry SM, Treatment of depression in dementia patients: a controlled clinical trial, *J Gerontol B Soc Sci* (1997) **52**:S159–S166.

Ueda D, Kawano H, Hasuo Y, Fujishima M, Prevalence and etiology of dementia in a Japanese community, *Stroke* (1992) **23**:798–803.

Valle R, Cultural and ethnic issues in Alzheimer's disease family research. Alzheimer's disease and family stress: directions for research 1989, *DHS Pub ADM* (1989) **89**:122.

Van Dijk PTM, Dippel DWJ, Habbema JDF, Survival of patients with dementia, *J Am Geriatr Soc* (1991) **39**:603–10.

Vedhara K, Cox NK, Wilcock GK et al, Chronic stress in elderly carers of dementia patients and antibody response to influenza vaccinations, *Lancet* (1999) **353**:627–31.

Vetter PH, Krauss S, Steiner O et al, Vascular dementia versus dementia of Alzheimer's type: do they have differential effects on caregiver's burden? *J Gerontol Soc Sci* (1999) **54B**:S93–S98.

Vitaliano PP, Russo J, Young HM et al, The screen for caregiver burden, *Gerontologist* (1991) **31**:76–83.

Wade DT, Legh-Smith J, Hewer RL, Effects of living with and looking after survivors of a stroke, *BMJ* (1986) **293**:418–20.

Wallsten SM, Elderly caregivers and care receivers. Facts and gaps in the literature. In: Nussbaum PD, ed, *Handbook of Neuropsychology and Aging* (Plenum Press: New York, 1997) 467–82.

Warlow CP, Dennis MS, van Gijn J et al, *Stroke. A Practical Guide to Management* (Blackwell Science: Oxford, 1996).

White L, Petrovich H, Ross WG et al, Prevalence of dementia on older Japanese-American men in Hawaii: the Honolulu–Asia aging study, *J Am Med Assoc* (1996) **276**:955–60.

Winblad B, Poritis N, Memantine in severe dementia: results of the 9M-Best Study (Benefit and efficacy in severely demented patients during treatment with memantine), *Int J Geriat Psychiatry* (1999) **14**:135–46.

Yeo G, Background. In: Yeo G, Gallagher-Thompson D, eds, *Ethnicity and the Dementias*, (Taylor & Francis: Bristol, 1996) 3–7.

Yoshitake T, Kiyohara Y, Kato I et al, Incidence and risk factors of vascular dementia and Alzheimer's disease in a defined elderly Japanese population: the Hisayama Study, *Neurology* (1995) **45**:1161–8.

chapter 26

The challenges in provision of longterm care and in understanding behavioral disorders in cerebrovascular disease and dementia

Edmond Chiu

'The provision of care for people suffering from dementia represents a considerable challenge to the research and clinical community. Examples of good practice abound but there is a dearth of empirical research to support what should properly be regarded as good practice and which improves the quality of care and the quality of life of patients and their carers.'

Alistair Burns, editorial introduction, *Intl J Geriatr Psychiatry* (1999) **14**:83

Introduction

Volume 14, Number 2 of the *International Journal of Geriatric Psychiatry* (1999) was mostly devoted to a collection of papers and critical commentaries presented at a symposium entitled 'What works in dementia care' held at the Centre for Social Research In Dementia at the University of Stirling, Scotland, in June 1998. The compelling need to be clear about what works in dementia care was ably demonstrated (Downs and Zarit, 1999), as was the very unsatisfactory state of the evidence-based research in dementia care.

However, it was argued that evidence-based practice, while laudable, is at present immature and would limit us to drug interventions which, while having a tradition of data collection through randomized controlled trials (RCTs), would not necessarily totally satisfy the objective of providing the best quality of life for people with dementia.

In the relative absence of hard evidence, the discussion of principles and consensus in the longterm care of people with dementia should proceed in order to provide a framework for debate and research. In this context, the discussion of the understanding of behavioral disorders in cerebral vascular disease and dementia is relevant, as the two areas frequently coexist. Indeed, behavioral disorder is a major risk factor that leads to early or premature institutionalization into longterm care (Colerick and George, 1986; O'Donnell et al, 1992), is present in up to 90% of patients in nursing homes (Finkel, 1998), and has a negative impact on the quality of life of patients and families (Finkel et al, 1996).

Principles of longterm care

The principles of longterm care of persons with dementia do not necessarily differentiate between subtypes of dementia and may be applied equally in dementia related to cerebral vascular disease as well as in other forms of dementia. The pathways of many types of dementia as progressive, deteriorating brain disease converge to a common final pathway when the longterm management is conceptualized, planned and implemented.

A study of official policy documents from each country of the European Union by the European Transnational Alzheimer's Study of the University of Glenmorgan was summarized by Marshall (1999) who identified five key principles emphasized by all member states. These are:

1. People with dementia should be enabled to remain at home for as long as possible.
2. Carers should receive as much help as possible in order to facilitate the above.
3. Sufferers should retain maximum control over the support they receive.
4. All relevant services should be co-ordinated at the local level.
5. Sufferers in institutional care should live in surroundings which are as 'homely' as possible.

Four key principles were emphasized by most member states:

1. There should be a systematic attempt to equate the provision of services with need.
2. Categorical care should be replaced by care which addresses the general need of sufferers.
3. Early diagnosis of dementia should be encouraged.
4. The needs of people with dementia are not addressed separately from the needs of older people in general at the national level.

To these key principles of policy may be added, although currently without supporting research evidence, the following:

1. Longterm care in dementia is care throughout the whole pathway of dementia, not just at the high dependency end of the disease process.
2. The style of longterm care emphasizes care throughout the whole life (continuity) and all of life (holistic).
3. Ability enhancement should have higher priority than disability minimization.
4. Care should be underpinned by a sense of optimistic humanity which embraces the person with dementia, despite the multiple negative impacts of the dementia processes on the individual.
5. The ultimate criterion of care outcome is best quality of life, and is translated to a decision-making approach valuing all activities that add to quality of life and eschews decisions which will detract from quality of life for the person with dementia.

What determines entry into longterm care?

Multidisciplinary assessment of the elderly is a well-established strategy to prevent inappropriate nursing home admissions (Kane et al, 1981; Quartararo et al, 1991; George, 1991). Behavioral disorders (Colerick and George 1986; O'Donnell et al, 1992), carer burden (Rabins et al, 1982), dementia, stroke, hip and other fractures (Temkin-Greenier and Meiners et al, 1995), and cognitive impairment in combination with functional decline (or higher level of dependence in activities of daily living) (Quartararo et al, 1995) are factors related to admission to longterm residential care.

In answer to the question of whether early intervention can reduce the number of elderly people with dementia admitted to institutions of longterm care, O'Connor et al (1991) offered a wide range of help, including financial benefits, physical aids, home helps, respite admissions, practical advice and psychiatric assessment. Their conclusion was that 64% of intervention subjects were admitted at the end of two years compared with 8% of the non-intervention (control) group. This study is at variance with the findings of Challis and Davies (1986) and Challis et al (1990), which indicated that the provision of specially tailored help reduced admission rates. However, the mentally frail elderly in these studies had higher admission rates to longterm care institutions compared with the physically frail elderly. O'Connor et al (1991) concluded that special assistance to the mentally frail elderly with dementia might actually increase rather than decrease the number admitted to institutions, particularly for those living alone.

Quality of life and quality of care in longterm facilities

It is an accepted axiom that quality of life is the ultimate test of any healthcare program. It is assumed that quality of life can only be achieved through quality of care in a longterm care environment. In 1987 Kane proposed a framework to merge the healthcare and social side of institutional care into a system that uses quality of life as its major outcome (Kane, 1987). She suggested a tripartite scheme, which integrates the healthcare component (medical care, nursing, rehabilitation and various specialized therapies), personal care (assistance with routines of living such as bathing, toileting, grooming, mobility and feeding) and the social milieu in which such care takes place (the physical/built environment, activities, rules and expectations).

The measure of achievement of such quality of care is in the outcome of functional capacity, emotional and social well-being, autonomy, freedom and choice; these should be well balanced and integrated with an acceptance of the progressive nature of the disease process that leads the patient into longterm care. Quality of life is a multidimensional concept and reflects a patient's retained abilities, preferences, interests and perceived satisfaction.

McCurdy (1998) after reading Kitwood's vignettes of nursing home experiences in the USA (Kitwood, 1997), was moved to propose the centrality of 'personhood' in dementia care to counter 'depersonalization' – a failure to treat the resident with dementia 'fully as a person'. The widespread belief that there is 'no cure, no help, no hope' for people with dementia shapes attitudes and behavioral responses to them and must be countered. It was argued that, despite underlying despair in both patients and carers, the need and capacity for spirituality are no less because of increasing dependence, declining verbal communication and cognitive impairment. A more expansive view of spirituality could recognize that 'connectedness' with others (Richards and Seicol, 1991) and the presence of supportive community-based care will help to maintain the dementia sufferer's sense of spirituality. The dignity of an individual as a spiritual being is grounded in 'the belief that others held us in high regard, should rest on the fundamental knowledge that intimates, care givers and even strangers think well of me and recognize . . . me to be as fully human as they are' (Holstein et al, 1997). The critique of Kitwood (1997) is that the minimalist interpretation of 'palliation' in dementia care, that led to the sense of hopelessness as reflected in such terms as 'the death that leaves the body behind' and 'keeping the patient comfortable', is not worthy of the true principles of palliative care. An essential task of providing quality care for quality of life is the cultivation of attitudes that are hopeful, open and receptive of spirituality and humanity in both the patient and the carer.

Quality environment for people with dementia

Marshall (1998, 1999) described design principles for people with dementia living in long-stay establishments. Buildings for people with dementia should:

- Make sense
- Help them to find their way
- Provide a therapeutic environment
- Provide a safe environment
- Provide good facilities for staff.

Marshall argued that good design is integral to good care, and technological development should provide new opportunity for increasing in dependence, dignity and privacy. There exists a remarkable international consensus on design for people with dementia, as summarized in Table 26.1 (Marshall, 1999). The application of such sound design principles can lead to further research into the efficacy in outcome for people with dementia who live in such environments. The application of these principles in other cultures may require the identification of different characteristics to those for developed or economically

Table 26.1 The consensus on principles and key design features

- Design should compensate for disability
- Design should maximize independence
- Design should enhance self-esteem and confidence
- Design should demonstrate care for staff
- Design should be orientating and understandable
- Design should reflect a balance of safety and autonomy
- Design should reinforce personal identity
- Design should welcome relatives and the local community
- Design should allow control of stimuli.

The consensus on design features includes

- Small
- Familiar, domestic, homely in style
- Plenty of scope for ordinary activities (unit kitchens, washing lines, garden sheds)
- Unobtrusive concern for safety
- Different rooms for different functions
- Age-appropriate furniture and fittings
- Safe outside space
- Single rooms big enough for lots of personal belongings
- Good signage and multiple cues where possible, e.g. sight, smell and sound
- Use of objects rather than color for orientation
- Enhanced visual access
- Controlled stimuli, especially noise.

advantaged Western societies. The increasing emphasis on people with dementia living in their own homes will call for the development of modifications of these design characteristics for homes and domestic dwellings.

The role of the primary care physician in longterm care

The primary care physician is increasingly taking a more important part in the longterm care of people with dementia. This has arisen from a combination of social policy imperatives to keep people at home as long as possible and the allocation of primary care physicians to nursing homes as the responsible physicians. In response to this, Jarvik and Wiseman (1991) offered a very practical approach using the mnemonic FICSM (Family, Intellectual Status, Continence, Sleep and Mobility) to help physicians address treatable problems associated with people with dementing illnesses. They also advocated that both the patient and the care-giver(s) should be evaluated at regular intervals.

Support and education for the patient's family includes the provision of accurate and understandable answers to their questions, referral to appropriate services and resources, treatment of disturbing behaviors, assistance in the negotiation of longterm placement and support through post-mortem investigations. It is important that the patient's intellectual status is observed through identification and treatment of delirium, depression and iatrogenic effects and that information be supplied regarding drug trials for cognitive impairments. Any continence issues should be discussed thoroughly, to be followed by investigation and retraining regimes. Sleep problems pose a considerable burden for both patients and carers, therefore counseling on sleep hygiene and the treatment of insomnia is very useful. Mobility impairment, which frequently accompanies aging, orthopedic disorders or stroke should be energetically investigated and treated. Prevention of mobility decline by early intervention through physiotherapy should be anticipated. Reduction of mobility side-effects of medication (akathisia, rigidity, falls, ataxia) by close surveillance of both prescribed and over-the-counter medication is necessary. Removal of hazards in the home and modifications to the built environment to prevent falls will require the services of an occupational therapist through referral by the primary care physician. This reinforces the idea that the primary care physician is in the best position to undertake case management to ensure that the total health, well-being and social circumstances be provided for in an integrated and comprehensive manner.

Such interventions should take into account the physical, psychological and social problems associated with dementia and will substantially increase mobility and improve the quality of life of both patient and carers.

Behavioral and psychological symptoms of dementia with cerebrovascular disease: a reconceptualization

Noncognitive behavioral changes in dementia have been a major management issue in longterm care and have been a subject for research efforts over many years.

In the last decade, due to the very vigorous activity of the IPA BPSD Task-force led by Sandy Finkel, the concept and description of Behavioral Psychological Symptoms of Dementia (BPSD) has advanced the understanding of behavioral phenomenology and neuropsychiatric symptoms in dementia (Finkel et al, 1996; IPA, 1998). This activity has encouraged more appropriate attitudes in caring for people with dementia and has provided the opportunity to examine more rational approaches to therapy and management.

However, as in all advances in science and clinical practice, questions are raised from such new activity thus driving the development of new conceptualizations. The very nature of the success of exploring BPSD leads to new data, which revealed that whilst current BPSD conceptualization addresses dementia in a generic approach but are so far not able to differentiate sufficiently between the types of dementia and therefore raises the question . . .

Are there differences in BPSD between different types of dementia?

An examination of the Cache County Study on Memory and Aging (Lyketsos et al, 2000) – in the comparison of study participants with AD to participants with VaD on frequency of individual NPI disturbances (Table 26.2) revealed differences between these two groups. In general, the prevalence of neuropsychiatric inventory (NPI) items are similar between AD and VaD. However, using a logistical regression model Lyketsos et al revealed that AD patients are more likely to have delusions while those with VaD are more likely to have depression. Although not reaching statistical significance, patients with VaD did seem to have a trend towards greater aggression than those with AD. This indicates the possibility that the pattern of BPSD in VaD may well be different to that of AD. It raises the question that there is a possible difference and whether the difference may lie in the nature of the overlapping neuropathological substrates of the two subtypes of dementia. Alzheimer's disease has predominantly alpha beta protein abnormality with increasingly recognized vascular contribution whereas VaD has a predominant vascular pathology although there is some overlap with concomitant occurrence of amyloid plaques and neurofibrillary tangles.

Amyloid plaques and neurofibrillary tangles are mainly distributed in temporal, parietal and frontal lobes and not recognized ante-mortem by neuroimaging techniques at this time. However, vascular lesions are increasingly being revealed by current neuroimaging technology.

Table 26.2 Cache County Study on Memory in Aging. Comparison of study participants with AD to participants with VaD on frequency of individual NPI disturbances

NPI items	AD	VaD
Delusion	23%	8%
Hallucinations	13%	13%
Depression	20%	33%
Anxiety	17%	19%
Apathy	29%	24%
Irritability	20%	18%
Elation	0.5%	2%
Aggressivity	23%	33%
Disinhibition	8%	11%
Aberrant motor behavior	17%	8%
Total NPI	59%	67%

Adapted with permission from Lyketsos et al (2000).

There is increasing evidence that late-life depression (with or without dementia) has a significant vascular contribution (Alexopoulos et al, 1997; Krishnan and McDonald, 1995; Krishnan et al, 1997). The existence of similar vascular pathology and risk factors both in Alzheimer's disease and VaD is supported by recent evidence. (Brown et al, 2000; Kivipelto et al, 2001). It raises the possibility that the domain differences in BPSD between AD and VaD may be real.

Assuming that to be the case further questions are raised:

- Does vascular burden confer specific BPSD?
- Does the subgroup of BPSD, which we can reconceptualize as behavioral psychological symptoms of VaD (BPSVaD), require different treatment options and strategies?

The localization paradigm of Penfield, Hughlings-Jackson, Brodman, Wernicke and others have historically contributed to our understanding of functional anatomy by:

- Stimulating one area of the brain during surgery and observing the result in motor function.

- Studying 'oblation' lesions of the brain as a major foundation of clinical neurology and behavioral neurology.
- By conducting follow-up post-mortem studies of neuropathology, correlating with clinical findings of natural oblation by the disease process.
- Study of 'Mental' symptoms from diseases of the hemispheres such as hemiplegia, chorea and convulsions.

If we were to apply such a paradigm to BPSVaD it may be anticipated that vascular lesions of the brain can now be identified with increasing sophistication by ante-mortem neuroimaging and other technologies. Through studies of vascular oblation (in location, type and severity) using the paradigm of localization the elucidation of the individual/clusters of symptoms may be possible. Vascular lesions may provide the opportunity or study window to increase and clarify our understanding of BPSD and BPSVaD.

In combination with this localization paradigm the increasing understanding of cerebral circuitries (Alexander et al, 1986) will add further opportunity to understanding vascular pathology and clinical expression of vascular burden on the brain.

With increasingly sophisticated neuroimaging and future investigational technology the identification and understanding of the location, nature and severity of vascular burden of the brain can be anticipated. The relationship with individual symptoms and symptom clusters embedded in existing and additional knowledge of functional neuroanatomy and neuropsychology will provide clinicians and neuropsychopharmacologists more rational strategies for improved treatment outcomes for our patients and their carers.

The final word is from Eric Kandel, Nobel Laureate (Kandel et al, 1991):

'There is a new excitement in neuro-science today, an excitement that is based on conviction that the proper conceptual and methodological tools – cognitive psychology, brain imaging techniques and neuro-anatomical methods are at last in hand to explore the origin of the mind. With these tools and this conviction comes the optimism that the principles underlying the biology of mental function will now be understood'.

This encourages both the clinician and the neuroscientist to proceed to explore BPSD as a symptom cluster that may have differing neuropathological substrates and using neuropsychological and neuroimaging techniques that will be available to us in the future to reconceptualize BPSD as symptom clusters that can be attributed to different types of dementia, thereby paving the way for the development of more specific and rational treatment strategies from knowledge of neuroscience, neuropsychopharmacology, cognitive neuropsychology and the development of nonpharmacological treatment modalities. A combination and collaboration of these domains of study will provide a better quality of life for persons with dementia and their carers.

Conclusion

In the area of longterm care for patients with dementia of all types there remain many unanswered research questions. Any evidence that may be available is derived from the study of patients with AD and not specifically VaD subjects. Whether studies in AD patients can be generalized to patients with non-Alzheimer's type dementia is a major issue awaiting clarification.

Another essential question requiring vigorous research is whether patients with cerebrovascular disease and dementia will respond to interventions (either pharmacological or nonpharmacological) in the same way as AD patients.

Grouping together all patients with dementia cannot clarify these questions. However, separating subjects with non-Alzheimer's subtypes from the AD group places the researchers in the invidious position of having small sample sizes lacking statistical power in quantitative studies. While multicenter studies may address the problem, this has considerable logistical difficulties, which will need to be overcome if we are to have a better understanding of the outcomes of interventions that target patients with cerebral vascular disease and dementia.

Qualitative methodology in combination with quantitative methodology may go some way towards resolving this dilemma. Woods (1999) suggested that while methodological, RCTs are not able to provide the answers to all the complex issues and the evaluation of consecutive single-case studies in terms of treatment failure and success will continue to be valuable. In clinical practice single-case methodology frequently provides the initial basis for the development of a hypothesis, which can then be tested and evaluated using group study methodology including RCTs.

With the improvements in the number of people surviving stroke (see Chapter 21), it is possible that some of these may proceed to develop VaD and thereby add to the pool of patients requiring longterm care. Therefore, more targeted research is needed into longterm care for patients of this group in order to provide the best quality of life for them through their pathway of dementia.

References

Alexander GE, Delong MR, Strick PL, Parallel organization of functionally segregated circuits linking basal ganglia and cortex, *Ann Rev Neurosci* (1986) **9**:357–81.

Alexopoulos GS, Meyers BS, Young RC et al, Vascular depression hypothesis, *Arch Gen Psychiatry* (1997), **54**:915–22.

Brown WR, Moody DM, Thore CR, Challa VR, Cerebrovascular pathology and Alzheimer's disease and leukoariosis, *Ann NY Acad Sci* 2000; **903**:39–45.

Challis D, Davies B, *Case Management in Community Care: An Evaluated Experiment in the Home Care of the Elderly* (Gower: Aldershot, 1986).

Challis D, Chessum R, Chesterman J et al, Case Management in Social and Health Care (University of Kent Personal Social Science Research Unit: Canterbury, 1990).

Colerick EJ, George LK, Predictors of institutionalisation amongst caregivers of patients with Alzheimer's disease, *J Am Geriatr Soc* (1986) **7**:493–8.

Downs MG, Zarit SH, What works in dementia care? Research evidence for policy and practice. Part I, *Int J Geriatr Psychiatry* (1999) **14**:83–5

Finkel SI, The signs of the behavioural and psychological symptoms of dementia, *Clinician* (1998) **16**:33–42.

Finkel SI, Costa e Silva J, Cohen G et al, Behavioural and psychological signs and symptoms of dementia: a consensus statement on current knowledge and implication for research and treatment, *Int Psychogeriatr* (1996) **8**(Suppl. 3): 497–500.

George S, Measures of dependency: the use in assessing the need for residential care for the elderly, *J Publ Health Med* (1991) **13**:178–81.

Holstein M, Reflections on death and dying, *Acad Med* (1997) **72**:850.

International Psychogeriatric Association, *BPSD Educational Pack* (Gardiner-Calwall: Macclesfield, UK, 1998).

Jarvik LF, Wiseman EJ, A checklist for managing the dementia patient, *Geriatrics* (1991) **46**:31–40.

Kandel E, Schwartz JH, Jessell TM, *Principles of Neural Science*, 3rd edn (Appleton & Lange: Norwalk, Connecticut, 1991) 16.

Kane RA. Quality of life in long-term institutions – is a regulatory strategy feasible? *Dan Med Bull* (1987) Suppl **5**:73–81.

Kane RI, Rubenstein LZ, Brook RH et al, Utilization review in nursing homes: making implicit level-of-care judgments explicit, *Med Care* (1981) **19**:3–13.

Kitwood T, *Dementia Reconsidered: The Person Comes First* (Open University Press: Philadelphia, 1997).

Kivipelto M, Helkala EL, Laakso MP et al, Midlife vascular risk factors and Alzheimer's disease in later life: longitudinal, population-based study, *BMJ* (2001) **322**:1447–51.

Krishnan KRR, McDonald WM, Arteriosclerotic depression, *Med Hypothesis* (1995) **44**:111–15.

Krishnan KRR, Hays JC, Blazer DG. MRI-defined vascular depression, *Am J Psychiatry* (1997) **154**:497–501.

Lyketsos CG, Steinberg M, Tschantz J et al, Mental and behavioral disturbances in dementia: findings from the Cache County Study on Memory in Aging. *Am J Psychiatry* (2000) **157**:708–14.

Marshall M, Better quality environment for people with dementia. In: Jacoby R, Oppenheimer K, eds, *Psychiatry of the Elderly* (Oxford University Press: Oxford, 1998).

Marshall M, What do service planners and policy makers need from research? *Int J Geriatr Psychiatry* (1999) **14**:86–96.

McCurdy DB, Personhood, spirituality and hope in the care of human beings with dementia, *J Clin Ethics* (1998) **9**:81–92.

O'Connor DW, Pollit PA, Brook CPB et al, Does early intervention reduce the number of elderly people with dementia admitted to institutions for long term care? *BMJ* (1991) **302**:871–5.

O'Donnell BF, Rachman DA, Barnes HJ et al, Incontinence and troublesome behaviour predict institutionalisation in dementia, *J Geriatr Psychiatry Neurol* (1992) **5**:45–52.

Quartararo M, O'Neill TJ, Tang G et al, Assessing the residential care needs of nursing home applicants, *Aus J Pub Health* (1991) **15**:222–7.

Quartararo M, Glasziou P, Kerr CB, Classification trees for decision-making in long term care, *J Gerontol* (1995) **50A**:M298–M302.

Rabins PV, Mace NL, Lucas MJ, The impact of dementia on the family, *JAMA* (1982) **248**:333–5.

Richards M, Seicol S, The challenge of maintaining spiritual connectedness for persons institutionalised with dementia, *J Relig Gerontol* (1991) **7**:38.

Temkin-Greenier H, Meiners MR, Transitions in long term care, *Gerontol* (1995) **15**:196–206.

Woods B, Promoting wellbeing and independence for people with dementia, *J Geriatr Psychiatry* (1999) **14**:97–109.

Index